Emotional Aftermath

of the

Persian Gulf War

Veterans, Families, Communities, and Nations

Emotional Aftermath

of the

Persian Gulf War

Veterans, Families, Communities, and Nations

EDITED BY

Robert J. Ursano, M.D.

Professor and Chairman, Department of Psychiatry
Uniformed Services University of the Health Sciences
F. Edward Hebert School of Medicine
Bethesda, Maryland

Ann E. Norwood, M.D.

Assistant Professor and Assistant Chair
Department of Psychiatry
Uniformed Services University of the Health Sciences
F. Edward Hebert School of Medicine
Bethesda, Maryland

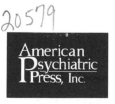

American
Psychiatric
Press, Inc.

Washington, DC
London, England

Note: The authors have worked to ensure that all information in this book concerning drug dosages, schedules, and routes of administration is accurate as of the time of publication and consistent with standards set by the U.S. Food and Drug Administration and the general medical community. As medical research and practice advance, however, therapeutic standards may change. For this reason and because human and mechanical errors sometimes occur, we recommend that readers follow the advice of a physician who is directly involved in their care or the care of a member of their family.

Copyright © 1996 American Psychiatric Press, Inc.
ALL RIGHTS RESERVED
Manufactured in the United States of America on acid-free paper
99 98 97 96   4 3 2 1
First Edition

American Psychiatric Press, Inc.
1400 K Street, N.W., Washington, DC   20005

Library of Congress Cataloging-in-Publication Data
Emotional aftermath of the Persian Gulf War: veterans, families,
    communities, and nations / edited by Robert J. Ursano and
    Ann E. Norwood. —   1st ed.
        p.   cm.
    ISBN 0-88048-652-X
    1. Persian Gulf War, 1991—Veterans—Mental health—United
States. 2. Persian Gulf War, 1991—Psychological aspects.
3. Military dependents—Mental health—United States.
4. Post-traumatic stress disorder. 5. War—Psychological
aspects. I. Ursano, Robert J., 1947–   . II. Norwood, Ann E.,
1953–   .
    [DNLM: 1. Stress Disorders, Post Traumatic—therapy.
2. Military personnel. 3. War—Middle East. 4. Syndromes.
5. Family—psychology. WM 170 P466 1996]
RC550.P47 1996
616.85'21—dc20
DNLM/DLC
for Library of Congress   95-33533
                                                                  CIP

British Library Cataloguing in Publication Data
A CIP record is available from the British Library.

Contents

Part III:
Preparation for the War

**Part V:
Conclusion**

Contributors

Paul T. Bartone, Ph.D.
Commander, U.S. Army Medical Research Unit—Europe, Heidelberg, Germany; Adjunct Assistant Professor, Department of Psychiatry, Uniformed Services University of the Health Sciences, F. Edward Hebert School of Medicine, Bethesda, Maryland

Brucinda L. Beach, Lic.S.W.–C.
Licensed Independent Clinical Social Worker, National Naval Medical Center, Bethesda, Maryland

Arthur S. Blank, Jr., M.D.
PTSD Team, Psychiatry Service, VA Medical Center, Minneapolis, Minnesota; Clinical Professor, Department of Psychiatry, Uniformed Services University of the Health Sciences, F. Edward Hebert School of Medicine, Bethesda, Maryland; Clinical Professor, Department of Psychiatry, Georgetown University School of Medicine, Washington, D.C.

George T. Brandt, M.D.
Assistant Professor of Psychiatry, Uniformed Services University of the Health Sciences, F. Edward Hebert School of Medicine, Bethesda, Maryland

Karen P. Hagen, R.N.
Navywide Ombudsman Advisor; Coordinator, Ombudsman Program and Command Family Support Team, National Naval Medical Center, Bethesda, Maryland

Harry C. Holloway, M.D.
Professor, Department of Psychiatry, Uniformed Services University of the Health Sciences, F. Edward Hebert School of Medicine, Bethesda, Maryland; Associate Administrator for Life and Microgravity Sciences and Applications, NASA Headquarters, Washington, D.C.

Elizabeth K. Holmes, Ph.D.
Chairman, Department of Leadership and Law, U.S. Naval Academy, Annapolis, Maryland; Assistant Professor, Department of Psychiatry, Uniformed Services University of the Health Sciences, F. Edward Hebert School of Medicine, Bethesda, Maryland

John T. Jaccard, M.D.
Medical Director, Medical Psychiatry Unit, Bristol Regional Medical Center, Bristol, Tennessee; Clinical Assistant Professor, Uniformed Services University of the Health Sciences, F. Edward Hebert School of Medicine, Bethesda, Maryland; Former Chief, Psychiatry Consultation/Liaison Service, Walter Reed Army Medical Center, Washington, D.C.

Peter S. Jensen, M.D.
Chief, Child and Adolescent Disorders Research Branch, National Institute of Mental Health; Associate Professor, Department of Psychiatry, Uniformed Services University of the Health Sciences, F. Edward Hebert School of Medicine, Bethesda, Maryland

Malcolm D. Johnson, M.S.
Chief of Current Operations, G3, 3d Infantry Division, Würzburg, Germany

Terence M. Keane, Ph.D.
Director, Behavioral Science Division, National Center for
PTSD, DVA Medical Center; Professor of Psychiatry, Tufts
University School of Medicine, Boston, Massachusetts

Ronald J. Koshes, M.D.
Chief Psychiatrist, The Center for Mental Health; Guest
Scientist, Walter Reed Army Institute of Research, Washington,
D.C.; Clinical Assistant Professor, Department of Psychiatry,
Uniformed Services University of the Health Sciences,
F. Edward Hebert School of Medicine, Bethesda, Maryland

Susan G. Larson, M.D.
Chief of Staff, Council of Deputies, National Capital Area;
Medical Director, TRICARE Northeast, Washington, D.C.;
Associate Professor of Clinical Psychiatry, Uniformed Services
University of the Health Sciences, F. Edward Hebert School of
Medicine, Bethesda, Maryland

Laurent S. Lehmann, M.D.
Associate Director for Psychiatry, Mental Health and
Behavioral Sciences Service, VA Central Office, Department of
Veterans Affairs, Washington, D.C.

David H. Marlowe, Ph.D.
Senior Scientist, Division of Neuropsychiatry, Walter Reed
Army Institute of Research, Washington, D.C.

James A. Martin, Ph.D, B.C.D.
Associate Professor, Graduate School of Social Work & Social
Research, Bryn Mawr College, Bryn Mawr, Pennsylvania

John M. Mateczun, M.D., M.P.H., J.D.
Principal Director (Clinical Services), Office of the Assistant
Secretary of Defense (Health Affairs); Associate Professor of
Clinical Psychiatry, Department of Psychiatry, Uniformed
Services University of the Health Sciences, F. Edward Hebert
School of Medicine, Bethesda, Maryland

Louis M. Mikolajek, M.S.
Professor, Boston University, Boston, Massachusetts

Ann E. Norwood, M.D.
Administrative Director, Center for the Study of Traumatic
Stress, and Assistant Professor and Assistant Chair,
Department of Psychiatry, Uniformed Services University of
the Health Sciences, F. Edward Hebert School of Medicine,
Bethesda, Maryland

Donna L. Ray, M.S.W.
Chief of the Family Support Division, Headquarters, U.S. Army
Europe

Robert A. Rosenheck, M.D.
Director, VA Northeast Program Evaluation Center, Evaluation
Division of the National Center for PTSD, VA Medical Center,
West Haven, Connecticut; Clinical Professor of Psychiatry, Yale
School of Medicine, Yale University, New Haven, Connecticut

James R. Rundell, M.D.
Associate Professor of Psychiatry, Uniformed Services
University of the Health Sciences, F. Edward Hebert School of
Medicine, Bethesda, Maryland; Program Director, National
Capital Military Psychiatry Residency, Washington, D.C.

Arieh Y. Shalev, M.D.
Associate Professor of Psychiatry, and Director, Center for
Traumatic Stress, Hadassah University Hospital, Jerusalem,
Israel

Jon A. Shaw, M.D.
Professor and Director, Division of Child and Adolescent
Psychiatry, University of Miami School of Medicine, Miami,
Florida

Zahava Solomon, Ph.D.
Professor and Chair, Chapel School of Social Work, Tel Aviv
University, Israel

Stephen M. Sonnenberg, M.D.
Clinical Professor of Psychiatry, Department of Psychiatry,
Uniformed Services University of the Health Sciences,
F. Edward Hebert School of Medicine, Bethesda, Maryland;
Clinical Professor of Psychiatry and Behavioral Sciences,
Baylor College of Medicine, Houston, Texas; Training and
Supervising Analyst, Houston-Galveston Psychoanalytic
Institute

Robert J. Ursano, M.D.
Professor and Chairman, Department of Psychiatry, Uniformed
Services University of the Health Sciences, F. Edward Hebert
School of Medicine, Bethesda, Maryland

Mark A. Vaitkus, Ph.D.
Deputy Commander and Research Psychologist, U.S. Army
Medical Research Unit—Europe, Heidelberg, Germany

Harold J. Wain, Ph.D.
Director, Psychiatry Consultation/Liaison Service, Walter Reed
Army Medical Center; Professor (Research), Department of
Psychiatry, Uniformed Services University of the Health
Sciences, F. Edward Hebert School of Medicine, Bethesda,
Maryland

Jessica Wolfe, Ph.D.
Director, Women's Health Sciences Division, National Center
for PTSD, DVA Medical Center; Associate Professor of
Psychiatry, Tufts University School of Medicine, Boston,
Massachusetts; Lecturer on Psychiatry, Harvard Medical School

Kathleen M. Wright, Ph.D.
Deputy Chief, Department of Military Psychiatry, Walter Reed
Army Institute of Research; Adjunct Assistant Professor,
Department of Psychiatry, Uniformed Services University of
the Health Sciences, F. Edward Hebert School of Medicine,
Bethesda, Maryland

Sandra A. Yerkes, M.D.
Training Director, Department of Psychiatry, National Naval
Medical Center; Teaching Fellow, Department of Psychiatry,
Uniformed Services University of the Health Sciences,
F. Edward Hebert School of Medicine, Bethesda, Maryland

Bruce L. Young, M.A.
National Center for PTSD, Boston, Massachusetts

Foreword

The Persian Gulf War raised new issues for maintaining the health of our fighting force and supporting the families of our military personnel. Operations Desert Shield and Desert Storm touched our entire nation—from the active forces to the reserves, from the East Coast to the West Coast, from our cities to our farms.

The focus of this book is unique. It addresses the issues affecting not only soldiers but also their families and their communities, with special attention to the experience of leaving for war, being left by loved ones for war, and returning home from war. This volume contains contributions from outstanding authors in the Department of Defense, Veterans Administration, National Institute of Mental Health, Israel Defense Forces, universities, and other institutions internationally renown for their work in trauma.

The Persian Gulf War presented many challenges to the nation and the Department of Defense. The rapid mobilization and deployment of reserve and National Guard personnel as well as active-duty servicemembers represented an enormous logistical challenge. The war showcased the importance of such logistical support for maintaining our fighting forces and our ability to return our military home. The potential use of chemical and biological warfare by Iraq was a serious threat, and the lessons learned in preparing for this threat must not be forgotten. These weapons may yet be used in a future conflict. The Gulf War was also unique in the role that technology played. Live television coverage, Patriot missiles, and "smart" bombs altered the experience of war for those in the Gulf and those at home. It is important to better understand the effects of these technological innovations on the fighting force and their families. I am particularly pleased to see attention given to the special needs of families and of reserve and National Guard members in the chapters that follow. These groups are critical to our nation's readiness.

The nation, including those who strive to understand the effects of war, must continue to work for and encourage initiatives that improve the quality of life of our total force. Providing the best medical and psychological care for military members and their families is central to the mental health and effectiveness of the fighting force. This book represents some of the finest authors and work done on the effects of war. It reflects an important commitment to ensuring that lessons learned are not forgotten and that our fighting forces and their families continue to receive the best support the nation can provide.

Dick Cheney

Preface

Nations go to war. Yet wars are about individuals, families, and communities. The Persian Gulf War was the story of nations at war and of a new technological warfare, and of the experience of that war as seen and heard instantaneously at home. It was a conflict that brought the United States, for the first time since World War II, to a "national" war, one in which all parts of the nation were involved. Communities in the cities and in the countryside anticipated the war, readied for it, and sent men and women from all branches of the armed forces into the combat theater.

The chaos of war is exemplified not only by what events transpire on the battlefield. Separation from loved ones, worries of home, anticipated terror of new weapons, adaptation to extreme environments, and eventual reunion and readaptation are all part of the stress of war. War is one of, but not the only, humanmade disaster. Much of the disaster literature is relevant to this broad conceptualization of the reverberating psychiatric and psychological effects of war. Understanding this broad view of war is necessary to best care for and help the individuals and communities affected by the demands of war. In the past, literature on the effects of war, particularly that from the Vietnam War era, focused on the chronic effects of combat. In this volume, through considering the Persian Gulf War, we hope to provide a broader view and, thus, a better basis from which to treat our patients and to conceptualize, intervene, and manage family and community stressors. With modern mobilization of troops and rapid air evacuation out of theater, the need to understand how war affects families and communities both in the leaving and in the return is critical. Similarly, determining how best to treat combat casualties—those with and without psychiatric illness—who are rapidly returned home still in the acute stage of their injuries is essential. We hope this volume will aid in this process both by providing the most up-to-date integration of the literature on the psychiatric and psychological effects of war and by presenting the data from the Persian Gulf War in particular as the paradigm of modern warfare, with its stressors and populations in need of help.

This volume is the result of the efforts of many. First, of course, are our contributors, who represent the cutting edge of clinical care and research as well as community interventions in times of war. They continue to bring together research knowledge, clinical care, and community leadership to help those on whom the war had an impact. In addition, we would like to particularly thank Drs. Harry Holloway, David Marlowe, James Zimble, and Nancy Gary for their support of and enthusiasm for this work and their ongoing interest in the care of those affected by war. Most important, however, are the soldiers, sailors, airmen, and marines, men and women, and their families and communities. In every generation, they bear the brunt of war. To them fall the terror and heartache of warfare. For most, this important part of their lives will fade in memory and yet will still mold their view of their past and future. For some, the pains of war will persist. We hope this volume will help those who care for them to better foster their health and also better prepare the next group of clinicians, researchers, and community leaders who must again think of the terror of war and its effects on soldiers and families, communities and nations.

Robert J. Ursano, M.D.
Ann E. Norwood, M.D.

Part I
Introduction

1 The Gulf War

Ann E. Norwood, M.D.
Robert J. Ursano, M.D.

War and the threat of war represent significant psychological trauma. Indeed, much of the literature on posttraumatic stress disorder (PTSD) stems originally from studies of soldiers, sailors, airmen, and Marines who were exposed to war and its attendant horrors. It is important to study the effects of war so that "lessons learned" can be applied in future wars and conflicts and a better understanding of the effects of other human-caused and natural disasters and traumas can be attained. In the case of the Persian Gulf War, because the war was relatively brief and the outcome militarily successful, we run the risk of complacency; it is tempting to rest on our laurels rather than to carefully analyze and record the lessons learned. During the Gulf War, American forces sustained 148 battle deaths and 145 nonbattle deaths (as a result of motor vehicle accidents, etc.); 467 American servicemembers were wounded in action (U.S. Department of Defense 1991). Although the forecasts of Iraqi chemical and biological warfare, which would result in tens of thousands of American dead, did not come to pass, such warfare, the use of which we so feared in the Gulf War, could well be the scenario of the next war. The U.S. military has also found itself increasingly involved in humanitarian missions that, despite their name, still expose our forces to the stress and trauma of combat. It is likely that American servicemembers, their families, and our nation will continue to grapple with the injuries and deaths of its service-

3

members operating in these contingencies. The knowledge of psychological and behavioral responses to war—of families, communities, and nations, as well as of individuals—will be needed in the future.

Although many researchers in this field have concentrated on the effects of combat and its sequelae, it is important to recognize that combat is not the only traumatic stressor inherent in war; nor are those persons directly affected by combat its only victims. PTSD is only one of several possible psychological outcomes following trauma. Substance abuse, depression, generalized anxiety disorder, and adjustment disorders are some of the other psychiatric disorders that have been associated with traumatic exposure (Ursano et al. 1994). Moreover, individuals exposed to trauma do not always develop psychiatric illness. In the Gulf War, combat-related stressors included "friendly fire" incidents, tank battles, air strikes, and other potentially lethal events. Fear of capture, injury, and death was a common concern of those sent to the combat theater. In the course of the war and its aftermath, many personnel saw the bodies of dead Iraqis and Kuwaitis. The debilitated condition of the Iraqi enemy prisoners of war (POWs) and of ethnic minorities such as the Kurds was also distressing to many. As is true of all wars, witnessing the results of atrocities was especially troublesome.

Increasingly, we appreciate the ever-expanding reverberations of trauma. In studying the effects of war, investigators first explored the direct victims of combat: combatants and civilian casualties. Although these direct victims of trauma are often readily discernible, there are also hidden victims. Trauma impacts the victims' friends and loved ones, rescue workers and medical personnel, colleagues/co-workers, communities, and social groups. Witnesses of traumatic events are also vulnerable to psychological sequelae. Research on terrorism and the effects of conventional war on indirect victims has been of relatively recent origin.

Similarly, the study of war's effects on families has been relatively limited. The first published report on families' reactions to war was Reuben Hill's (1949) observations on families' responses to World War II. His observations led him to develop the ABCX model of family stress crisis. During the Vietnam War era, families of military personnel who were either POWs or missing in action (MIA) were studied (McCubbin and Patterson 1983). Most recently, the effects of soldiers' PTSD on families and spouses have been reported. Solomon (1993) found increased somatic and psychiatric distress in the wives of Israeli veterans with diagnoses of PTSD or combat stress reaction. There is a relative dearth of contemporary work on the longitudinal stressors of war on families. Special populations, such as reserve families, single-parent households, and joint service marriages, may be particularly vulnerable. In one of the few studies on Desert Storm, Rosen and colleagues (1993) reported the results of questionnaires in which parents were asked to rate their children's responses to Operation Desert Storm. Sadness was a common complaint for both girls and boys. From 42% to 64% of children between the ages of 3 and 12 years were described by their parents as being sad or tearful. Discipline problems at home were reported to occur fairly frequently with boys but infrequently with girls. Both boys and girls demanded more attention from the nondeployed parent.

Children of deploying parents were not the only ones who worried about the war. There were reports of children throughout the United States who feared terrorist attacks and/or did not realize that they were geographically distant from where hostilities were taking place. War affects an entire nation, before, during, and after hostilities.

The mobilization of reservists for Desert Storm exerted a substantial burden on many small communities in America. Deployment resulted in some small towns losing major figures in their communities such as business and civic leaders, teachers, and health care providers. The burden experienced by these communities was compounded by the ambiguity and uncertainty surrounding when (and if) these individuals would return. The impact of war on these relatively neglected populations is an area that future research must address.

In addition to considering a broader array of populations—

both those directly and those indirectly affected by war—it is important to dissect war into its component traumatic stressors. Too often, we focus narrowly on combat-related stressors, forgetting that threat to life and exposure to death, injury, and the grotesque are not the only stressors that cause the pain and suffering of combat. Separation of family members; fear of capture, injury, and death; shifts in family roles; disruption of the normal routine; increased financial pressures; fear of terrorist attacks—all are part of the experience of nations, communities, and families during time of war. It is helpful to conceptualize the stressors of war along the following time line: predeployment, deployment, sustainment, hostilities, reunion, and reintegration (Figure 1–1).

Applying this time line to different populations increases our ability to identify the multitude of war stressors encountered by various individuals and groups. For example, the stressors encountered by active-duty soldiers along this continuum differ substantially from those experienced by family members of reserve units during the same periods. Similarly, the experience for families of active-duty personnel who were being deployed to the Gulf differs from that of those who were stationed abroad and of those who lived on bases and posts within the U.S. The identification of populations at risk and of the relevant biopsychosocial stressors can further our understanding of the factors that render certain individuals relatively more vulnerable or more resilient to the development of psychological sequelae

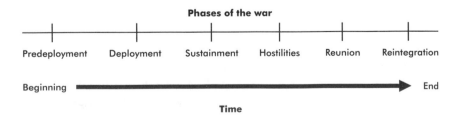

Figure 1–1. Phases of war, which call for different psychological support.

to war. Specific interventions can then be targeted toward specific individuals and populations, either to inoculate them against the effects of particular stressors or to increase their ability to cope successfully.

Based on the regularity with which we find ourselves involved in armed conflicts, the psychological legacy of war merits study in its own right. In addition, however, although direct exposure to war is not a common part of most Americans' experience, exposure to significant traumatic stressors is. An estimated 6% to 7% of the American population is exposed to some sort of significant trauma each year (Norris 1988). Thus, although the odds of American civilians being directly impacted by a war seem low, it is possible that they will be subject to, or witness, a natural disaster, motor vehicle accident, physical assault, or other traumatic event. The extent to which findings from research on war can be generalized to other traumatic stressors must always be carefully assessed. But such findings can offer important considerations for all health care providers. The study of psychological reactions to war, then, holds broader implications for the understanding of other types of trauma.

In this volume the authors focus on the stressors associated with the Persian Gulf War and on the populations and time phases of the war that are often overlooked. We do not focus on combat psychiatry. Rather, the psychiatric and psychological effects seen before and after combat—in those about to leave for war and in those returning from war, as well as in their children and families—are highlighted, as are the potential long-term effects as suggested by studies of previous war veterans. Whenever possible, attempts are made to quantify the nature of the stressor and the individual or community response to the trauma.

Stressors of the Persian Gulf War

The pace of the Gulf War buildup was unprecedented in military history. Iraq invaded Kuwait on August 2, 1990. On August 7, the U.S. began moving air forces to the region, the Eighty-Second Airborne Division from Ft. Bragg began deploying, and the first prepositioned ship departed for the Gulf from Diego Garcia. On August 22, President Bush signed an executive order placing 48,000 American reservists on active duty by September 1. By August 18, there were 50,000 Americans in the Gulf theater. With the addition of reservists, the number of American servicemembers reached 150,000 by September 15, 1990. Within the next month another 60,000 Americans arrived in the theater. On November 14, Secretary of Defense Cheney activated 72,500 reservists and extended the current call-up from 90 to 180 days. Approximately 2 weeks later, Secretary Cheney authorized the call-up of an additional 63,000 reservists and guard members, raising the total to 188,000. By Christmas 1990, there were over a quarter of a million U.S. military personnel in the Gulf. By the beginning of the air war on January 17, 1991, there were over 300,000 American troops deployed. Over half a million Americans were deployed to Southwest Asia when the ground war began on February 24 ("Tracking the Storm" [Chronology] 1991).

The Gulf War brought both old and new threats to American forces (Table 1–1). A number of stressors were unique to living in the desert. As in other areas of military medicine, strong emphasis was placed on prevention through educating soldiers and command about these dangers. High priority was placed on acclimatizing soldiers as rapidly as possible. The first stressor to overcome was jet lag after the long flights to Southwest Asia. Familiar and well-publicized threats included venomous snakes and scorpions indigenous to Southwest Asia. From a medical perspective, however, the largest predictable threat was heat

Table 1–1.   Major stressors of the Persian Gulf War

Threat of chemical/biological warfare	Desert environment
	Jet lag
Threat of mass casualties (up to 50% losses predicted)	Cultural isolation
	Media

injury. Air temperature in the summer can exceed 115°F. Sand receiving full sun is usually 30 to 45° hotter than the air and can reach temperatures of 150°F. Command emphasis was placed on educating soldiers to force fluids—for example, instructing them to drink even when they were not thirsty, because by the time a person experiences thirst, he or she is $1\frac{1}{2}$ quarts below the optimal physiological level. Television news was filled with images of soldiers carrying bottles of spring water.

Heat is not the only environmental hazard. The desert can also become very cold in the winter; the wind chill at night drops well below freezing. Protection of skin and eyes from sand and dust was imperative. The wearing of contact lenses was prohibited except in areas that were air-conditioned and protected from sand. Sunglasses and goggles were distributed for eye protection. Soldiers were urged to use extra caution in securing tent pegs and other objects that could be turned into missiles by heavy winds.

Medical authorities were educated on the types of problems they might encounter over the course of the deployment. In the first few weeks of deployment, diarrheal diseases were expected. The dusty environment was expected to precipitate acute respiratory illness. Medical authorities were cautioned to be vigilant within the first month for the development of febrile illnesses caused by viral respiratory diseases, arboviruses such as sandfly fevers or dengue, enteric diseases, hepatitis A and E, and rickettsial diseases.

After several weeks of deployment, illnesses in soldiers could herald other diseases such as hepatitis B, leishmaniasis, and parasitic infections. Medical personnel were also instructed to watch for psychological problems; both health problems and the strain of preparing for battle might manifest themselves in acting out of tensions. It should be remembered, too, that psychological factors can influence the development of physical illness. For example, noncompliance with preventive measures, such as malaria prophylaxis or use of sunscreens and proper clothing to prevent sunburn, generates nonbattle injury casualties that are truly psychological casualties.

The experience of U.S. personnel in Saudi Arabia differed strikingly from that of Vietnam War veterans with regard to the social outlets available to them. Servicemembers in Saudi Arabia were culturally isolated: troops were given orders not to fraternize with local people. In accord with the religious dictates of the host countries, alcohol was prohibited.

Living conditions were harsh for U.S. personnel in Saudi Arabia. Hot showers were an infrequent luxury. Cots were usually lined up side by side in buildings, an arrangement that afforded virtually no privacy or quiet. Although living aboard ship provided a few more amenities, lack of privacy, fear of chemical/biological attack, and other stressors were part of everyday life for naval personnel (Dinneen et al. 1994).

The threat of chemical and biological warfare was a major consideration throughout the war. During the Iran-Iraq War and in attacks on the Kurdish minority in Iraq, Saddam Hussein had used mustard gas, nerve agents, and T-2 toxin. At the time of the war, Iraq was believed to have a 2,000- to 4,000-ton arsenal of chemical weapons, consisting predominantly of mustard gas but also including the nerve agents sarin and tabun. It was estimated that Iraq had the capability of annually producing more than 700 tons of mustard gas and 50 tons each of sarin and tabun. Moreover, Iraqi delivery systems were capable of striking distances up to 530 miles (Knudson 1991). Intelligence agencies reported that Iraq had been conducting research on biological agents, including anthrax, botulism, cholera, typhoid, equine encephalitis, and tularemia (Knudson 1991).

The Persian Gulf War also offered the world glimpses of high-technology warfare in the coming millennium. In addition, the war showcased the ways in which media coverage of warfare has changed. The media not only reports the war but also observes and participates in it. The media has changed not only the way in which the public learns about the war but also the very ways in which wars are fought. For example, the television display of the battered American aviator held as a POW by the Iraqis helped galvanize public support for the war.

The Gulf War: Technological Advances and Their Implications for Future Wars

The Persian Gulf War represented the largest military deployment since World War II (Salomon and Bankirer 1991). It was a new, fast-paced, "high tech" war that differed from past wars both in terms of the armament employed and in the ways in which the news of the war was conveyed to the public back home. The Vietnam War has been characterized as the first "television war"; the Gulf War, then, was the first war that was televised "live." Beginning with the initial reports of a radar blip indicating that U.S. warships were headed for Baghdad, television brought the war as it unfolded into the living rooms of America. Many Americans, especially military spouses, became "news junkies." One military spouse noted, "I watch ABC while I tape CBS, then *MacNeil/Lehrer*. I get *Christian Science Monitor* and the *World Monitor*. Also the *Louisville Courier-Journal* and *USA Today*. And I watch CNN" (Kantrowitz 1990, p. 33). Satellite technology also brought closer and more rapid communication from soldiers to their families, allowing soldiers to "phone home" from the combat theater. As in previous wars, mail provided a key link with home. Often, soldiers exchanged audiotapes with their families back home in an effort to bridge the distance.

In many important ways the Gulf War bears a closer resemblance to World War II than it does to either the Korean War or the Vietnam War. The Gulf War, like World War II, was characterized by clear-cut objectives, whereas the objectives in the Korean and Vietnam Wars were not so clear. Other similarities included the massive deployment of multilateral forces in World War II and the Gulf War. In the Gulf War, in contrast to the Korean and Vietnam Wars, the U.S. and the host countries shouldered the vast majority of the personnel commitment (Summers 1992).

As in World War II, large numbers of reservists were activated. The first reservists were called up by Secretary Cheney on

August 23, 1990 ("Tracking the Storm" [Chronology] 1991). Between August 1990, the time of Iraq's invasion of Kuwait, and March 1991, approximately 227,000 reservists and National Guard members were called up; an additional 10,700 volunteered for service (see Dunning, Chapter 8, this volume). Approximately 7% of the American forces in the Gulf were women; 43% of the American forces were married, and the average age was 28 (U.S. Department of Defense 1991). The mobilization of reservists permeated the fabric of American society. Involvement of individuals from communities across the nation highlighted the fact that the war was going on. The decision to call up the reserves was considered by some to be a pivotal event in galvanizing public opinion to support the strategy in the Gulf.

Another important distinction was that both the Gulf War and World War II were successful offensive wars. Fear of provoking the Soviet Union and China changed American policy in the 1950s from its historic policy of "rollback and liberation" to a policy of "containment" (Summers 1992). This policy of containment was also used in Vietnam. Under a policy of containment, the most successful outcome is a stalemate; this carries implications for national sentiment and popular support. The move away from containment to a policy that allowed the possibility of victory was made possible by the resolution of the Cold War. Because war with the Soviet Union was no longer an issue, a multinational coalition could be forged (Summers 1992).

The logistical support provided by the military was the largest supply effort since World War II (Salomon and Bankirer 1991). Although airlift played a minor role in World War II, it contributed significantly to the success of the Allied forces. By January 11, 1991, the Military Airlift Command (MAC) had flown more than 10,000 missions, carrying more than 370,000 passengers and more than 346,000 tons of cargo ("Tracking the Storm" [Chronology] 1991). Over the course of the war, the MAC flew more than 15,800 missions and moved more than half a million passengers and almost half a million tons of supplies (Summers 1992). Ships, as they had during World War II, carried the bulk of supplies. The sealift consisted of some 250 ships that carried, in total, 9 million tons of equipment and fuel (Summers 1992). The Allied forces had a combined strength of more than 1,500 combat aircraft (Van Voorst 1991, p. 34); between January 17, 1991, the initiation of the air war, and January 27, 1991, the coalition flew more than 18,500 bombing sorties, losing 23 planes ("Tracking the Storm" [Chronology] 1991). American forces fielded almost 1,000 M1A1 tanks, which were capable of outrunning and outgunning any Iraqi tanks (Van Voorst 1991, p. 35).

Perhaps the most striking feature of the Gulf War in comparison with past wars was the compression of time and space because of the increased pace of battle and the increased accuracy and range of weapons (RisCassi 1993). The speed with which personnel and equipment were moved to Southwest Asia was extraordinary. The impressive logistical support provided during Desert Storm, in comparison with that provided in other recent American wars, is documented in Table 1–2.

It is not just that the pace was fast, but that it was unremitting. Modern military operations are continuous (Peters 1993). A key innovation contributing to the 24-hour waging of war has been night-vision equipment. This advantage was pressed in the

Table 1–2. Army deployment in the first 90 days of four wars

	World War II	Korean War	Vietnam War	Persian Gulf War
Passengers	138,060[a]			
Via ship		—[b]	82,800	1,453
Via air		32,357	85,562	183,030
Supplies and equipment: tons shipped	836,060	979,833	1,300,000	1,071,317
Supplies and equipment: tons airlifted	—[b]	—[b]	38,564	175,668

[a]Mostly by ship.
[b]Not available.
Source.   Adapted from "Tracking the Storm" [Chronology] 1991.

Gulf by using nighttime air raids and tank maneuvers in fighting the Iraqis. Interestingly, the only major change in weapons used since World War II "involved space, stealth, and the mating of nuclear power and missiles with submarines" (Bodnar 1993, p. 8). The tremendous advantage we have gained in terms of military capability is in large part a result of the revolution in military sensors and communications. Combat efficiency has increased as a result of our ability to collect, analyze, and respond to sensor data and then, based on these data, to launch "smart" weapons. With the exception of satellites, communications hardware is not better than that used in the Vietnam War (Peters 1993). However, in the Gulf War, satellites were important. They provided critical intelligence, communications, and location data for friendly forces. Although similar numbers of troops had been used in other invasions, their movements had always been programmed ahead of time. In Desert Storm, technological advances allowed close monitoring of the battlefield and continual fine-tuning (Bodnar 1993). However, despite the advances, problems occurred. For example, navigation difficulties, inaccurate target identification, lack of fire discipline, and the confusion of battle contributed to "friendly fire" casualties among tank units (Fontenot 1993).

Changes in Demographics of the Military Since the Vietnam War

There have been several major demographic changes in the military since the Vietnam War and earlier wars as a result of policy changes within the Department of Defense and changes in cultural values. Some of these differences are summarized in Table 1–3. Perhaps the most significant policy changes, which in turn have caused other changes, were the replacement of the draft by an "all volunteer" force and the broadening of fields open to women. Women now account for 11% of active-duty personnel in the armed forces—up from 2% in 1972. From 1951 to 1975, being a parent, getting married, or becoming

Table 1–3. Differences in the American military between the Gulf War and the Vietnam War

Vietnam War	Gulf War
Draftees	All-volunteer force
No reserves	Reserves activated
2% women; limited jobs	10% women; wider variety of jobs
High alcohol/drug use	Lower alcohol/drug use
Ground war	Air war highlighted
Conventional weapons	High-technology weapons (e.g., "smart" bombs)

pregnant was grounds for terminating servicewomen's employment. Therefore, the Gulf War represents the military's first experience with the deployment of large numbers of active-duty mothers and wives. More than 33,300 military women were deployed to the Gulf. The Army deployed 26,000 female soldiers to the theater during Desert Storm. These women functioned in varied roles: flying helicopters, commanding air defense batteries and military police, and performing medical, administrative, intelligence, and transportation duties (Maginnis 1992). Over the course of the war, 11 Army women died, 5 of them killed in action (Becraft 1991); 21 female soldiers were wounded in action, and two women were Iraqi POWs (Maginnis 1992).

The Air Force deployed 3,800 women to Southwest Asia; women piloted and crewed aircraft that were involved in aeromedical evacuation, reconnaissance, and transport missions. The Navy deployed 2,500 women who served on a wide variety of ships, worked in construction units, staffed hospitals, and flew aircraft. The Marine Corps sent 1,000 women to the theater in combat support roles. The Coast Guard also was represented by women during Desert Storm; 13 women participated in port security operations (Becraft 1991).

Women lived under the same austere conditions as their male counterparts. Generally, either women had separate showers or special times were set aside for their use of the showers. Hygiene concerns proved inconsequential for the most part

(U.S. General Accounting Office 1993), although sanitary napkins and tampons were initially in short supply.

Today's military members are better educated. In the Army, the percentage of recruits who enlisted with at least a high school education rose from 64% in 1979 to 93% by 1988. Another important change has been in the amount of substance use and abuse in today's military compared with the military during the era of the Vietnam War. For example, in 1990 the Army reported that fewer than 1% of drug tests were positive. In compliance with the request of the host countries that alcohol not be used, there was dramatically less alcohol (and other substances) use during the Gulf War than in previous wars.

The reduction in the size of the military and other considerations have also changed military doctrine toward increasing reliance on augmentation from the reserves. This increased involvement of the reserves results in an entire nation's experiencing being engaged in war, as in the Persian Gulf, rather than just a segment of society—the military—being engaged in war. As a result, whether reservist and National Guard troops were more likely to develop PTSD was an important question in the Persian Gulf War. Similarly, the chance that their families would be more adversely affected was of concern. Reserve and National Guard units tend to have less well developed family support structures in place, which may place their families at higher risk of psychological sequelae, but they also are very cohesive units that have lived and worked together for years.

Just as today's military members have changed, so too have the members' families (Table 1–4). The military has seen a dramatic increase in the number of single-parent families and dual-

Table 1–4.   Changes in the military family since the Vietnam War

More single-parent families
More dual-career couples
Higher percentage of married soldiers
More "temporary" military families (because of activation of
    reserves)

career couples since the Korean War and the Vietnam War. Some 75% of officers and 60% of enlisted personnel are married; roughly half of their spouses work outside the home (Brant 1993). During the Gulf War, there were over 32,000 children affected by the deployment of their single parents. These children represent approximately 8.2% of all children (390,283) of deployed active-duty, reserve, and National Guard personnel (U.S. Department of Defense 1992).

Sadly, about 140 American children lost one of their parents during the Persian Gulf War (Dunnigan and Bay 1992, p. 342).

Combat Psychiatry in the Gulf War

The principles of combat psychiatry that were applied during the Gulf War, involving proximity, immediacy, and expectancy, were originally developed during World War I. Nonpathological labels (e.g., "combat fatigue"), simple interventions, and treatment in non-hospital-based facilities were used to promote recovery and return to duty (McDuff and Johnson 1992). The principles had been well tried in the context of previous wars and conflicts, and the Gulf War afforded the Army the opportunity to use its combat stress control (CSC) teams for the first time on a major scale. During the Gulf War, psychiatric care for the Army Seventh Corps (roughly 100,000 soldiers) was provided by the 531st Psychiatric Detachment. Mental health personnel were located at three different sites. One psychiatrist, 1 psychologist, 1 social worker, and 5 to 8 enlisted mental health counselors were assigned to each forward combat division. During the Gulf War, each of the 400-bed evacuation hospitals located at the rear of the corps was also supported by a psychiatrist and nursing personnel. These evacuation hospitals could be augmented by additional psychiatric personnel to create a 20-bed psychiatric unit. Mental health assets at the corps level consisted of a 48-person detachment including 5 psychiatrists, 6 social workers, 2 psychiatric nurses, 1 psychologist, 1 field officer, and 33 enlisted mental health counselors (McDuff and Johnson 1992). These multidisciplinary teams provided education and consultation to commanders and medical staff and performed psychiatric interventions (Hales 1992).

The Army reported extremely low evacuation of psychiatric casualties from the theater, equivalent to only 2.7 per 1,000 evacuations per year (Hales 1992). Follow-up studies by the Department of Veterans Affairs indicate that approximately 9% of Persian Gulf returnees reported symptoms scoring in the PTSD range on the Mississippi Scale for Combat-Related PTSD (Keane et al. 1988) in the first 6 to 9 months after returning. As many as 34% have experienced other forms of psychological distress since their return from Southwest Asia (Rosenheck et al. 1992). In the National Vietnam Veterans Readjustment Study, 31% of the male veterans and 27% of the female veterans were reported to have met criteria for PTSD at some time since their war zone deployment (Kulka et al. 1990), and 14% reported current PTSD symptomatology. The low rate of combat stress in the Gulf War may be a result of the war's brevity and successful outcome; time to train and adapt to hostilities; reduced alcohol or drug use; the no-replacement policy; older, better-educated, and better-trained troops; and favorable public opinion to bolster morale before going and upon return (Hales 1992).

The mental health community has also changed since the Vietnam War era. PTSD is now well recognized as a psychiatric condition. Progress has been made in identifying and treating persons affected by trauma. Finally, advances in telecommunications have enabled satellite broadcasts and conference calls as means of promoting interactive continuing education on PTSD (see Chapter 10, this volume, by Blank and Lehmann). Mental health professionals can be linked with PTSD experts and have access to the medical literature throughout the world.

In this book, the effects of the Gulf War on various populations—active-duty military, reservists, and their children and families—are explored. The unique and expected stressors of the war are discussed. The threat of terrorism and chemical/biological warfare, although not carried out in this war, remains a serious challenge for future military operations. The psychological stressors before, during, and after war and the resulting psychiatric morbidity are discussed at length in this book, based on both our past knowledge and new data from the Persian Gulf War. The contributions in this book serve as a summary of the effects of the Persian Gulf War and a textbook for psychiatric care and interventions in the broader perspective of modern-day warfare and affected populations.

References

Becraft CH: Women in the U.S. Armed Services: The Persian Gulf War. Washington, DC, Women's Research & Education Institute, March 1991

Bodnar JW: The military technical revolution: from hardware to information. Naval War College Review, Summer 1993, pp 7–21

Brant BA: Vanguard of social change? Military Review, February 1993, pp 12–19

Dinneen MP, Pentzien RJ, Mateczun JM: Stress and coping with the trauma of war in the Persian Gulf: the hospital ship USNS Comfort, in Individual and Community Responses to Trauma and Disaster: The Structure of Human Chaos. Edited by Ursano RJ, McCaughey BG, Fullerton CS. Cambridge, UK, Cambridge University Press, 1994, pp 306–329

Dunnigan JF, Bay A: From Shield to Storm: High-Tech Weapons, Military Strategy, and Coalition Warfare in the Persian Gulf. New York, William Morrow, 1992

Fontenot G: Fright night: Task Force 2/34 Armor. Military Review, January 1993, pp 38–52

Hales RE: Taking issue: psychiatric lessons from the Persian Gulf War. Hosp Community Psychiatry 43:769, 1992

Hill R: Families Under Stress: Adjustment to the Crises of War Separation and Reunion. Westport, CT, Greenwood Press, 1949

Kantrowitz B: Somebody in Saudi Arabia loves me. Newsweek, November 19, 1990, pp 32–33

Keane TM, Caddell JM, Taylor KL: Mississippi Scale for Combat-Related Posttraumatic Stress Disorder: three studies in reliability and validity. J Consult Clin Psychol 56:85–90, 1988

Knudson GB: Operation Desert Shield: medical aspects of weapons of mass destruction. Mil Med 156:267–271, 1991

Kulka RA, Schlenger WE, Fairbank JA, et al: Trauma and the Vietnam War Generation. New York, Brunner/Mazel, 1990

Maginnis RL: The future of women in the Army. Military Review, July 1992, pp 21–33

McCubbin HI, Patterson JM: The family stress process: the double ABCX model of adjustment and adaptation, in Social Stress and the Family. Edited by McCubbin HI, Sussman M, Patterson JM. New York, Haworth Press, 1983, pp 7–37

McDuff DR, Johnson JL: Classification and characteristics of Army stress casualties during Operation Desert Storm. Hosp Community Psychiatry 43:812–815, 1992

Norris FH: Toward establishing a database for the prospective study of traumatic stress. Presentation at the National Institute of Mental Health Workshop "Traumatic Stress: Defining Terms and Instruments," Uniformed Services University of the Health Sciences, Bethesda, MD, 1988

Peters R: The movable fortress: warfare in the twenty-first century. Military Review, February 1993, pp 62–72

RisCassi RW: Doctrine for joint operations in a combined environment: a necessity. Military Review, June 1993, pp 20–37

Rosen LN, Westhuis DJ, Teitelbaum JM: Children's reaction's to the Desert Storm deployment: initial findings from a survey of Army families. Mil Med 158:465–469, 1993

Rosenheck R, Becnel H, Blank AS Jr, et al: Returning Persian Gulf Troops: First Year Findings. VA Northeast Program Evaluation Center (NEPEC), The Evaluation Division of the National Center for PTSD, VA Medical Center, West Haven, CT, 1992

Salomon LE, Bankirer H: Total Army CSS providing the means for victory. Military Review, April 1991, pp 3–8

Solomon Z: Combat Stress Reaction: The Enduring Toll of War. New York, Plenum, 1993

Summers H: Full circle: World War II to the Persian Gulf. Military Review, June 1992, pp 38–48

Tracking the storm [Chronology]. Military Review, September 1991, pp 65–81

Ursano RJ, Fullerton CS, McCaughey BG: Trauma and disaster, in Individual and Community Responses to Trauma and Disaster: The Structure of Human Chaos. Edited by Ursano RJ, McCaughey BG, Fullerton CS. Cambridge, UK, Cambridge University Press, 1994, pp 3–28

U.S. Department of Defense: Desert Storm. Defense 91, September/October 1991, pp 56–59

U.S. Department of Defense: DoD Report on Title III of the Persian Gulf Conflict and Supplemental Authorization and Personnel Benefits Act of 1991, Public Law 102-25, in Family Policy and Programs: Persian Gulf Conflict. Washington, DC, U.S. Department of Defense, 1992

U.S. General Accounting Office: Women in the Military: Deployment in the Persian Gulf War (NSIAD-93-93). Washington, DC, U.S. General Accounting Office, July 1993

Van Voorst B: Advantage: the Alliance. Time, January 21, 1991, pp 34–35

Part II
Stressors of the Persian Gulf War

2

War and Homecomings: The Stressors of War and of Returning From War

Sandra A. Yerkes, M.D.
Harry C. Holloway, M.D.

No generation of Americans has escaped the experience of soldiers preparing for battle, leaving loved ones behind, participating in conflict, and then returning home. These rituals of war were repeated during the recent Persian Gulf conflict. In this chapter we review the factors that shape the consequences of homecoming for the serviceperson and for his or her receiving environment. In particular, we review the issues that the primary practice physician and psychiatric clinician need to know to understand with empathy the story the returnee tells. If the physician understands the context of homecoming from war, he or she can better listen to the returnee's story and reach a proper diagnosis and treatment plan.

Throughout history, many mythic tales have dealt with the homecoming of returning veterans, seen as returning saviors or avenging destroyers. *The Odyssey* describes Odysseus' killing of suitors in a homecoming that was as violent as the Trojan War. *The Orestia* of Aeschylus presents the violent murder of Agamemnon and the leaders of the Greek forces upon their return home from Troy. His wife, Clytemnestra, has come to love another, and with that other, she kills Agamemnon. More recent examples include Spencer Tracy's character in *Bad Day at Black Rock* (returning savior) and the Special Forces Team of *Lethal Weapon* (avenging destroyers). Such powerful myths and stories promote the belief that there is justice in the world and embody the cognitive processes associated with this belief.

These myths, as well as media images of sociocultural events (e.g., antiwar movements, movements that represent war as a religious crusade, etc.), economic conditions, stress exposure, and new romantic/sexual relationships that can occur during a deployment, are critical in determining what homecoming is like and the consequences of returning home from war. Veterans, families of veterans, and other members of society are affected during war by their assumptions, expectations, observations, and suffering, and by those with whom they share their experiences. The consequences of these experiences eventually show up in personal tales, historical accounts, attitudes, and behaviors.

The demographic characteristics of the returnee also have an impact on homecoming. The young returnee drafted out of school is seen differently by society than the older returnee who had an established place in society before the war. The unmarried returnee lacks the support provided by a spouse. The married returnee may have immediate responsibilities to provide economic security to others. The career military veteran returning to the security of a highly cohesive military unit may be more supported than, for example, the reservist who, in the absence of a support network, returns to a large city that is experienced as impersonal and uncaring. The need to feel and be supported is a significant factor in maintaining the mental health of veterans. Studies of returnees from Vietnam showed that those who remained in active-duty units had relatively lower rates of psychological distress than those who returned to civilian life (Stretch 1986a, 1986b). This could be an effect of self-selection as well as the former group's having increased social supports.

During Operation Desert Storm and Provide Comfort, approximately 500,000 servicemembers were deployed to the Persian Gulf area. In total, 216,871 reservists were called to active duty, and 106,047 reservists were deployed to the Gulf. The mean age of the deployed enlisted individuals was mid-20s; the mean age of the officers was early 30s. Of the reservists, about half were married to civilians, and 13,387 were single parents (U.S. Department of Defense 1991).

Each of these demographic qualities is likely to critically influence the individual's homecoming. For instance, 254,611 of the deployed active-duty troops were lower ranking (E1 to E4). Rank is a good indicator of the economic resources available to military members and their families during the deployment. Being a reservist indicated a high probability that the individual suffered an unexpected career disruption. Prior planning, character structure, and chance alone determined whether deployment was an intolerable burden or a welcome adventure.

The Fantasy of Homecoming

No matter when homecoming occurs, it is preceded by the expectation of what it will be. The process of creating this expectation (i.e., the fantasy of homecoming) begins at the time of deployment and continues until homecoming. The media prepared the population for a bloody war in the Persian Gulf. The unreliability of high-tech weapons systems was emphasized, and the experienced nature of the Iraqi Army was reported repeatedly. High casualty rates were expected, and dangers posed by weapons of mass destruction and terror, such as chemical weapons, were discussed by a wide variety of experts. The psychological consequences of participating in battle were discussed, and conditions such as posttraumatic stress disorder (PTSD) were explained by numerous experts.

For the veteran, the expectations of the return home are influenced by the circumstances at home at the time of departure, communications with home during the conflict, and the circumstances of the war's termination. The fantasy of homecoming is created jointly by the expectations of the veteran and by those of the receiving environment. Both the veterans and their families expected a terrible war in the Gulf, with many physically and emotionally traumatic consequences for those who served. At the war's end, the Iraqi Army had experienced massive trauma and almost complete destruction, but the trauma for the Allied forces was both less than and different from that which had been anticipated. The United States returnees observed the destruction of a much feared but overmatched enemy force and the massive ecological disaster imposed by that force for revenge. For many combat soldiers, the end of the war meant the end of an important identity as a warrior irrespective of whether they returned to civilian jobs or to the routine of a peacetime military unit. Such a loss of identity may be profound for those unable to find a new identity upon their return.

During war, the expectations of home are shaped by the types and frequency of communication (i.e., telephone, letter, audiotape), the interpersonal nature of the communication (the writer's desire to write), the family's and society's ability to support the veteran from afar, the media's portrayal of the conditions at home (e.g., American society's unrest seen by soldiers in the Vietnam War), and the information about home relayed by the veteran's command. At the time of the veteran's departure for war, the circumstances at home have a direct impact on the communications with home during the war. For example, unsettled finances, hurt feelings, and earlier instances of infidelity affect what is said and how it is communicated. Leaving home at a time of unresolved conflicts can result in hurtful discussions and angry feelings, whereas leaving home on good terms enhances the communications. Soldiers are encouraged by their command to believe that they will come home intact physically and psychologically and that their families will be safe. They are led to believe that society will be appreciative of the sacrifices they are making. These expectations and the assumption that they will return victorious are used by the command to motivate soldiers and enhance performance. Upon the war's end, the veterans' expectations of homecoming are shaped by assumptions of what society owes them for their sacrifices and by society's perception of the veterans as victors or losers.

Society, as well as the young soldier, vIews participation in battle as an adult activity. The adolescent who leaves his or her family to fight in war achieves a new identity as soldier/warrior and completes the process of separation and individuation. The soldier anticipates that his or her family will accept and adjust to new behaviors and habits (e.g., use of alcohol and/or tobacco, staying out late) and that society will accord him or her adult status.

For the returning American soldier, the fantasy of homecoming has traditionally included an expectation of various "rewards" such as free land, education, and veterans' bonuses. Although free land is no longer an incentive for veterans, favorable mortgage loans, educational benefits, and monetary bonuses continue to exist and are part of the anticipated reward fantasized by the soldier.

Often soldiers assume that women will be more responsive to them if they have been in combat. The perception that one will be admired or seen as more handsome and masculine if one participates in battle is used in recruiting efforts and as motivation during training. The increasing presence of women in the military and on the battlefield diminishes the power of these beliefs as women and men work side by side for military victory. The belief by some in society that women who are combatants are more masculine generates negative attitudes toward them and their positions in the military. That the battle experience will somehow make them less sexually desirable has long been an undercurrent of popular opinion in both civilian and military populations.

As battle technology advances and brute strength alone no longer dictates who will be victorious, these assumptions regarding a combatant's sexual attractiveness are slowly fading. What new assumptions will replace the old is not yet known, leaving uncertainty as to how men and women warriors will be perceived upon returning home from future conflicts.

For a soldier anticipating a return to an economically deprived community or family, the fantasy of a homecoming marked by poor employment opportunities, overwhelming financial responsibilities, or financial destitution may motivate him or her not to return. The veteran's fantasy of homecoming may then include going to a new place where, the veteran unrealistically believes, all of his or her needs will be met.

The stage in life of the returning veteran, in many cases correlated with age, is also important to the meaning of homecoming and how it is anticipated. The veteran who is returning to his or her family of origin (father and mother) looks forward to being independent, whereas the veteran who is returning to his or her own family expects to reintegrate into the family and resume predeployment roles. Children are a central factor in the expectation of homecoming. They represent continuity and connections to the future for a person who is risking his or her life and whose own future is uncertain.

The Fantasy of the Receiving Environment

The expectations (psychological state) created by the conditions of deployment have a critical impact on the way veterans are viewed when they return home. A common fantasy of deployment is that the departing veteran will return victorious. Building upon past victories, news articles, editorials, and television and radio commentary inundate the country that is anticipating victory. With defense budgets consuming billions of taxpayers' dollars, victory in war is not just desired, but demanded. Soldiers are sent off to war amid marching bands and promises of wonderful reunions after their victory.

Prior homecomings and past societal traumas influence each subsequent homecoming. The public's view of the conflict will be projected upon war participants at the time of their return. Distant wars fought on foreign shores generate different attitudes regarding conflict than do local wars, in which the possibility of direct attack of civilian populations is present. With current technology, what was once considered distant is becoming increasingly closer in military terms. Missile attacks can strike hundreds of miles from the launching site, destroying areas once thought to be safe by virtue of their distance from the battlefield. When security and safety are not guaranteed by the end of battle and the return of troops, society's expectation of homecoming changes.

For the family, the fantasy of homecoming assumes that everything will be as it was before the war and that nothing will have changed. However, the deployment of a family member creates a painful void within the family system that is eventually filled (or denied) so that life can go on. Economic support is established as family members who are not accustomed to working take on jobs. New friendships and relationships are made or existing ones strengthened in order to meet emotional and companionship needs. New roles within the family and social system are taken on to replace those lost through the departure of the soldier. The family assumes that their experiences at home and the soldier's activities on the battlefield will be easily assimilated by each other at the time of reunion and that the pre-war roles will be resumed. The fact that new roles and re-sponsibilities may not be given up quickly upon homecoming is not anticipated. The idealization of a "perfect homecoming" at the time of deployment does not allow the family or the soldier to envision a future marked by, for example, loss of work when a temporary worker is released to make room for a returning soldier, provision of care to a wounded or disabled family member, or the dissolution of established relationships.

The crucial factor in society's anticipated homecoming is the anticipated economic status of the family and society at that time. A prosperous and expanding economy, such as that which followed World War II, in which there are considerable unfilled consumer needs and a surplus of jobs, welcomes the veteran with available employment, support, and assistance during the transition. On the other hand, a devastated economy will not welcome returning veterans, regardless of whether the soldiers were victorious, if it has difficulty absorbing them, as was the situation in Germany, Japan, and Russia immediately following the end of World War II.

The U.S. did not use a draft to augment its forces during the Gulf War. Instead, it called upon more than 100,000 reservists to temporarily leave their jobs and fight. These individuals had their normal occupational career patterns disrupted. For many, the disruption may have provided an escape from boredom, but it also created profound anxiety that they might not have a job upon their return. Not knowing how long they would remain at war or how their employers would handle personnel shortages in their absence led them to worry about their civilian jobs. Employers bound by law and moral responsibility were anxious about maintaining unfilled positions while their employees served in the Persian Gulf. Many reservists who were self-employed suffered considerable financial loss as a result of their military service. These concerns undoubtedly had an impact on the fantasies of homecoming envisioned by reservists and their employers.

The Reality of Homecoming

The Veteran and Society

The response of the veteran to homecoming is influenced and determined by the role and status of the veteran in the military and the status granted the veteran in society. Because the privileged elite in the U.S. have historically been deferred from military service, the nonelite and unprivileged may achieve positions of responsibility that might be unavailable to them in civilian life. Those who have found prestige, honor, and enhancement of self-esteem through their military position may be disappointed when the same prestige is not available to them in their civilian role. (For example, Civil War veterans were not welcomed in some communities where they were feared as individuals who had killed and were reported to drink and swear [Wecter 1944].) However, some returning veterans who held low-status positions in the military return to high-status positions in society, positions obtained through family connections or through completing courses of study that allow entry into those positions. Homecoming might be viewed by the former as a loss of status and by the latter as a gain. For some individuals, civilian positions may be less exciting than military positions, and the transition to a civilian role may result in a psychic loss.

Many military personnel are led to believe that if they act appropriately during battle, they will not suffer injury. If they are injured, they may blame themselves, be stigmatized by others, or be identified as heroes. The distinction between hero and failure is not an objective one. Rather it is based on political and ideological factors in the receiving (home) social group. If the soldier is not victorious (as in the Vietnam War) or becomes a casualty or prisoner of war, the outcome is much more ambiguous. Monetary, material, and emotional rewards may be denied, and the psychological stigma associated with being a "loser" may be placed on the returning soldier.

The quality of demobilization is often the first indication of how society will welcome the veteran home. The homecoming experience contributes substantially to the veteran's appraisal of the military and the society that sent him or her into battle. For example, the end of World War II was marked by parades, speeches, and special veteran educational experiences as whole units were returned home and discharged back to their civilian lives. The country felt elated at winning the war, and veterans were welcomed back as heroes. Conversely, returning Vietnam War veterans came home from Southeast Asia individually when their military service was completed. No parades or speeches welcomed them home; instead they were confronted with a society bitterly opposed to the war. The wearing of military uniforms in public often prompted insults and harassment by certain segments of the civilian population. Frequently these veterans spent many days living in impersonal barracks waiting for their discharge paperwork. Once discharged, they were confronted by social changes and a shift in cultural values as well as the unmet expectation of rewards for their military service. Many felt slighted, betrayed, invalidated, and used by America (Fleming 1985).

The roles in which society chooses to place returned veterans affect the process of homecoming. Victors and heroes receive public acknowledgment and praise for their sacrifice. They are entitled to the "spoils of war" and societal support. Losers are not entitled to public recognition, and their sacrifices are quickly forgotten by society, which may view them as being responsible for the loss. For returning Vietnam War veterans, society's reaction caused only feelings of being unappreciated, distrust of government and authority, cynicism, concern with humanistic values with an overlay of hedonism, and existential malaise (Fleming 1985).

The economic and social support given the veteran is a public acknowledgment of the veteran's worth. Vietnam veterans were traumatized by the indifference they found when they returned. One veteran is quoted by Fleming (1985, p. 123) as saying, ". . . you will find this in all Vietnam veterans—this rage within them that's a reaction to the reaction we got when we came home." Formal organizations (such as the Veterans Administration, American Legion, and Veterans of Foreign Wars) and informal networks of veterans help the veteran reintegrate into society through monetary assistance, job opportunities, networking for educational and training opportunities, and social support. Community supports can reduce the likelihood of psychiatric disease in returnees and provide a valuable resource for the treatment of those who are ill.

As mentioned previously, returning veterans must compete at the time of homecoming with civilians and other returning veterans for jobs. Temporary workers hired during conflicts have traditionally been released from employment to make room for returning veterans. Following World War II, "temporary" female workers were released from industrial positions to make jobs available for returning male GIs. The impact of homecoming for the released female workers, thus, was one of displacement and hardship as they were forced to seek other means of support. Such dramatic employment shifts have not occurred in recent wars but remain a potential problem should the draft be reinstituted. For those civilian populations living through a war fought in their own territory, accommodating returning soldiers and their needs for jobs, education, retraining, and rehabilitative medical care presents a considerable burden that may be impossible to provide if the society's finances and resources have been exhausted by the war.

In the past, those veterans who have fought in distant wars have lived an experience difficult to comprehend by those left behind. Since the Korean War, the battlefield experience has been a part of nightly television, and anyone can experience the selected sound and video images of the battlefield correspondent. Strangely, there is no evidence that this has increased the empathy of those who have never been in combat. Despite the images communicated about war by television, an increased understanding of the plight of the combat soldier does not seem to get through.

As military policy allows women to assume a greater role in combat operations, society's expectations of the military, women, and war will inevitably change. During the Gulf War, female soldiers were extensively singled out for interviews, sometimes concurrently with their families at home. Millions watched on television as families struggled to contain their emotions and fears for their mothers and wives. How did society view these media forays into the private lives of its military members? What expectations and apprehensions were generated as the possibility of mothers and wives being killed, captured, tortured, and maimed was brought into every home? Hopes for loving family reunions at homecoming were voiced daily by families waiting expectantly for Mom to return, always with the unspoken possibility of loss through death. These video images and commentary carried powerful messages and were used by various organizations, such as advocates and opponents of women's serving in combat, to propel their own political agendas.

Another problem for the receiving environment is how to reestablish empathic bonds with the returning veteran. That is, how can the population open itself to experiencing the pain, helplessness, and hopelessness associated with the traumatic experiences? Frequently, one way to close out or isolate oneself

from such experiences is to maintain that the veteran who suffered the trauma can be understood only by another veteran
who suffered the same experience. This mode of isolating nonveteran from veteran allows one to avoid the necessity of developing a method of communication, and it reinforces a personal
conviction of specialness in the veteran. This specialness can
exist at both the cognitive and affective levels. The veteran's
avoidance of communication with nonveterans may protect
against pain at the price of isolating the veteran.

Reunion With Family

Once the fanfare of return to country and community, if such
takes place, is over, the process of reintegration into the family
truly begins. The family itself may be a conduit for the societal
attitude toward the veteran and the resources that society
makes available to him or her. Families can be extremely important in helping veterans reintegrate and reestablish themselves
in society. However, the expectation that the family will help
can also cause severe disappointments when that expectation is
not met.

The returning veteran cannot help but be affected by the
experience of going to war and contemplating and witnessing
death. Similarly, the process of working with men and women
from different cultures and sharing hardships with others who
previously were viewed as different, inferior, or dangerous influences the veteran's understanding of the world and challenges the lessons learned in the past through family and
community. These life experiences can result in the assignment
of new priorities and attitudes that counter those previously
held. The returning veteran may have difficulty adjusting to
a family that has also changed. The empathic bonds of family,
friends, and community that were established before deployment may not be easily reestablished with the "changed" veteran. The veteran, likewise, may be unable to understand his or
her community and family.

The veteran's family is influenced by the time at which the deployment and the homecoming occur within the family's life cycle and the length of the deployment. The initial loss of the veteran at the time of deployment is mourned, and then the role previously filled by the veteran is assumed by someone else. The birth of children, family traumas and triumphs, and other life events are missed by the deployed soldier and are only partially shared through whatever means of communication are available. The longer the deployment, the longer intimate participation in the family is denied. At the time of reunion, the newly assumed roles and the accompanying power may not be so easily given up. Women's self-esteem, reliance, and earning power increase as they take on the responsibilities previously assumed by the male soldier (Wecter 1944). Powerful emotional struggles may be played out as a new equilibrium of power is established within the family. Families that learned to live without the veterans must now include them (Borus 1977) and learn to live with them as they are, perhaps physically or mentally changed.

Younger veterans deploying as adolescents are in the process of separating from their families; after the war they return to their families to complete the separation process, a transitional situation that often is relatively chaotic. Other veterans acquire families in the course of the war and return home with them. Irrespective of which stage in the family life cycle the deployment occurs, the family is certain to struggle with the change in the veteran upon return.

The family's experience at home, coping with society and the local community, differs dramatically from the veteran's experiences. With few shared deployment experiences between them, each is seen as a stranger in the other's world. The veteran is often isolated from the family's experience and may wish to return to the "family" of military buddies who shared the battle experience and "understand" the veteran's feelings. The idealized relationships within combat units are remembered and used as a comparison for new family relationships (Borus 1977).

As the family struggles to reassign roles, it is generally supported by the medical, social, and behavioral systems and groups in the community that provide strategies and rituals to help the family cope during crisis (Milgram 1986). Wives' clubs and networks understand what waiting wives and children go through and plan special events and seminars to help them deal with changes that are well known to members. Such groups may be unprepared and thus unable to meet the needs of select segments of the military population when homecoming involves groups such as mothers returning to their families, nonmarried individuals returning to partnerships, and ethnic minorities returning to their families. These families must deal with their homecomings alone, having no models for reintegrating the military member into the family.

Although women have always been associated with armies in the field, the inclusion of women in the military has introduced new issues to homecoming. The gender specificity of the receiving environment influences the family's expectations. In past wars, American women were left behind to care for homes and children. During the Gulf War, many men were left behind with the children as their wives packed their duffel bags and deployed to the Gulf. A male spouse of a female veteran must deal with the reversal of conventional roles. Traditional support networks frequently have difficulty including "Mr. Moms" into what has until recent years been the "Wives' Club." Although a change in terminology to "Key Volunteers" has removed the feminine appellation, these groups continue to be organized by wives to support wives. Male participation in these organizations is an infrequent event, which can cause social awkwardness and generalized discomfort when they attend meetings.

Unmarried partnerships, which are not recognized by military support systems, society, and sometimes even the extended families of the involved individuals, are a relatively silent segment of both the civilian and the military populations. Whether these partnerships are composed of straight or gay couples, the traditional societal and military supports for families are not available to them.

Children have always been affected by war and the departure of family members. In the case of a prolonged deployment, the veteran returns to his or her children as a stranger. This is a critical issue in the difficulties and problems encountered in parenting. Rapid developmental changes in the child are not directly experienced by the returning parent, and a gap occurs in the continuity of the parenting experience. This gap is just as disconcerting for the child as for the parent. The normal holding environment for a child is influenced, in part, by parental coordination and authority. When veterans return, the emotional resources of the children and parents are challenged. The return of one's mother from battle is a relatively new cultural experience, the impact of which is unknown at this time. Continued research is required to evaluate its potential impact upon future generations.

Impact of the Strangeness of War

The development of *Gulf War syndrome*, characterized by multiple symptoms that appear related to different causal agents ranging from parasitic infections, to sensitivities to multiple chemicals, to the consequences of traumatic experience, is another problem confronting veterans of the Gulf War. The causal agents, whether they are leishmaniasis, exposure to the toxins resulting from burning oil wells, and/or the experience of combat, are beyond the usual experience of veterans, their society, and their physicians. The cause of Gulf War syndrome is under intensive study. There may yet be a single explanation, or perhaps a limited number of explanations, for the problems affecting a portion of the Gulf War veterans.

It is useful to recall past experiences of soldiers who have been exposed to "strange" tropical diseases in "unusual" environments. Jerome Frank (1946) described how physicians and patients responded to exposure to schistosomiasis in the Philippines (an illness caused by a very small fluke trematode). Numerous symptoms and problems were attributed to this disease. On the one hand, soldiers were told that the disease should not be a source of much concern, and on the other hand, armed forces radio got the message out that all should avoid walking in swamps, where they might be infected with the deadly condition.

Servicemembers in the Gulf War were warned of the terrible weapons that would be deployed against them. They were given vaccines to protect them against biological agents that, as it turned out, were not used. Some groups in the U.S. held that giving these "experimental" vaccines was unethical. High-tech detectors of chemical agents gave positive readings, but these readings were thought to be false positives. The sky was dark with smoke from oil fires, but testing systems were reported to indicate that no one was exposed to excessive smoke. Perceived discrepancies between soldiers' observations and information provided by official sources about possible exposure to toxic agents generated anxiety and mistrust for some. Research on individuals exposed to the uncertainty associated with the Three Mile Island accident demonstrated symptom patterns (e.g., increased somatic symptoms, anxiety) that lasted for 10 years and that were correlated with elevations of norepinephrine and epinephrine (Baum 1983, 1986). Perhaps the same sort of phenomena have contributed to development of Gulf War syndrome.

In situations like those experienced by the Gulf War veteran, there are at least two groups that are operating at high levels of uncertainty: veterans and their physicians. Both veterans and their physicians are quite uncertain about what processes may be involved in causing the symptoms associated with the Gulf War. Given the stigmatizing nature of attributing the symptoms to stress or psychiatric illness, there is an appropriate reluctance to making an unwarranted attribution of causality. The attribution to other causes is at high risk of being imprecise at best and encouraging an inappropriate validation of illness at worst.

The resultant sense of uncertainty on the part of the caregiver makes both the caregiver and the patient feel helpless. This mutual helplessness seldom encourages a therapeutic alliance between the two. It does encourage premature closure of investigations and conflict about inappropriate labeling and denial of care. These interactions are particularly dangerous to the patient and to the long-term integrity of the caregivers. In this situation the physicians are challenged to exercise all of the diagnostic and therapeutic tools available with compassion and disciplined curiosity for the patient's benefit. If the veteran is to benefit, the two primary rules of care in this situation must be two of the oldest: do no harm and relieve suffering.

Conclusions

History records how our veterans returned from war, but little has been written about the emotional impact of homecoming on veterans, families, and society. This is surprising in light of the influence these events have upon attitudes toward the military and toward future conflicts, and for family interactions that reverberate throughout future generations. The fantasy of homecoming is shaped by many factors and may not reflect the reality of the actual event. As our military forces become more demographically heterogeneous, including more women and minorities in nontraditional roles, support institutions endorsed by the military and society must assess the needs of these groups and create strategies to make homecoming a smooth transition to postdeployment roles for veterans, families, and society.

When searching for the meaning of homecoming, we must define the concept of home. What is home and what does it mean? In the transactional definition of the word, the internal object "home" is generated from both the internal expectations of the veteran, the family, and community members and the transactions between the individual and his or her social environment. What relationships are present between immediate and extended family members, and how are they acted upon? How do these networks interact, and what expectations do members contribute to the overall expectations of the family? What empathic bonds are present, and how will they change as a result of the experience of a family member's going to war?

How does the receiving "home" open itself to experiencing the helplessness, hopelessness, pain, and trauma of the veteran's experience? In what way will the fantasy of home interact with the reality of the experience? For each soldier, sailor, aviator, and marine, these questions must be asked and assessed to understand the meaning and impact of homecoming for that specific individual.

References

Baum A: Emotional, behavioral, and physiological effect of chronic stress at Three Mile Island. J Consult Clin Psychol 51:565–572, 1983

Baum A: Biopsychosocial effects of disasters: Three Mile Island. Bethesda, MD, Department of Psychiatry, Uniformed Services University of the Health Sciences, 1986

Borus FB: Reentry: adjustment issues facing the Vietnam returnee. Arch Gen Psychiatry 28:501–506, 1977

Fleming RH: Post Vietnam syndrome: neurosis or sociosis? Psychiatry 48:122–139, 1985

Frank J: Emotional reactions of American soldiers to an unfamiliar disease. Am J Psychiatry 102:631–640, 1946

Milgram NA: Stress and Coping in the Time of War. New York, Brunner/Mazel, 1986

Stretch RH: The Factors Associated With Post-Traumatic Stress Disorder Among Active Duty Army Personnel. Washington, DC, Walter Reed Army Institute of Research, updated 1986a

Stretch RH: Incidence and etiology of post-traumatic stress disorder among active duty Army personnel. Journal of Applied Social Psychology 16:464–481, 1986b

U.S. Department of Defense: Desert Storm. Defense 91, September/October 1991, pp 56–59

Wecter D: When Johnny Comes Marching Home. Boston, MA, Houghton-Mifflin, 1944

3

Psychiatric Responses to War Trauma

James R. Rundell, M.D.
Robert J. Ursano, M.D.

Military personnel live and work in a culture that is unique in our society. War-related stressors are unique in human experience. During Operations Desert Shield/Desert Storm, for instance, apart from the unequaled experience of being in actual combat, there were also the associated stressors of anticipating combat, being in the confined environment of gear designed to protect against chemical warfare, and, for some, the handling of dead bodies that hours before had been buddies, peers, or enemies (Brooks et al. 1983; Carter and Cammermeyer 1985; McCarroll et al. 1993a).

Some people exposed to combat develop psychiatric disorders (Centers for Disease Control 1988; Helzer et al. 1987; Kulka et al. 1990; Rundell et al. 1989; Ursano 1981; Ursano et al. 1987; Yager et al. 1984). Others show no long-term effects (Rundell et al. 1989; Ursano 1981), and still others report psychological growth (Borus 1973; Sledge et al. 1980; Ursano 1981; Van Putten and Yager 1984).

Historically, psychiatric signs and symptoms observed in soldiers after combat were called "nostalgia," "shell shock," or "war neurosis" (Sargent and Slater 1940; War Office 1922). Our diagnostic nomenclature now identifies a number of disorders that have been well documented after combat and other disaster trauma. Among servicemembers exposed to combat, some will have acute stress disorder (ASD) or posttraumatic stress disorder (PTSD). Depression, substance-related disorders, anxiety disorders, adjustment disorder, somatoform disorders, and psychosomatic disorders may also occur. The coexistence of two or more psychiatric disorders is the rule.

During Operations Desert Shield/Desert Storm, for the first time, significant numbers of women were deployed to serve in combat support roles that resulted in exposure to combat itself. The notion that a nation's wives and mothers will be exposed to combat situations on a large scale is new, but such deployment is a phenomenon that will expand in future wars. Never before in the history of United States military operations have so many fathers and mothers with young children been so abruptly deployed for such an extended period.

Because the Gulf War was brief, the number of combat stress disorder casualties was fewer than had been feared (Rosenheck et al. 1991). However, combat stress–related symptomatology was not infrequent. A 1991 survey of 26 Gulf War veterans revealed a number of PTSD symptoms: startle response (62%), irritability (50%), reliving experiences (35%), feeling on edge (35%), and nightmares (31%) (Rosenheck et al. 1991). Twenty-three percent of this group scored in the PTSD range on the Mississippi Scale for Combat-Related PTSD (Keane et al. 1988).

Exposure of civilians to war trauma is the norm for most countries. For example, in the early 1990s, 90% of casualties during the war in the republics of the former Yugoslavia were civilians. This incidence of civilian casualties is in contrast to the estimated 5% civilian casualty rate during World War I (Sivard 1991). Strategies to terrorize civilian populations, such as systematic use of rape, are underreported. During recent wars, these methods have been used to undermine community bonds and weaken resistance to aggression (Swiss and Giller 1993).

Acute stress disorder and PTSD are both common posttraumatic psychiatric disorders. The National Vietnam Veterans Readjustment Study (NVVRS) has provided some of our best data on the long-term psychiatric effects of combat (Kulka et al. 1990,

1991). In the NVVRS, investigators examined the lifetime and current prevalences of psychiatric disorders among a national sample of Vietnam War veterans. This sample included those who served in Vietnam, other Vietnam War–era veterans, and matched civilian control subjects. The investigators estimated psychiatric disorder rates with a number of measures, including the Structured Interview for DSM-III-R (SCID). For male theater veterans with high levels of combat/war-zone stress exposure, there were markedly higher rates for most psychiatric disorders compared with the rates found for other male veterans or civilians. Higher current psychiatric illness rates were also found for female veterans exposed to high levels of "war zone stress" compared with other theater female veterans, nontheater female veterans, or civilian women.

It is important to recall that veterans with psychiatric illness are also more likely to have physical problems because of combat injuries. Such medical problems must always be a part of the psychiatric assessment and care.

The data on psychiatric disorders in veterans of the Gulf War are still limited. However, the literature on war trauma clearly indicates a number of disorders that the clinician must consider. In this chapter we discuss the psychiatric disorders—acute, delayed, and chronic—that frequently appear in persons exposed to war trauma. We also address, specifically, the data on Gulf War veterans.

Psychiatric Illness After War

Acute Stress Disorder

Curiously absent from DSM-III (American Psychiatric Association 1980) and DSM-III-R (American Psychiatric Association 1987) was a diagnostic category for acute responses to traumatic events such as war. In DSM-IV (American Psychiatric Association 1994), acknowledgment is made to the spectrum of responses to exposure to traumatic events by inclusion of the diagnosis acute stress disorder (Table 3–1). Symptoms of ASD occur within 4 weeks of a traumatic event and last between 2 days and 4 weeks. The symptoms cannot be due to the direct effects of a substance or a general medical condition or to an exacerbation of a psychiatric disorder that was present before exposure to the event.

Glass (1955) defined "combat stress disorder" (i.e., ASD) as "a temporary period of persistent failure of the supportive or defensive forces to sustain the individual against the opposing pressures of functional disorganization" (p. 233). More recent experience confirms that sustained combat-related ASD has adverse effects on postwar functioning (Solomon and Mikulincer 1987). These adverse effects include increased rates of somatic complaints following the war (Solomon et al. 1987a, 1987b). The risk of ASD associated with combat is related to social support, particularly perceived support from officers, and to loneliness (Solomon and Benbenishty 1986; Solomon et al. 1986a, 1986b).

Each branch of the service is associated with stressors specific to that branch that have the potential to produce special areas of unique ASD vulnerability. For example, Army and Marine service personnel are exposed to close combat on relatively large scales. Navy personnel have the unique inability to evade direct threats (the "sitting duck" feeling). Similarly, in the Air Force, a number of factors may contribute to ASD vulnerability: the passive nature of combat duties, the relatively small amount of combat skills training for most Air Force personnel, lack of experience with mass casualty situations, family proximity to potential operational areas, and base/personnel immobility (Rundell et al. 1990). Fortunately, during Operations Desert Shield/Desert Storm, the duration of the conflict was so short, there were relatively few cases of ASD (Rosenheck et al. 1991).

It is important to differentiate *primary* war trauma victims from *secondary* war trauma victims. Types of stressors and response syndromes may differ between these two groups, and treatment and coping strategies may also vary. For example, health assistance workers (Bartone et al. 1989) at sites of military or combat traumatic events, as well as body handlers in military morgues (McCarroll et al. 1993a, 1993b; Ursano et al. 1988), may become secondarily exposed to war trauma. Stressors associated with body handlers include anticipation (especially in the case of inexperienced workers), multiple sensory stimuli (especially odors), handling of victims' personal effects, and identification with victims (McCarroll et al. 1993a, 1993b).

It has been traditional to attempt to treat ASD casualties in a rapid manner near the combat area with the expectation of return to duty. During World War II, this approach and doctrine resulted in a high return to duty among psychiatric combat casualties (Glass 1947). This tradition has formed the basis of combat casualty care planning during every war since that time (Jones and Hales 1987; Solomon and Benbenishty 1986). For example, the Israeli Army discharged only 6% of its ASD casualties following the 1973 Yom Kippur War (Solomon et al. 1986a, 1986c). Eighty percent of those eligible for combat among the soldiers with ASD actually took part in the 1982 Lebanon War, and only 1% of those soldiers had recurrent ASD episodes. In contrast, during the Korean War, combat stress (i.e., ASD) casualties were frequently evacuated to Japan and treated with medications, "nonconvulsive shock therapy," and/or brief psychotherapy; placed in convalescent units; and evacuated back to the U.S. (Glass 1953, 1954). Fifty-nine percent of Israeli soldiers who developed combat stress reaction (a condition somewhat similar to ASD) during the 1982 Lebanon War developed PTSD within 1 year, compared with only 16% of soldiers without combat stress reaction (Solomon et al. 1987a, 1987b). This finding suggests that early attention to combat stress reaction may significantly prevent future psychiatric morbidity. In future wars, the decision whether to return a soldier, sailor, or aviator to duty following short-term treatment versus evacuation for more comprehensive treatment will be more difficult. Such decisions will depend upon the availability of air evacuation, the nature of the symptoms, whether a person's unit can be located, the needs of the unit, the availability of treatment resources near the "front," sociocultural contexts, and psychiatric predisposition.

Table 3–1.   Diagnostic criteria for acute stress disorder

A.   The person has been exposed to a traumatic event in which both of the following were present:
   (1)   the person experienced, witnessed, or was confronted with an event or events that involved actual or threatened death or serious injury, or a threat to the physical integrity of self or others
   (2)   the person's response involved intense fear, helplessness, or horror
B.   Either while experiencing or after experiencing the distressing event, the individual has three (or more) of the following dissociative symptoms:
   (1)   a subjective sense of numbing, detachment, or absence of emotional responsiveness
   (2)   a reduction in awareness of his or her surroundings (e.g., "being in a daze")
   (3)   derealization
   (4)   depersonalization
   (5)   dissociative amnesia (i.e., inability to recall an important aspect of the trauma)
C.   The traumatic event is persistently reexperienced in at least one of the following ways: recurrent images, thoughts, dreams, illusions, flashback episodes, or a sense of reliving the experience; or distress on exposure to reminders of the traumatic event.
D.   Marked avoidance of stimuli that arouse recollections of the trauma (e.g., thoughts, feelings, conversations, activities, places, people).
E.   Marked symptoms of anxiety or increased arousal (e.g., difficulty sleeping, irritability, poor concentration, hypervigilance, exaggerated startle response, motor restlessness).
F.   The disturbance causes clinically significant distress or impairment in social, occupational, or other important areas of functioning or impairs the individual's ability to pursue some necessary task, such as obtaining necessary assistance or mobilizing personal resources by telling family members about the traumatic experience.
G.   The disturbance lasts for a minimum of 2 days and a maximum of 4 weeks and occurs within 4 weeks of the traumatic event.
H.   The disturbance is not due to the direct physiological effects of a substance (e.g., a drug of abuse, a medication) or a general medical condition, is not better accounted for by Brief Psychotic Disorder, and is not merely an exacerbation of a preexisting Axis I or Axis II disorder.

Source.   Reprinted from American Psychiatric Association: *Diagnostic and Statistical Manual of Mental Disorders,* 4th Edition. Washington, D.C., American Psychiatric Association, 1994, pp. 431–432. Copyright 1994, American Psychiatric Association. Used with permission.

In addition, the meaning of the specific traumatic event will also affect the psychiatric outcome of decisions about whether or not to return to duty (Ursano et al. 1992).

Acute maladaptive reactions to combat, such as ASD, may lead to recovery or may blend imperceptibly into acute or chronic PTSD. Longitudinal follow-up of combat veterans who had experienced ASD at the time of combat (Belenky 1987; Solomon 1988, 1993) suggests that the risk for future PTSD is associated with both the extent/intensity of the ASD episode and the nature/intensity of the combat experiences. Fortunately, most combat veterans experience diminished psychiatric signs and symptoms with passage of time (Solomon and Mikulincer 1988).

Posttraumatic Stress Disorder

Traumatic nightmares, reliving of events, detachment, numbness of responses to the external world, guilt, sleep disturbance, and exaggerated startle response have been observed in various controlled studies of combat veterans with PTSD (Atkinson et al. 1984; Egendorf et al. 1981; Laufer et al. 1985; Pearce et al. 1985). The symptoms are often grouped into two clusters: 1) intrusive thoughts and symptoms of reexperiencing the trauma, and 2) symptoms of avoidance and denial (Horowitz et al. 1980; Laufer et al. 1985). Delayed PTSD is reported but does not appear to be common. The DSM-IV diagnostic criteria for PTSD are presented in Table 3–2. Suicide attempts in combat veterans with PTSD represent a significant source of morbidity even decades after combat (Hedin and Haas 1991). Factors significantly relating to suicide attempts in PTSD patients have been reported to include guilt about combat actions, survivor guilt, depression, anxiety, and severity of PTSD symptoms.

The symptoms of PTSD have been described in veterans from World War II (Van Dyke et al. 1985; N. S. White 1983), the Korean War (Thienes-Hontos 1983), recent Middle East conflicts (Belenky et al. 1983), and Operation Desert Storm (J. R. Rundell and M. R. Fragala, unpublished data, 1993). PTSD has also been

Table 3–2.   Diagnostic criteria for posttraumatic stress disorder

A. The person has been exposed to a traumatic event in which both of the following were present:
 (1) the person experienced, witnessed, or was confronted with an event or events that involved actual or threatened death or serious injury, or a threat to the physical integrity of self or others
 (2) the person's response involved intense fear, helplessness, or horror.   **Note:** In children, this may be expressed instead by disorganized or agitated behavior
B. The traumatic event is persistently reexperienced in one (or more) of the following ways:
 (1) recurrent and intrusive distressing recollections of the event, including images, thoughts, or perceptions.   **Note:** In young children, repetitive play may occur in which themes or aspects of the trauma are expressed.
 (2) recurrent distressing dreams of the event.   **Note:** In children, there may be frightening dreams without recognizable content.
 (3) acting or feeling as if the traumatic event were recurring (includes a sense of reliving the experience, illusions, hallucinations, and dissociative flashback episodes, including those that occur on awakening or when intoxicated).   **Note:** In young children, trauma-specific reenactment may occur.
 (4) intense psychological distress at exposure to internal or external cues that symbolize or resemble an aspect of the traumatic event
 (5) physiological reactivity on exposure to internal or external cues that symbolize or resemble an aspect of the traumatic event
C. Persistent avoidance of stimuli associated with the trauma and numbing of general responsiveness (not present before the trauma), as indicated by three (or more) of the following:
 (1) efforts to avoid thoughts, feelings, or conversations associated with the trauma
 (2) efforts to avoid activities, places, or people that arouse recollections of the trauma
 (3) inability to recall an important aspect of the trauma
 (4) markedly diminished interest or participation in significant activities
 (5) feeling of detachment or estrangement from others
 (6) restricted range of affect (e.g., unable to have loving feelings)
 (7) sense of a foreshortened future (e.g., does not expect to have a career, marriage, children, or a normal life span)

Table 3–2. Diagnostic criteria for posttraumatic stress disorder *(continued)*

D. Persistent symptoms of increased arousal (not present before the trauma), as indicated by two (or more) of the following:
   (1) difficulty falling or staying asleep
   (2) irritability or outbursts of anger
   (3) difficulty concentrating
   (4) hypervigilance
   (5) exaggerated startle response
E. Duration of the disturbance (symptoms in Criteria B, C, and D) is more than 1 month.
F. The disturbance causes clinically significant distress or impairment in social, occupational, or other important areas of functioning.

Specify if:
   Acute: if duration of symptoms is less than 3 months
   Chronic: if duration of symptoms is 3 months or more

Specify if:
   With delayed onset: if onset of symptoms is at least 6 months after the stressor

Source. Reprinted from American Psychiatric Association: *Diagnostic and Statistical Manual of Mental Disorders,* 4th Edition. Washington, D.C., American Psychiatric Association, 1994, pp. 427–429. Copyright 1994, American Psychiatric Association. Used with permission.

identified in victims of traumatic events not related to combat (Modlin 1983), such as floods (Rangell 1976), fires (Adler 1943; McFarlane 1986), volcanoes (Shore et al. 1986), accidents at sea (Leopold and Dillon 1963), the Holocaust (Chodoff 1963), rape (Nadelson et al. 1982), and kidnappings (Terr 1983).

In the NVVRS (Kulka et al. 1990), investigators found that an estimated 15.2% of all male Vietnam War theater veterans met the criteria for current PTSD at the time the data were compiled. This represents about 479,000 American men. Among female Vietnam War theater veterans, the frequency of current PTSD was 8.5%, or about 610 current cases. For both men and women, current PTSD prevalence rates for theater veterans were consistently higher than for veterans of a comparable era who did not serve in the theater (2.5% male, 1.1% female). About one-half of the men in the NVVRS study who had ever met the criteria for PTSD (49.2%), and just fewer than one-third of the women (31.6%), still met the criteria at the time of the study, more than 10 years after the war. These data indicate the frustrating chronicity of PTSD for many patients (Yehuda et al. 1992; Zeiss and Dickman 1989). Preliminary studies of Gulf War veterans during the first year after return indicate that approximately 9% of veterans had symptoms that were diagnosed as PTSD (Rosenheck et al. 1991).

A positive association has been reported in the literature between PTSD symptom severity and each of the following factors: 1) the degree of trauma experienced, 2) the duration of trauma experienced, and 3) having been wounded (Blake et al., in press; Branchey-Buydens et al. 1990; Frye and Stockton 1982; Green et al. 1990a, 1990b; Kulka et al. 1990; Penk et al. 1981; Shore et al. 1986; Yager et al. 1984). Although individual subjective meaning and vulnerability play important roles in producing symptoms, the degree of war trauma is the best predictor (Ursano 1987). One of the most severe combat-related experiences studied has been the prisoner-of-war experience among World War II Pacific theater veterans. Prisoners of war (POWs) from this theater of the war still, 40 years after their release, have symptoms that would meet the diagnosis for PTSD (Page 1992).

A traumatic event such as war has many different aspects that complicate cause-and-effect analysis (Laufer et al. 1985; Ursano et al. 1987). The qualitative and quantitative differences between the stress of combat and that of noncombat situations, or the stress of perpetrating abusive violence and that of being wounded, are not well defined. In one recent study (Goreczny and Griger 1992), it was found that Vietnam War veterans had more posttraumatic psychiatric problems than World War II veterans or Korean War veterans. These differences could not be explained by the presence or absence of combat exposure. Other military factors (e.g., degree of combat exposure, predisposition, or sociocultural factors) may be responsible for the higher incidence of problems among Vietnam War veterans.

Additional comorbid psychiatric disorders are common in patients with PTSD. Prevalences vary among studies because of methodological differences and variability in the diagnostic criteria used, but rates of both depression and substance abuse appear to be high.

In addition to having excess psychiatric comorbidity, patients with PTSD are at higher risk for having a variety of medical problems (White and Faustman 1989). In one study of inpatient veterans with PTSD, 60% appear to have significant medical problems, and 42% had multiple medical problems. In this sample of patients, 8% had medical or surgical sequelae from combat-related physical trauma (White and Faustman 1989).

Depression

Depression may be underestimated as a posttraumatic psychiatric illness, especially in the first months after combat. Both controlled and uncontrolled studies of psychiatrically ill veterans who were examined shortly after their return from Vietnam reveal depression to be a common diagnosis. In one report, 15% of 106 combat veterans referred for psychiatric evaluation after their return to the U.S. received a rigorously defined diagnosis of depression (Fox 1972). Except for adjustment disorder, depression was the most frequent diagnosis. Strange and Brown (1970) found depression in 62% of returning psychiatrically ill Vietnam veterans, compared with 44% of psychiatrically ill men who served in the military but not in Vietnam during the years of the war. Paykel (1978) found a sixfold greater risk of suicide and a twofold greater risk of depression following traumatic life events such as combat.

In a national sample (Jordan et al. 1991), about 3% of Vietnam veterans were found to have current depressive episodes as defined by Diagnostic Interview Schedule criteria; Vietnam War veterans who had experienced higher war-zone stress were, as a group, seven times more likely to have current depression than were veterans who had been exposed to low- or moderate-stress war-zone experiences. The veterans who had been exposed to low- or moderate-stress experiences were, as a group, no more likely to have current depression than were Vietnam War era veterans who had not been sent to Vietnam or matched civilian control subjects. Rates of depression are similar for women veterans. Helzer and co-workers (1976) reported significant differences in the frequency of depression between a group of Vietnam veterans who had experienced combat and a group who had not. During the 12 months after their return from Vietnam, 11% of the combat veterans exhibited symptoms that met the criteria for a depressive episode, compared with 3% of the noncombat veterans. Combat retained its predictive value for depression even when preservice and postservice variables were controlled for. At follow-up 3 years later, Helzer and associates (1979) found that the correlation between combat and depression was no longer present. That finding suggests that the risk for posttraumatic depression may be time-specific or episodic.

Helzer's findings are consistent with those of Green and associates (1983), who found that the frequency of moderate to severe depression in survivors of the Beverly Hills Supper Club fire declined from 22% at 1-year follow-up to 11% after 2 years, and with Breslau and Davis's finding (1986) that exposure to war-related trauma in the Vietnam War did not predict a current diagnosis of major depression in 69 veterans. In contrast, Hearst et al. (1986) showed that suicide—and, by association, depression—continues to be more frequent in men who were eligible for the military draft between 1970 and 1972 than in draft-exempt men of the same age, who were less likely to have been exposed to the trauma of war.

Patients with PTSD frequently report depressive symptoms (Hovens et al. 1992). Three diagnostic criteria—loss of interest in activities, sleep disturbance, and concentration impairment—are shared by major depressive episode and PTSD, according to DSM-IV. Patients with ASD may also have symptoms and signs that are diagnostic criteria for major depression: difficulty sleeping, poor concentration, and restlessness. In various studies,

8% to 51% of PTSD patients have concurrent depression or had depression in the past. PTSD patients have also been reported to have significantly more depression than normal control subjects on the Beck Depression Inventory, the Zung Depression Scale, and the Minnesota Multiphasic Personality Inventory (MMPI) (Fairbank et al. 1983). In addition, depression is a frequently recorded diagnosis for psychiatric patients who subsequently receive a diagnosis of PTSD (Birkhimer et al. 1985; Haley 1978).

Substance-Related Disorders

Alcohol Use Disorders

The association between combat and substance-related disorders is weaker than that between combat and other posttraumatic psychiatric illnesses. Substance-related disorders, PTSD, and depression frequently occur together, and cause-and-effect relationships are not entirely clear. However, substance-related disorders are more likely than PTSD or depression to be secondary psychiatric disorders after combat. Therefore, psychiatric treatment of substance-related disorders in people who have been exposed to combat may constitute only a partial treatment of their war-related psychiatric response. When multiple diagnoses exist, it is important to recognize and treat each one.

In a national Vietnam War veteran study, alcohol abuse or dependence appear to have been more common in Vietnam War–era veterans exposed to higher-stress war-zone experiences than in those exposed to low- or moderate-stress war-zone experiences (17.2% vs. 8.8%) (Jordan et al. 1991). However, factors other than combat war stress level may be more important. For example, Boscarino (1979) found that being male and being unmarried were each more important than being a veteran of the war in Vietnam in accounting for greater current alcohol consumption, when comparison was made with an unmatched control group. On the other hand, Yager et al. (1984) showed a correlation between combat and later alcohol consumption.

They found that daily drinking was four times more prevalent among veterans of heavy combat than among veterans exposed to light or no combat. However, the authors did not control for preservice drinking and drug use.

Helzer (1984) found that preservice drinking problems and drug use were more powerful predictors than combat of later problem drinking or alcoholism among Vietnam War veterans. Combat itself explained only 2% of the variance in later alcohol use. When there is particularly severe war trauma, however, there is a suggestion that risk for heavy postwar alcohol use is high. Three different groups of former POWs (World War II European and Pacific theaters and Korean War) all had higher-than-expected death because of liver cirrhosis (Keehn 1980).

Excessive consumption of alcohol frequently accompanies PTSD (Birkhimer et al. 1985; Boehnlein et al. 1985; Hogben and Cornfield 1981; Laufer et al. 1985; Shen and Park 1983; van der Kolk 1983; Walker 1982) and posttraumatic depression (Helzer et al. 1976, 1979). Alcohol use disorders after combat trauma may be a secondary ("organic") psychiatric disorder or a form of self-medication for depression or PTSD (Birkhimer et al. 1985; Helzer et al. 1976; Lacoursiere et al. 1980; Nace et al. 1978; van der Kolk 1983). Alcohol may suppress nightmares, diminish autonomic activity, and foster more pleasant, nontraumatic fantasies (van der Kolk 1983).

Precise cause-and-effect relationships among coexisting posttraumatic alcohol misuse, PTSD, and depression are unknown. There are no studies that have controlled for the presence of PTSD or depression when analyzing posttraumatic alcohol abuse or dependence. There are only two studies that have controlled for daily or problem drinking when analyzing the association between trauma and PTSD (Laufer et al. 1985) or depression (Helzer et al. 1976). In both of these studies, associations between trauma, PTSD, and depression remained significant, which suggests that even when trauma is followed by daily or problem drinking, the drinking cannot fully explain the presence of PTSD or depression after war trauma.

Other Substance Use Disorders

In the Gulf War, strict cultural prohibitions contributed to much lower rates of substance abuse than in other wars. The development of or return to substance abuse after return home from the Gulf is, however, a more complicated issue. Data in this area are not yet available. Among Vietnam War veterans, soldiers who abused opiates and marijuana were more likely to do so during their tours in Vietnam than they were to have done so before their arrival in that combat theater (Holloway 1974; Robins 1973, 1974; Robins et al. 1974). However, this association has not been conclusively demonstrated for the use of barbiturates, amphetamines, cocaine, and LSD (Goodwin et al. 1975; Stanton 1971).

Drug use greatly declined among Vietnam War veterans after their return home (Boscarino 1979; Goodwin et al. 1975; Nace et al. 1977, 1978; Robins et al. 1974). Current drug use diagnoses can be made in only about 2% of all Vietnam War–era veterans 20 to 30 years after the war (Jordan et al. 1991). After controlling for demographic variables, Boscarino (1979) found no significant difference between Vietnam War veterans' postservice drug use and drug use in a general population comparison group. Indeed, Yager et al. (1984) conducted a study of 1,342 men who had been of military age during the Vietnam War and found that drug use by noncombat Vietnam War veterans did not exceed nonveterans' drug use during the years after the war. However, combat veterans who participated in abusive violence, such as actions against civilians, mistreatment of POWs, or use of unnecessarily cruel weapons, reported substantially more postservice marijuana and heroin use than did other combat veterans, noncombat veterans, or nonveterans. More individuals in the group who had participated in abusive violence, compared with other groups, also reported signs and symptoms of PTSD, a finding that again raises the question of self-medication. Of individuals with PTSD, 16% to 50% may also have diagnoses of drug abuse or dependence (Behar 1984; Davidson et al. 1985; Escobar et al. 1983; Sierles et al. 1983).

Depression is associated with drug use among Vietnam War veterans (Nace et al. 1977, 1978). A group of depressed Vietnam War veterans reported significantly more use of amphetamines, barbiturates, and opiates during the war and more use of opiates an average of 28 months after their return to the U.S. than was reported by a matched group of nondepressed veterans. Helzer et al. (1976) demonstrated an association between depression in Vietnam War veterans and postservice use of barbiturates, amphetamines, and opiates. Like patients who have PTSD or depression and who also abuse alcohol, psychiatrically ill victims of war trauma may turn to drugs to self-treat their symptoms or may be subject to increased risk for other psychiatric disorders because of their drug use, or both.

Controlling for postservice marijuana use in Vietnam veterans who have PTSD has not been shown to affect the correlation between war trauma and PTSD (Laufer et al. 1985). In addition, in one study, when depressed Vietnam veterans showed more frequent drug use, the level of combat intensity was associated with the depression, not the drug use (Helzer et al. 1976). These findings suggest that PTSD symptoms and depression do not occur secondary to drug use, but the studies did not address the issue of self-medication.

Often forgotten is the abuse of cigarettes—a concern during the Gulf War. Shalev et al. (1990) found higher cigarette use in Israeli PTSD patients than in a combat control group.

Anxiety Disorders

Jordan et al. (1991), in their study of lifetime and current psychiatric diagnoses in male Vietnam veterans who had been exposed to either high- or low/moderate-stress war-zone experiences, male Vietnam War–era control subjects, and male civilian control subjects, found that the veterans who been exposed to high-stress combat experiences were, as a group, more likely to have generalized anxiety disorder (lifetime and current) than were the individuals in the other groups. Among women in the same categories, no significant group differences were found. Current panic disorder was found to be more likely in Vietnam War veterans who had been exposed to high-stress combat experiences than in male and female veterans who had been exposed to low- or moderate-stress experiences. Lifetime diagnoses of panic disorder were found to be more common only in female veterans who had been exposed to high-stress experiences.

Anxiety syndromes, panic disorder, and phobias are frequently present in PTSD patients at both the symptom and the disorder levels (Birkhimer et al. 1985; Davidson et al. 1985; Escobar et al. 1983; Fairbank et al. 1983; Horowitz et al. 1980; Hovens et al. 1992; Sierles et al. 1983; Ursano 1987). In a study of 66 PTSD patients by Horowitz and co-workers (1980), 75% of the patients reported feeling fearful, and 48% had spells of terror or panic. Most also reported palpitations, dizziness, hot or cold spells, paresthesias, headaches, chest pain, or tremulousness. Before the inception of DSM-III, anxiety reaction, anxiety state, and anxiety neurosis were by far the most frequent diagnoses given psychiatrically hospitalized or disabled World War II and Korean War veterans (Beebe 1975; Grinker 1945). In one study of Pacific theater World War II former POWs, anxiety disorders were the most common psychiatric diagnoses (Goldstein et al. 1987).

Somatoform and Psychophysiological Disorders

Somatoform disorders and psychophysiological disorders were reported after the Mount St. Helens volcanic eruption (Adams and Adams 1984), after the Chowchilla kidnapping incident (Terr 1983), in Holocaust survivors (Chodoff 1963; Eaton et al. 1982), after accidents at sea (Leopold and Dillon 1963), and in combat veterans (Beebe 1975; Belenky et al. 1983; Escobar et al. 1983; Grinker 1945; Horowitz et al. 1980; Strange and Brown 1970). Upper gastrointestinal symptoms were particularly common in those groups. Conversion disorders accounted for 22% of the psychiatric casualties that occurred among Israeli forces present in Lebanon in 1982 (Belenky et al. 1983).

Shalev (1988) has found that reporting of somatic symptoms among Israeli combat veterans (of the 1982 Lebanon War) with combat stress reaction (i.e., ASD) was significantly higher 3 years after the war than among age-matched war veterans without ASD or any other psychiatric history. He also studied combat veterans with and without PTSD (Shalev et al. 1990) and found that subjects with PTSD reported significantly more physical symptoms but did not differ from control subjects on their physical examination and laboratory test findings. These findings have been replicated by others (Solomon 1988).

Nonspecific somatic symptoms such as weight loss and fatigue were more common in World War II Pacific theater former POWs and in Korean War former POWs than in veterans of the same eras who had not been POWs (Beebe 1975). Dutch Resistance fighters during World War II were found to have more cardiovascular disease risk factors, and particularly type A behaviors, than matched control subjects who had not been exposed to combat-related trauma (Falger et al. 1992). Causes of mortality during long-term follow-up studies of former POWs from World War II and Korea revealed excess rates of death from tuberculosis, trauma, and hepatic cirrhosis (Keehn 1980).

The influence of stress and physical deprivation on immune functions is now well documented (Chrousos and Gold 1992; Khansari et al. 1990; Kiecolt-Glaser and Glaser 1991). Dekaris and co-workers (1993) assessed immune reactivity in Croatian men who had just been released from a war prison camp by Serbians following the 1992 conflict between Serbian and Croatian militias in the former Yugoslavia. The ratio of CD4 to CD8 lymphocytes was decreased in returned POWs compared with in healthy matched control subjects. In vitro natural killer cell cytotoxic activity and phagocytic functions of ingestion and digestion were also signficantly depressed. Serum interferon, serum cortisol, and prolactin were signficantly lowered.

The nature of the so-called Operation Desert Storm syndrome, or Gulf War syndrome, requires study. This syndrome, consisting of widely varying symptoms, may represent true organic illness or be related to somatic symptom reports after other wars. Further study is needed.

Antisocial Behavior

Studies of violence and other antisocial behaviors occurring after trauma are inconclusive. Lifetime rates of antisocial personality disorder were found to be higher among Vietnam War–era veterans exposed to high-stress war-zone experiences (16.6%) than among same-era veterans exposed to low- or moderate-stress war-zone environments (7.1%) (Jordan et al. 1991). However, precombat antisocial behavior must be controlled for to address the etiology issue. Controlled studies of Vietnam War veterans find a modest difference between combat veterans and noncombat veterans with regard to attitudes toward the use of violence (Brady and Rappoport 1973; Egendorf et al. 1981). However, a propensity to act on hostile impulses has yet to be demonstrated. Strange and Brown (1970) found that among hospitalized psychiatric inpatients, Vietnam War veterans who experienced combat were more likely than other Vietnam War–era military veterans (20% vs. 8%) to verbalize aggressive threats. However, the authors also found that direct behavioral expression of aggressive conflicts was not more common. Fox (1972) reported that 52% of psychiatrically ill Vietnam War returnees reported fears of acting violently but that only 16% had actually done so.

McFall and associates (1991) demonstrated that PTSD, per se, does not appear to be associated with risk of arrests for antisocial conduct. However, Yager and co-workers (1984) showed that veterans who had experienced heavy combat had an overall arrest rate per combat scale unit about 23% higher, and a conviction rate about 12% higher, than those of veterans who had experienced little or no combat. The actual number of arrests was four times higher in men who had been exposed to heavy combat, but most of those arrests were for nonviolent offenses. The data from Yager et al.'s study were adjusted for preservice arrest history and other juvenile problems but were not controlled for history of postservice substance abuse.

In the study by Yager and co-workers (1984), daily drinking was also significantly correlated with level of combat, a finding that leaves unanswered the question of whether posttraumatic violence is more strongly associated with the psychological effects of the trauma itself or with substance use disorders.

Adjustment Disorder

During psychiatric evaluations of combat veterans who had recently returned from Vietnam, 57 of 106 men who were found to be psychiatrically ill had adjustment disorder (Fox 1972). Ursano and associates (1981), in a study of groups of U.S. Air Force personnel who had been POWs during the Vietnam War before and after 1969, demonstrated that 17% to 18% of the sample had symptoms diagnosed as adjustment disorder or experienced marital or occupational maladjustments upon repatriation from Vietnam. At 5-year follow-up, 9% to 16% of the sample had those syndromes. These syndromes were the most common psychiatric diagnoses made in the study.

In the same study, Ursano and associates found that 3% of 325 POWs (Vietnam War) had neurotic disorders at repatriation, and 8% of 253 had neurotic disorders at follow-up 5 years later. Crystallization or exacerbation of neuroses has also been reported in veterans of other wars (Beebe 1975; Grinker 1945; Helzer et al. 1979) and in victims of collisions at sea (Hoiberg and McCaughey 1984). Obsessiveness, oppositional behavior, free-floating anxiety, dysthymia, hypochondriasis, passivity, and dependency have all been reported following traumatic events (Chodoff 1963; Grinker 1945; Modlin 1983). Development of neuroses following combat exposure appears to be associated with age; older persons who had been exposed to combat during World War II were less resilient and had higher rates of neuroses 10 years after their combat experiences than did younger persons (Brill et al. 1953).

Other Psychiatric Disorders

Other psychiatric syndromes and disorders diagnosed acutely and chronically after combat exposure include dissociative identity disorder (Bremner et al. 1992), dissociative amnesia (Fisher 1945), factitious disorder with predominantly psychological symptoms (Stegman and Blanford 1992), and malingering (Stegman and Blanford 1992).

Personality Change

Individuals exposed to war trauma also report changes in life goals and plans and orientations that are much more subtle than those that can be described in our current diagnostic nomenclature. The direction of such personality change—toward health or toward pathology—depends not only on the nature and severity of the traumatic event but also on the meaning and significance of the event, the individual vulnerabilities, and the biopsychosocial context before, during, and after the trauma (Holloway and Ursano 1984, 1985; Ursano and Holloway 1985a, 1985b). As time passes, the psychological meaning of recalled trauma is subject to reorganization, with changes in life circumstances and biopsychosocial contexts (Holloway and Ursano 1984; Ursano and Holloway 1985a, 1985b; Ursano et al. 1992). Traumatic events enter into our lexicon of life events by which we see, describe, and interpret our life experience. Recognizing personality change as an outcome of trauma is really a statement that the brain is subject to change by the environment in multiple ways, and trauma is one input to the brain that may lead to subtle as well as more dramatic changes (Kolb 1987; P. B. Watson et al. 1988).

Factors Associated With Psychiatric Disorders Following War-Related Trauma

The incidence of psychiatric disorders after combat is positively associated with the degree and duration of war trauma experienced, with witnessing or participation in atrocities, and with being wounded (Jordan et al. 1991; Kulka et al. 1990, 1991; Sutker et al. 1991; Ursano et al. 1981).

Posttraumtic psychiatric syndromes occur in all cultures and in all types of armed forces. During the Vietnam War, psychiatric casualties occurred in equivalent numbers and under similar circumstances for both American and South Vietnamese soldiers (Bourne and San 1967). Cultural factors may, however, influence the nature of the psychiatric response. Bourne and San (1967) noted that Americans tended to manifest more personality-related symptoms than did the South Vietnamese, who tended to exhibit more anxiety and somatoform disorders.

In addition to combat severity, other factors contribute to the risk of psychiatric disorder following combat. Psychiatric predisposition and sociocultural support are important determinants of acute, chronic, and delayed reactions to combat stress. Bremner and associates (1993) suggested an association between history of childhood physical abuse and combat-related PTSD among Vietnam veterans. In a small but unique sample for which data were available before the Vietnam War, after level of combat exposure was considered, premilitary personality attributes, as measured by the MMPI scales hypochondriasis, psychopathic deviate, masculinity-femininity, and paranoia, also contributed to the prediction of vulnerability to lifetime PTSD symptoms in men who had been exposed to combat (Schnurr et al. 1993).

A number of pretrauma risk factors for the diagnosis of PTSD have also been suggested by other authors (see Davidson and Foa 1993). These factors include family psychiatric illness, parental poverty, childhood abuse history (sexual and physical), early-life separation or divorce of parents, childhood behavior disorder, prior physical illness, neuroticism, introversion, pretrauma adverse life events, low education, pretrauma psychoactive substance use, and early separation from parents. It is very important to note that the best predictors found in any study depend greatly on the nature of the sample, the severity of life threat experienced, and the stage of illness (acute vs. chronic) that is studied. There is likely an interaction between traumatic events themselves and predispositional factors in chronic post-traumatic psychiatric illness (Davidson and Foa 1993). Predictors of ASD that resolve may be quite different but have been rarely studied.

World War II was, in general, a conflict for which there was a great deal more popular support at home than there was for the Vietnam War. Comparison of groups of demographically similar veterans from those two conflicts and in degree of exposure to combat differ significantly with regard to findings of long-term psychiatric disability (Davidson et al. 1990). Vietnam veterans were more likely than World War II veterans to have experienced more severe PTSD symptoms, depression, survivor guilt, occupational impairment, derealization, suicidal ideation, panic disorder, and early age at onset of alcoholism. In one study, patients with the particular psychiatric predisposition of "neurotic" or introverted personality were more likely than patients without these personality characteristics to develop chronic PTSD (Davidson et al. 1987).

In the National Vietnam Veterans Readjustment Study (Kulka et al. 1990), perhaps the best and most extensive methodological study on combat responses, investigators assessed a number of potential predisposing factors for psychiatric illness. These factors included demographic characteristics, socioeconomic status, family relationships, psychiatric history, childhood behavioral problems, childhood health problems, marital status, education, non-Vietnam War military history, and health and psychiatric status at the beginning of Vietnam War service. Consideration of these factors in data analyses changed prevalence risk for a number of groups studied. However, even after controlling for predisposing factors, current PTSD prevalence among theater veterans who had been exposed to high levels of war-zone stress was much higher than that among those exposed to low or moderate levels (18 percentage points difference for men, and 13 percentage points difference for women) (Kulka et al. 1990).

There have been few studies of relative contributions of premilitary, military, and postmilitary risk factors to postwar psychiatric diagnoses (C. G. Watson et al. 1988). The few data that exist suggest that the relative contribution of these factors depends on the type of disorder. For example, posttraumatic panic disorder and PTSD may be more heavily related to war stressors, including threat to life and exposure to grotesque death, than substance-related disorders (Green et al. 1990a). Persistent substance-related disorders may be relatively more associated with the presence of premilitary psychiatric predisposition. In a unique study, Rosenheck et al. (1992) showed that the contribution of the meaning of the war trauma experience was significant in chronic PTSD even after war-zone exposure was controlled for. Such studies, which first control for life threat experiences and then specify acute versus chronic conditions, offer important new information relevant to treating psychiatric disorders that occur after exposure to war-related trauma.

Future Research for Clinical Care

Resilience

The majority of persons exposed to combat trauma do not develop psychiatric illness. The study of resilience will help us better predict under what conditions and in which people posttraumatic psychiatric illness may develop.

Demographic Differences

There may be differences in the symptomatic expression of various psychiatric syndromes and disorders among different ethnic, cultural, educational, and socioeconomic groups.

Relationship Between Acute Stress Disorder and Other Posttraumatic Psychiatric Illnesses

Individuals who develop combat stress syndromes (i.e., ASD) may be predisposed to development of other psychiatric illnesses in the aftermath of trauma. With the formal recognition of the important psychiatric disorder ASD in DSM-IV, the opportunity exists for research of this question. If associations between ASD and other posttraumatic psychiatric disorders exist, opportunities present themselves for effective primary, secondary, and tertiary prevention efforts.

Posttraumatic Depression

Long-term follow-up studies of posttraumatic depression are needed for us to further clarify the natural course and duration of this syndrome.

Relationship Between Posttraumatic Stress Disorder and Other DSM-IV Anxiety Disorders

Studies are needed to determine the relationship of PTSD to other anxiety disorders. Similar neurobiological pathology may underlie these disorders. Requiring special attention is the relationship between PTSD and panic disorder and generalized anxiety disorder. Similarly, a better understanding of the frequent comorbidity among PTSD, depression, and substance abuse is needed, as well as increased insight into the differences between acute and chronic PTSD.

Transgenerational Effects of Combat Trauma

The effects of exposure to combat trauma on families have been very incompletely studied. There is anecdotal evidence which suggests that offspring of combat veterans can develop mood disorders, psychological distress, guilt, and other aspects of "secondary traumatization" (Rosenheck 1986). Preventive interventions in returning combat veterans could potentially make significant positive impacts on family and individual functioning in subsequent years. Retrospective and prospective research needs to be conducted in this area.

Adjustment Disorder

Adjustment disorder can serve as the paradigm of posttraumatic psychiatric illness. Systematic research on adjustment disorder is almost totally lacking. Initial studies should determine whether adjustment disorder, like ASD, is associated with development of more severe psychiatric illness and whether early treatment can diminish the consequences of such an association.

Physiological Responses to Trauma

Studies of the physiological and neuroanatomic responses to combat trauma hold promise of further clarifying the impact of chronic stress on physical health and neuropsychiatric development. The basic question of how external events effect internal biological changes remains unanswered. Such studies should examine the relationship between acute and chronic trauma and immunosuppression, chronic sympathetic nervous system arousal, and alterations in central nervous system anatomy and physiology (P. B. Watson et al. 1988).

The design of future studies must be sensitive to the differences between acute and chronic disorders, regardless of the disorder studied. Clarifying factors that contribute to chronicity is an important area that has been neglected in current scientific literature (Ursano et al. 1992). Factors that prevent psychiatric disorders following war trauma (i.e., recovery) need study in their own right. Researchers also need to be more sensitive to the nature of the population being studied. For example, addressing the contributions of life threat in a population with minimal combat exposure does not allow a sufficient test of this hypothesis. Unless such factors are considered, results are not interpretable.

Conclusions

Exposure to combat is always a major life change event. Most who are exposed to combat trauma will adjust well. Acute stress disorder and posttraumatic stress disorder are not the only psychiatric disorders that arise following the combat experience. Mood disorders, anxiety disorders, substance-related disorders, somatoform disorders, adjustment disorder, personality changes, and psychophysiological disorders also occur. Former military personnel who meet the criteria for one postcombat psychiatric disorder, as a rule, also meet the criteria for at least one other psychiatric disorder. The relationship of one disorder with another is not clear. For example, among combat veterans, depression is associated with more drug use; however, the level of combat intensity is associated with the depression, not the drug use (Helzer et al. 1976). Substance-related disorders following combat exposure may, therefore, be at least partially a form of self-medication.

Factors that are important when one is considering treatment possibilities for former service personnel who develop postcombat psychiatric disorders include psychiatric predisposition, sociocultural influences, the level of combat-related exposure, the meaning of the traumatic event to the person, underlying medical sequelae of combat, and the nature and context of postcombat life events.

All conflicts and wars are unique. Operations Desert Shield/ Desert Storm had a number of characteristics of psychiatric importance that may have been present in other wars but were particularly acute for Gulf War veterans. First, Gulf War veterans had unique deployment stressors (Rosenheck et al. 1991). Women and parents of small children were deployed away from their families in unprecedented numbers. As in all wars, military families were exposed to substantial stress. Second, the duration between notification and deployment was very short. Third, sobriety among deployed American forces was universally enforced, and the long-term impact of this on future substance misuse is unknown. Fourth, the actual ground combat phase of the war was relatively brief. There was little time for an ASD to develop. Fifth, the accuracy of weapons was unusually high and the types of weapons particularly threatening, and consequently the fear of such weapons was especially great. Missiles were guided to targets with pinpoint accuracy, and chemical and biological warfare was a persistent threat.

Operations Desert Shield/Desert Storm, Operation Restore Hope, and the experiences of combatants in the former Yugoslavia reinforce the notion that the nature of postcombat psychiatric syndromes is evolving. Modern conflicts result in more exposure of civilians to combat-related stress, the deployment of women into harm's way, the increased potential for exposure of combat support personnel (including medical personnel) to combat, and the exposure to toxic and contained environments (e.g., chemical and biological warfare, gear used to protect against such warfare). Further research is needed to better prepare mental health professionals to treat postcombat acute, chronic, and delayed psychiatric disorders, with which they are increasingly likely to be confronted in the coming decades.

References

Adams PR, Adams GR: Mount Saint Helen's ashfall: evidence for a disaster stress reaction. Am Psychol 39:252–260, 1984

Adler A: Neuropsychiatric complications in victims of Boston's Coconut Grove disaster. JAMA 123:1098–1101, 1943

American Psychiatric Association: Diagnostic and Statistical Manual of Mental Disorders, 3rd Edition. Washington, DC, American Psychiatric Association, 1980

American Psychiatric Association: Diagnostic and Statistical Manual of Mental Disorders, 3rd Edition, Revised. Washington, DC, American Psychiatric Association, 1987

American Psychiatric Association: Diagnostic and Statistical Manual of Mental Disorders, 4th Edition. Washington, DC, American Psychiatric Association, 1994

Atkinson RM, Sparr LF, Sheff AG, et al: Diagnosis of posttraumatic stress disorder in Vietnam veterans: preliminary findings. Am J Psychiatry 141:694–696, 1984

Bartone PT, Ursano RJ, Wright KM, et al: The impact of a military air disaster on the health of assistance workers. J Nerv Ment Dis 177:317–328, 1989

Beebe GW: Follow-up studies of World War II and Korean War prisoners. Am J Epidemiol 101:400–422, 1975

Behar D: Confirmation of concurrent illnesses in posttraumatic stress disorder. Am J Psychiatry 141:1310, 1984

Belenky GL: Varieties of reaction and adaptation of combat experience. Bull Menninger Clin 51:64–79, 1987

Belenky GL, Tyner CF, Sodet FJ: Israeli Battle Shock Casualties: 1973 and 1982. Washington, DC, Walter Reed Army Institute of Research, 1983

Birkhimer LJ, DeVane LC, Muniz CE: Posttraumatic stress disorder: characteristics and pharmacological response in the veteran population. Compr Psychiatry 26:304–310, 1985

Blake DD, Cook JD, Keane TM: Posttraumatic stress disorder and coping in veterans seeking medical treatment. J Clin Psychol (in press)

Boehnlein JK, Kinzie D, Ben R, et al: One-year follow-up of posttraumatic stress disorder among survivors of Cambodian concentration camps. Am J Psychiatry 142:956–959, 1985

Borus JF: Reentry II: "making it" back in the States. Am J Psychiatry 130:850–854, 1973

Boscarino J: Current drug involvement among Vietnam and non-Vietnam veterans. Am J Drug Alcohol Abuse 6:301–312, 1979

Boscarino J: The impact of combat on later alcohol use by Vietnam veterans. J Psychoactive Drugs 16:183–191, 1984

Bourne PG, San ND: A comparative study of neuropsychiatric casualties in the United States Army and the Army of the Republic of Vietnam. Mil Med 132:904–909, 1967

Brady D, Rappoport L: Violence and Vietnam: a comparison between attitudes of civilians and veterans. Human Relations 26:735–752, 1973

Branchey-Buydens L, Noumair D, Branchey M: Duration and intensity of combat exposure and posttraumatic stress disorder in Vietnam veterans. J Nerv Ment Dis 178:582–587, 1990

Bremner JD, Southwick SM, Brett E, et al: Dissociation and posttraumatic stress disorder in Vietnam combat veterans. Am J Psychiatry 149:328–332, 1992

Bremner JD, Southwick SM, Johnson DR, et al: Childhood physical abuse and combat-related posttraumatic stress disorder in Vietnam veterans. Am J Psychiatry 150:235–239, 1993

Breslau N, Davis GC: Chronic stress and major depression. Arch Gen Psychiatry 43:309–314, 1986

Brill NQ, Beebe GW, Loewenstein RL: Age and resistance to military stress. U.S. Armed Forces Medical Journal 9:1247–1266, 1953

Brooks FR, Ebner DG, Xenakis SN, et al: Psychological reactions during chemical warfare training. Mil Med 148:232–235, 1983

Carter BJ, Cammermeyer M: Emergence of real casualties during simulated chemical warfare training under high heat conditions. Mil Med 150:657–665, 1985

Centers for Disease Control: Centers for Disease Control Vietnam Experience Study: health status of Vietnam veterans, I: psychosocial characteristics. JAMA 259:2701–2707, 1988

Chodoff P: Late effects of the concentration camp syndrome. Arch Gen Psychiatry 8:323–333, 1963

Chrousos GP, Gold PW: The concepts of stress and stress system disorders. JAMA 267:1244–1252, 1992

Davidson JRT, Foa EB: Posttraumatic Stress Disorder: DSM-IV and Beyond. Washington, DC, American Psychiatric Press, 1993

Davidson JRT, Swartz M, Storck M, et al: A diagnostic and family study of posttraumatic stress disorder. Am J Psychiatry 142:90–93, 1985

Davidson JRT, Kudler HS, Smith R: Personality in chronic posttraumatic stress disorders: a study of the Eysenck Inventory. Journal of Anxiety Disorders 1:295–300, 1987

Davidson JRT, Kudler HS, Saunders WB: Symptom and comorbidity patterns in World War II and Vietnam veterans with posttraumatic stress disorder. Compr Psychiatry 31:162–170, 1990

Dekaris D, Sabioncello A, Mazuran R, et al: Multiple changes of immunologic parameters in prisoners of war: assessments after release from a camp in Manjaca, Bosnia. JAMA 270:595–599, 1993

Eaton WW, Sigal JJ, Weinfield M: Impairment in Holocaust survivors after 33 years: data from an unbiased community sample. Am J Psychiatry 139:773–777, 1982

Egendorf A, Kadushin C, Loafer R, et al: Legacies of Vietnam: Comparative Adjustment of Veterans and Their Peers. Washington, DC, U.S. Government Printing Office, 1981

Escobar JI, Randolph ET, Puente G, et al: Posttraumatic stress disorder in Hispanic Vietnam veterans: clinical phenomenology and sociocultural characteristics. J Nerv Ment Dis 171: 585–596, 1983

Fairbank JA, Keane TM, Malloy PF: Some preliminary data on the psychological characteristics of Vietnam veterans with posttraumatic stress disorders. J Consult Clin Psychol 51:912–919, 1983

Falger PRJ, Op den Velde W, Hovens JE, et al: Current posttraumatic stress disorder and cardiovascular disease risk factors in Dutch Resistance veterans from World War II. Psychother Psychosom 57:164–171, 1992

Fisher C: Amnesic states in war neuroses: the psychogenesis of fugues. Psychoanal Q 14:437–468, 1945

Fox RP: Post-combat adaptational problems. Compr Psychiatry 13:435–443, 1972

Frye JS, Stockton RA: Discriminant analysis of posttraumatic stress disorder among a group of Vietnam veterans. Am J Psychiatry 139:52–56, 1982

Glass AJ: Effectiveness of forward neuropsychiatric treatment. Bulletin of the U.S. Army Medical Department 7:1034–1041, 1947

Glass AJ: Psychiatry in the Korean Campaign, Part I. U.S. Armed Forces Medical Journal 10:1387–1401, 1953

Glass AJ: Psychiatry in the Korean Campaign, Part II. U.S. Armed Forces Medical Journal 11:1563–1583, 1954

Glass AJ: Principles of combat psychiatry. Mil Med 15:27–33, 1955

Goldstein G, Van Kammen W, Shelly C, et al: Survivors of imprisonment in the Pacific theater during World War II. Am J Psychiatry 144:1210–1213, 1987

Goodwin DW, Davis DH, Robins LN: Drinking amid abundant illicit drugs. Arch Gen Psychiatry 32:230–233, 1975

Goreczny AJ, Griger ML: A comparison of combat and non-combat veterans from three wars. Paper presented at the annual meeting of the American Psychological Association, Washington, DC, August 1992

Green BL, Grace MC, Lindy JD, et al: Levels of functional impairment following a civilian disaster: the Beverly Hills Supper Club fire. J Consult Clin Psychol 51:573–580, 1983

Green BL, Grace MC, Lindy JD, et al: Risk factors for PTSD and other diagnoses in a general sample of Vietnam veterans. Am J Psychiatry 6:729–733, 1990a

Green BL, Grace MC, Lindy JD, et al: War trauma and symptom persistence in posttraumatic stress disorder. Journal of Anxiety Disorders 4:31–39, 1990b

Grinker RR: Psychiatric disorders in combat crews overseas and in returnees. Med Clin North Am 29:729–739, 1945

Haley SA: Treatment implications of postcombat stress response syndromes for mental health professionals, in Stress Disorders Among Vietnam Veterans. Edited by Figley CR. New York, Brunner/Mazel, 1978, pp 254–267

Hearst N, Newman TB, Hulley SB: Delayed effects of the military draft on mortality: a randomized natural experiment. N Engl J Med 314:620–624, 1986

Hedin H, Haas AP: Suicide and guilt as manifestations of PTSD in Vietnam combat veterans. Am J Psychiatry 5:586–591, 1991

Helzer JE: The impact of combat on later alcohol use by Vietnam veterans. J Psychoactive Drugs 16:183–191, 1984

Helzer JE, Robins LN, Davis DH: Depressive disorders in Vietnam returnees. J Nerv Ment Dis 163:177–185, 1976

Helzer JE, Robins LN, Wish E, et al: Depression in Vietnam veterans and civilian controls. Am J Psychiatry 136:526–529, 1979

Helzer JE, Robins LN, McEvoy L: Posttraumatic stress disorder in the general population: findings of the Epidemiologic Catchment Area survey. N Engl J Med 317:1630–1634, 1987

Hogben GL, Cornfield RB: Treatment of traumatic war neurosis with phenelzine. Arch Gen Psychiatry 38:440–445, 1981

Hoiberg A, McCaughey BG: The traumatic aftereffects of collision at sea. Am J Psychiatry 141:70–73, 1984

Holloway HC: Epidemiology of heroin dependency among soldiers in Vietnam. Mil Med 139:108–112, 1974

Holloway HC, Ursano RJ: The Vietnam veteran: memory, social context, and metaphor. Psychiatry 47:103–108, 1984

Holloway HC, Ursano RJ: Vietnam veterans on active duty: adjustment in a supportive environment, in The Trauma of War: Stress and Recovery in Vietnam Veterans. Edited by Sonnenberg SM, Blank AS Jr, Talbott JA. Washington, DC, American Psychiatric Press, 1985, pp 321–338

Horowitz MJ, Wilner N, Kaltreider N, et al: Signs and symptoms of posttraumatic stress disorder. Arch Gen Psychiatry 37:85–92, 1980

Hovens JE, Op den Velde W, Falger PRJ: Anxiety, depression, and anger in Dutch Resistance veterans from World War II. Psychother Psychosom 57:172–179, 1992

Jones FD, Hales RE: Military combat psychiatry: a historical review. Psychiatric Annals 17:525–527, 1987

Jordan BK, Schlenger WE, Hough R, et al: Lifetime and current prevalence of specific psychiatric disorders among Vietnam veterans and controls. Arch Gen Psychiatry 48:207–215, 1991

Keane TM, Caddell JM, Taylor KL: Mississippi Scale for Combat-Related Posttraumatic Stress Disorder: three studies in reliability and validity. J Consult Clin Psychol 56:85–90, 1988

Keehn RJ: Follow-up studies of World War II and Korean Conflict prisoners, III: mortality to January 1, 1976. Am J Epidemiol 111:194–211, 1980

Khansari DN, Murgo AJ, Faith RE: Effects of stress on the immune system. Immunol Today 11:170–175, 1990

Kiecolt-Glaser JK, Glaser R: Stress and immune function in humans, in Psychoneuroimmunology. Edited by Ader S, Felgen DL, Cohen N. Orlando, FL, Academic Press, 1991, pp 849–867

Kolb LC: A neuropsychological hypothesis explaining posttraumatic stress disorders. Am J Psychiatry 144:989–995, 1987

Kulka RA, Schlenger WE, Fairbank JA, et al: Trauma and the Vietnam War Generation: Report of Findings From the National Vietnam Veterans Readjustment Study. New York, Brunner/Mazel, 1990

Kulka RA, Schlenger WE, Fairbank JA, et al: Assessment of posttraumatic stress disorder in the community: prospects and pitfalls from recent studies of Vietnam veterans. J Consult Clin Psychol 59:547–560, 1991

Lacoursiere RB, Godfrey KE, Ruby LM: Traumatic neurosis in the etiology of alcoholism: Vietnam combat and other trauma. Am J Psychiatry 137:966–968, 1980

Laufer RS, Brett E, Gallops MS: Symptom patterns associated with posttraumatic stress disorder among Vietnam veterans exposed to war trauma. Am J Psychiatry 142:1304–1311, 1985

Leopold RL, Dillon H: Psychoanatomy of a disaster: a long-term study of posttraumatic neuroses in survivors of a marine explosion. Am J Psychiatry 119:913–921, 1963

McCarroll JE, Ursano RJ, Fullerton CS: Traumatic responses to the recovery of war dead in Operation Desert Storm. Am J Psychiatry 150:1875–1877, 1993a

McCarroll JE, Ursano RJ, Wright KM, et al: Handling bodies after violent death: strategies for coping. Am J Orthopsychiatry 63:209–214, 1993b

McFall ME, Mackay PW, Donovan DM: Combat-related PTSD and psychosocial adjustment problems among substance-abusing veterans. J Nerv Ment Dis 179:33–38, 1991

McFarlane AC: Posttraumatic morbidity of a disaster: a study of cases presenting for psychiatric treatment. J Nerv Ment Dis 1:4–14, 1986

Modlin HC: Traumatic neurosis and other injuries. Psychiatr Clin North Am 6:661–682, 1983

Nace EP, Meyers AL, O'Brien CP, et al: Depression in veterans two years after Vietnam. Am J Psychiatry 134:167–170, 1977

Nace EP, O'Brien CP, Mintz J, et al: Adjustment among Vietnam veteran drug users two years postservice, in Stress Disorders Among Vietnam Veterans. Edited by Figley CR. New York, Brunner/Mazel, 1978, pp 71–128

Nadelson CC, Notman MT, Zackson H, et al: A follow-up study of rape victims. Am J Psychiatry 139:1266–1270, 1982

Page WF: The Health of Former Prisoners of War. Washington, DC, National Academy of Sciences, 1992

Paykel E: Contribution of life events to causation of psychiatric illness. Psychol Med 8:245–254, 1978

Pearce KA, Schauer AH, Garfield NJ, et al: A study of posttraumatic stress disorder in Vietnam veterans. J Clin Psychol 41:9–14, 1985

Penk WE, Robinowitz R, Roberts WR: Adjustment differences among male substance abusers varying in degree of combat experience in Vietnam. J Consult Clin Psychol 49:426–437, 1981

Rangell L: Discussion of the Buffalo Creek disaster: the course of psychic trauma. Am J Psychiatry 133:313–316, 1976

Robins LN: A Follow-Up of Vietnam Drug Users (Special Action Office Monogr, Ser A, No 1). Washington, DC, U.S. Government Printing Office, 1973

Robins LN: The Vietnam Drug User Returns (Special Action Office Monogr, Ser A, No 2). Washington, DC, U.S. Government Printing Office, 1974

Robins LN, Davis DH, Goodwin DW: Drug use by U.S. Army enlisted men in Vietnam: a follow-up on their return home. Am J Epidemiol 99:235–249, 1974

Rosenheck R: Impact of posttraumatic stress disorder of World War II on the next generation. J Nerv Ment Dis 174:319–326, 1986

Rosenheck R, Becnel H, Blank AS Jr, et al: War Zone Stress Among Returning Persian Gulf Troops: A Preliminary Report. VA Northeast Program Evaluation Center (NEPEC), The Evaluation Division of the National Center for PTSD, VA Medical Center, West Haven, CT, 1991

Rosenheck R, Becnel H, Blank AS Jr, et al: Returning Persian Gulf Troops: First Year Findings. VA Northeast Program Evaluation Center (NEPEC), The Evaluation Division of the National Center for PTSD, VA Medical Center, West Haven, CT, 1992

Rundell JR, Ursano RJ, Holloway HC, et al: Psychiatric responses to trauma. Hosp Community Psychiatry 40:68–74, 1989

Rundell JR, Ursano RJ, Holloway HC, et al: Combat stress disorders and the U.S. Air Force. Mil Med 155:515–518, 1990

Sargent W, Slater E: Acute war neuroses. Lancet 2:1–20, 1940

Schnurr PP, Friedman MJ, Rosenberg SD: Premilitary MMPI scores as predictors of combat-related PTSD symptoms. Am J Psychiatry 150:479–483, 1993

Shalev A: Somatic diseases and somatic complaints following combat stress reaction. Presentation at "Trauma, Disaster, and Stress," a symposium presented at the annual meeting of the American Psychiatric Association, Montreal, Canada, May 1988

Shalev A, Bleich A, Ursano RJ: Posttraumatic stress disorder: somatic comorbidity and effort tolerance. Psychosomatics 31:197–203, 1990

Shen WW, Park S: The use of monoamine oxidase inhibitors in the treatment of traumatic war neurosis: case report. Mil Med 148:430–431, 1983

Shore JH, Tatum EL, Vollmer WM: Psychiatric reactions to disaster: the Mount St Helen's experience. Am J Psychiatry 143:590–595, 1986

Sierles FS, Chen JJ, McFarland RE, et al: Posttraumatic stress disorder and concurrent psychiatric illness: a preliminary report. Am J Psychiatry 140:1177–1179, 1983

Sivard RL: World Military and Social Expenditures, 14th Edition. Washington, DC, World Priorities, 1991

Sledge WH, Boydstun JA, Rabe AJ: Self-concept changes related to war captivity. Arch Gen Psychiatry 41:411–413, 1980

Solomon Z: Somatic complaints, stress reaction, and posttraumatic stress disorder: a three-year follow-up study. Behav Med 14:179–185, 1988

Solomon Z: Combat Stress Reaction: The Enduring Toll of War. New York, Plenum, 1993

Solomon Z, Benbenishty R: The role of proximity, immediacy, and expectancy in frontline treatment of combat stress reaction among Israeli soldiers in the Lebanon War. Am J Psychiatry 143:613–617, 1986

Solomon Z, Mikulincer M: Combat stress reactions, posttraumatic stress disorder, and social adjustment: a study of Israeli veterans. J Nerv Ment Dis 175:277–285, 1987

Solomon Z, Mikulincer M: Psychological sequelae of war: a two-year follow-up study of Israeli combat stress reaction casualties. J Nerv Ment Dis 176:264–269, 1988

Solomon Z, Benbenishty R, Spiro S: Front-Line Treatment of Israeli Combat Stress Casualties: An Evaluation of Its Effectiveness in the 1982 Lebanon War. Tel Aviv, Medical Corps, Department of Mental Health, The Israeli Defense Forces, 1986a

Solomon Z, Mikulincer M, Hobfoll SE: Effects of social support and battle intensity on loneliness and breakdown during combat. J Pers Soc Psychol 51:1269–1276, 1986b

Solomon Z, Oppenheimer B, Noy S: Subsequent military adjustment of combat stress reaction casualties: a nine-year follow-up study. Mil Med 151:8–11, 1986c

Solomon Z, Mikulincer M, Kotler M: A two-year follow-up of somatic complaints among Israeli combat stress reaction casualties. J Psychosom Res 31:463–469, 1987a

Solomon Z, Weisenberg M, Schwarzwald J: Posttraumatic stress disorder among frontline soldiers with combat stress reaction: the 1982 Israeli experience. Am J Psychiatry 144:448–454, 1987b

Stanton MD: Drug use in Vietnam, a survey among Army personnel, in Technical Report for the Department of Defense Task Group Convened to Recommend Appropriate Revisions to DOD Policy on Drug Abuse, Appendix 2. Washington, DC, U.S. Government Printing Office, 1971, pp 2141–2156

Stegman RL, Blanford RV: Combat experiences: identification of false reports and judgments about trauma. Paper presented at the annual meeting of the American Psychological Association, Washington, DC, August 1992

Strange RE, Brown DE: Home from the war: a study of psychiatric problems in Vietnam returnees. Am J Psychiatry 127:488–492, 1970

Sutker PB, Winstead DK, Galina ZH, et al: Cognitive deficits and psychopathology among former prisoners of war and combat veterans of the Korean conflict. Am J Psychiatry 148:67–72, 1991

Swiss S, Giller JE: Rape as a crime of war: a medical perspective. JAMA 270:612–615, 1993

Terr LC: Chowchilla revisited: the effects of psychic trauma four years after a school-bus kidnapping. Am J Psychiatry 140:1543–1550, 1983

Thienes-Hontos P: Stress disorder symptoms in Vietnam and Korean War veterans: still no difference. J Consult Clin Psychol 51:619–620, 1983

Ursano RJ: The Vietnam era prisoner of war: precaptivity personality and the development of psychiatric illness. Am J Psychiatry 138:315–318, 1981

Ursano RJ: Posttraumatic stress disorder: the stressor criterion. J Nerv Ment Dis 175:273–275, 1987

Ursano RJ, Holloway HC: Military psychiatry, in Comprehensive Textbook of Psychiatry/IV, 4th Edition, Vol 2. Edited by Kaplan HI, Sadock BJ. Baltimore, MD, Williams & Wilkins, 1985a, pp 1900–1909

Ursano RJ, Holloway HC: Perspectives on posttraumatic stress disorder (letter). Am J Psychiatry 142:1526, 1985b

Ursano RJ, Boydstun JA, Wheatley RD: Psychiatric illness in U.S. Air Force Vietnam prisoners of war: a five-year follow-up. Am J Psychiatry 138:310–314, 1981

Ursano RJ, Wheatley RD, Carlson EH, et al: The prisoner of war: stress, illness, and resiliency. Psychiatric Annals 17:532–535, 1987

Ursano RJ, Ingraham L, Saczynski K, et al: Psychiatric responses to death and body handling. Paper presented at the annual meeting of the American Psychiatric Association, Montreal, Canada, May 1988

Ursano RJ, Tzu-Cheg K, Fullerton CS: Posttraumatic stress disorder and meaning: structuring human chaos. J Nerv Ment Dis 180:756–759, 1992 van der Kolk BA: Psychopharmacological issues in posttraumatic stress disorder. Hosp Community Psychiatry 34:683–692, 1983

Van Dyke C, Zilberg N, McKinnon JA: Posttraumatic stress disorder: a 30-year delay in a World War II veteran. Am J Psychiatry 142:1070–1073, 1985

Van Putten T, Yager J: Posttraumatic stress disorder: emerging from the rhetoric. Arch Gen Psychiatry 141:694–696, 1984

Walker I: Chemotherapy of traumatic war stress. Mil Med 147:1029–1033, 1982

War Office: Report to the War Office Committee of Enquiring Into "Shell Shock." London, War Office, 1922

Watson CG, Kucala T, Manifold V, et al: The relationships of posttraumatic stress disorder to adolescent illegal activities, drinking, and employment. J Clin Psychol 44:592–598, 1988

Watson PB, Hoffman L, Wilson GV: The neuropsychiatry of posttraumatic stress disorder. Br J Psychiatry 152:164–173, 1988

White NS: Posttraumatic stress disorder. Hosp Community Psychiatry 34:1061–1062, 1983

White P, Faustman W: Coexisting physical conditions among inpatients with post-traumatic stress disorder. Mil Med 154:66–71, 1989

Yager T, Loafer R, Gallops M: Some problems associated with war experience in men of the Vietnam generation. Arch Gen Psychiatry 41:327–333, 1984

Yehuda R, Southwick SM, Giller EL Jr: Exposure to atrocities and severity of chronic posttraumatic stress disorder in Vietnam combat veterans. Am J Psychiatry 149:333–336, 1992

Zeiss RA, Dickman HR: PTSD 40 years later: incidence and person-situation correlates in former POWS. J Clin Psychol 45:80–87, 1989

4 The Effects of War and Parental Deployment Upon Children and Adolescents

Peter S. Jensen, M.D.
Jon A. Shaw, M.D.

In recent years we have witnessed increasing awareness of the effects of stressful and traumatic events upon children and adolescents. Although most research has focused upon natural disasters or discrete human-initiated acts of violence such as rape, kidnapping, and sniper shooting, the recent events in Operations Desert Shield and Desert Storm have heightened awareness and concerns about the effects of war upon children and adolescents. In this chapter we specifically address the effects of war-related stressors on children and adolescents, drawing specifically upon the events of Operation Desert Storm when appropriate. War-related stressors include both direct effects (i.e., those stemming from clear, unequivocal exposure to life-threatening situations, violent injury, and violent death, as are seen in conditions of acute and chronic war settings) and indirect effects (e.g., the effects of parental separation, loss, and absence). Of particular concern in the recent conflict in Iraq was the number of American families in which both parents were military members and were sent overseas, forcing them to leave their children under the care of a primary caretaker who, in many cases, was not familiar to the children.

What are the psychological consequences of war and armed conflict on children and adolescents? How do children experience the exposure to injury and death of loved ones, bodily and life threats, loss of family and community, and the sense of danger and uncertainty that suddenly pervades their lives? The context of war, given its broad scope, imposes an enormous diversity of stressors, not only upon its active participants but also upon its more passive bystanders, such as children and families. Exposure to war, with its multiple stressors, may constitute a significant interference with children's development. Yet their cognitive immaturity, plasticity, and adaptive capacities have often veiled the effects of war in a certain obscurity. Garmezy and Rutter (1985) noted that, not infrequently, children's response to stress is such that their "behavior disturbances appear to be less intense than might have been anticipated." In part for these reasons, there is a conflicting and controversial literature in which the existence, frequency, and configuration of psychological and psychiatric morbidity in children exposed to war are debated.

Much of our understanding of the effects of war upon children is based on relatively few studies. Much of the United States literature, particularly that from the Vietnam War era, has focused on the effects of war and soldier-father absence upon spouses. Thus, there have been relatively few studies of the effects of military action per se on children, and most relevant reports have been limited to clinical-descriptive approaches. One might reasonably assume that the effects of exposure to war on children may be similar to the effects of overwhelming, disastrous life events on adults and children (e.g., posttraumatic stress disorder [PTSD]). Applying PTSD constructs to children of war-torn settings, a number of authors have described the children of war as manifesting regressive behaviors, episodic aggression, psychophysiological disturbances, guilt, grief reactions, changes in school performance, personality changes, and various depressive and anxiety symptoms (Arroyo and Eth 1985;

Baker 1990; Chimienti et al. 1989; Shaw and Harris 1989).

However, although war is undoubtedly "stressful" for children, the concept of PTSD (as usually employed) may have limited applicability to the full understanding of the effects of war upon children. War usually represents a chronic, enduring condition, in which the entire context and social fabric may be dramatically altered. Entire nations and cultures may be disrupted, whereas most events leading to PTSD occur under much more limited circumstances. The dramatic contextual changes of war may result in conditions in which the stressful events and circumstances seem normative, with the possibility that the child may become somewhat acclimated to these new surroundings. Furthermore, the meanings of war's stressful events and processes are often embedded in a larger national context that is bound up with patriotism, heroism (e.g., Desert Storm, for the children of multinational forces personnel who were mobilized), or even stigma (e.g., the Vietnam War, for U.S. personnel; or the Afghanistan occupation, for military personnel of the former Soviet Union). Such considerations likely have less relevance for the construct of PTSD.

When considering the effects of war upon children, even a fairly circumscribed action such as Desert Shield/Desert Storm, one should carefully examine the nature of the stressors themselves, including the actual damage to body or to property, loss of family and/or friends (or threats of such losses), and the geographic and psychological proximity of the war-related stressors. One should also carefully scrutinize the intrinsic adaptive capacities of the child and the social and community resources that he or she has at hand to deal with the stressful circumstances, so that the effects of war may be disentangled from those of other adverse or detrimental conditions.

Stress Severity and Populations of Study

Much of the previous work examining children who have been affected by war has encompassed four major groups (Table 4–1).

Drawing upon the importance of "proximity" from the PTSD literature, we have ordered war stressors in terms of the likely severity of the stressor or the degree of exposure to stressful/traumatic conditions (a similar approach was used previously by, for example, Stoltz [1951] and Pynoos et al. [1987]) (Table 4–1). In general, children of U.S. and multinational forces were not exposed directly to war (in contrast to Kuwaiti and Iraqi children), nor did many suffer permanent parental loss or prolonged parental imprisonment (as during the Vietnam War era). In the subsections that follow, we describe what is known about the effects of war on each of the populations listed in Table 4–1. We place greater emphasis upon the exposures implicit in the last two populations of interest—experiencing of "routine" parental absence and exposure to media, societal, and cultural factors—which were more characteristic of the experience of U.S. children whose parents were deployed during Operations Desert Shield/Desert Storm.

Direct Exposure to War

The literature describing the direct effects of war upon children first began to emerge during World War II. Dunsdon (1941) reported that children who remained under bombing attacks in Bristol, England, were 8 times more likely to demonstrate psychological distress compared with those who were evacuated to the countryside. Bodman (1941) observed that only 4% of schoolchildren exposed to air bombings in the general vicinity demonstrated psychological distress, whereas 61% of those children in a hospital hit by bombs showed signs of distress sev-

Table 4–1.   Populations of interest in the study of the effects of war-related trauma on children and adolescents

Children exposed directly to war
Children suffering parental loss or prolonged parental imprisonment
Children experiencing "routine" parental absence
Children exposed to media, societal, and cultural factors

eral weeks after the incident. More recently, Chimienti and co-workers (1989) noted that children in Lebanon exposed to war conditions of shelling, destruction of home, death, and forced displacement were 1.7 times more likely to manifest regression, depression, and aggressive behaviors. Saigh (1991) found that 24 of 72 Lebanese adolescents exposed to major war-related stressors met the diagnostic criteria for PTSD.

However, depending upon the intensity of the exposure, direct exposure to war events does not appear to always bear a one-to-one relationship with psychological and behavioral consequences for children. For example, in a study of the dreams and sleep habits of Israeli youth in a border town subject to terrorist activities, it was found that the exposed youth slept longer and had fewer bad dreams, and had fewer daydreams about violent themes, the enemy, and other wartime themes, than did nonexposed children (Rofe and Lewin 1982). Similarly, Ziv and Israeli (1973) discovered that children from frequently shelled kibbutzim were no different from those from nonshelled kibbutzim on measures of anxiety.

Whereas massive exposure to wartime trauma seems likely to overwhelm many children's defenses, some evidence suggests that moderate degrees of exposure may result in self-protective, adaptive, cognitive styles that allow effective functioning. Minimal degrees of threat may not invoke these protective mechanisms for some children. It seems likely that the child's age and developmental level, as well as family and community factors, may mediate the strength and nature of these effects.

Parental Loss or Extended Imprisonment

There are few systematic studies of the effects of parental loss and bereavement upon children and adolescents during times of war, much less during the recent Operation Desert Storm. Although it is reasonable to expect that the effects of parental loss and the process of bereavement upon children under these conditions may be similar to those upon children who lose their parents during peacetime conditions, the context and meaning of the loss may have unique significance. For example, to the grieving child, the lost parent (usually father) may be regarded as a hero, or the child may feel that the father's death was due to some kind of failure on the father's part. Circumstances in which the larger national community also shares the grief and respect for the lost one may result in different consequences for bereaved children. A continuing study of 25 Israeli children who lost their father to military action when they were 2 to 10 years of age indicates the sustained effect of parental death on the psychological health of these children. Fifty percent of these children continued to have significant behavioral and emotional problems 3.5 years after the father's death (Elizur and Kaffman 1982, 1983). Unfortunately, these studies were uncontrolled, rendering it difficult to compare the effects of parental loss due to military action with parental loss and bereavement under other circumstances, as well as to the situation of children who did not lose their parents.

A few studies are available that have examined the effects of parental separation on families of prisoners of war. As one would expect, the family of the prisoner of war fares poorly during his or her absence. Understandably, the determination of effects of prolonged husband-father or wife-mother absence per se in this select population is difficult, because many other changes occur to these families in addition to the individual's imprisonment (e.g., the family's ever-present fears for his or her safety and their reasonable doubts about his or her eventual return). In one study of families of prisoners of war 1 year after reunion, McCubbin and Dahl (1976) found that children in these families scored significantly lower on personal and social adjustment on the California Test of Personality when their scores were compared with standardized norms. Interestingly, the father's increasing length of absence was associated with better child adaptation, suggesting that with increasing lengths of father absence, children (and possibly wives) are able to develop partially compensatory adaptive strategies to cope with the separation and absence caused by the father's prisoner-of-war experience.

Parental Deployment and Absence

Operations Desert Shield/Desert Storm were relatively short-lived; consequently, one would expect that the effects of this military action upon children whose parents were deployed were relatively mild. Along this line, previous studies of U.S. military families suggest that "routine" wartime father absence (i.e., not due to being held prisoner of war) does not necessarily produce uniform, adverse effects upon children. Hill (1949) and Boulding (1950), studying randomly selected Iowa World War II veterans and their families with extensive interviews at the war's end, found that good marital adjustment and the degree of family affection before separation predicted good reunion adjustment. Families that only *partially* "closed ranks" (i.e., kept the absent father's role and importance central to the family emotional environment, yet got on with the business at hand) suffered more during his absence but did better at reunion than those families that *completely* "closed ranks" at the time of father separation (as if to shut out the reality of the father's absence). Individual instances occurred in these studies in which a family did not have a good "track record" before the father's departure but was nonetheless poised for a developmental spurt: some families "rose to the challenge" and used the period of father absence as one of significant growth and development. Thus, effects of parental absence during wartime may be variable and may not always be deleterious.

Several studies during the Vietnam War documented significant effects (both positive and negative) of father absence upon children, particularly boys. Hillenbrand (1976) studied boys and girls in a sixth-grade classroom in a school for children of military families and demonstrated that cumulative father absence (defined as the total amount of time separated from the child and family up to that point in the child's life) was associated with higher IQ scores in first-born boys. But for younger boys with older siblings, "early-beginning" father absence was related to increased aggression and dependency, as well as higher verbal than math scores. Nice (1978) studied the personal adjustment of children 1 to 4 months before the wartime deployment of their fathers aboard a U.S. Navy aircraft carrier, and again 1 to 3 months after their fathers' return. During the course of their father's absence, children demonstrated significant gains on standardized personality tests. Although such findings were not hypothesized a priori, similar findings were described by other researchers (e.g., Garmezy 1974), who noted the "steeling" effect of certain life challenges that can facilitate growth and adaptation.

We are unaware of any published studies that examined the effects of Desert Shield/Desert Storm upon children. However, our overall review of the military parental absence literature (pre–Desert Storm) indicates that relatively brief parental absences during wartime situations (as occurred in Desert Storm) are associated with modest, temporary behavioral and emotional symptoms in family members, particularly in wives and sons. The reunion and reintegration process is critical to the resolution of these difficulties. Absence of greater length or frequency, or absence under combat or wartime conditions, may exert more persistent effects. The data at hand suggest that absence effects are mediated by preexisting father-family relationships; the age, sex, and order of siblings; the meanings of the absence to the family; the extent of danger to which the father is exposed; and how the mother copes with the father's absence. Under some circumstances, the absence of the father for military reasons may be associated with adaptive outcomes and enhanced personality development.

One relatively unique factor that affected a number of children during Desert Storm was related to the recent increase in two–military parent families, as well as the increase in female active-duty parents. Some degree of media attention was focused on children whose parents were both deployed, a situation that resulted in the children's being placed with family members or other persons during the deployment. Obviously, these are important phenomena and deserve further study, but we have been unable to locate any systematic literature on the effects of these absences (female military parent absence or dual-parent absence) on children. However, it seems likely that these conditions result in greater disruption to children's emotional equilibrium than instances of the historically more common and traditionally sanctioned father absence.

Media, Societal, and Cultural Effects

Although the total length of deployment for most U.S. personnel during Operations Desert Shield/Desert Storm was less than the 12-month overseas "hardship" tour commonly experienced by many military families, the degree of media attention, reflected by the 24-hour news coverage, was unprecedented in U.S. military history. Many families found themselves riveted to the hourly television programming, waiting to hear any piece of new information. The live coverage of bombing attacks in Baghdad, the video footage of cruise missiles finding their targets, and the daily briefings by U.S. commanders in Bahrain provided an immediacy and reality to the conflict that absorbed national attention. Certainly, this absorption in the events of the war provided by such exhaustive coverage could have been no more pronounced than in the watchful spouses and families of deployed servicemembers. In one instance, one spouse of a deployed servicemember who (like many others) found herself spending long hours watching the live broadcasts was approached by her 3-year-old daughter: the little child turned off the television and announced to her mother, "It makes me sad when you watch TV." This child had to deal not just with the temporary absence of her father and her fears for his safety, but also with the preoccupation, sadness, anxiety, and temporary loss of her mother.

Clearly, exposure to wartime conditions may result in subtle but perhaps important shifts in interactions within families. Cohen and Dotan (1976) studied the wartime and postwar communication patterns of a stratified random sample of married Israeli women with 6- to 18-year-old children. Their findings indicated that the wartime stress resulted in increased mother-child conversations and time spent together watching television. These effects were greater for families of a higher-socio-economic background. Although these "ripple effects" of war on the waiting families and society have been described by many observers, there have been few studies of these phenomena.

Effects of War

Psychopathology

A common concern raised by researchers since World War II and continuing into the present has been the potentially specific effects of wartime conditions on the emergence of child and adolescent antisocial behavior and delinquency (Alcock 1941; Cook 1941). In more recent years, a number of authors (e.g., Fee 1980) have suggested that chronic warlike conditions in Northern Ireland result in children's development of antisocial behavior. However, most lines of evidence do not provide support for the notion of profound effects of war or sectarian violence on development of aggression and violence in children. McWhirter and colleagues (McWhirter 1983) studied 3- to 16-year-old Belfast children and asked them about their perceptions of causes of death in their society. These children's perceptions indicated that they attribute death more to sickness and old age than to violence; these perceptions paralleled official death statistics. Because of the evidence that children may become acclimated to these chronic, low-to-moderate levels of violence, and because of evidence that children's responses to such difficulties tend to be short-lived, more recent research has shifted the focus from psychopathology to social awareness, values, and attitudes.

Values and Attitudes

Growing evidence indicates that wartime stresses, particularly at the low to moderate levels experienced by most children in a major or global conflict, have more important effects in shaping children's attitudes and perceptions than in determining any direct expressions of psychopathology. For example, Ziv and co-workers (1974) compared children who had been exposed to wartime stress with children who had not had such exposure. Children's peer relationships, levels of aggression, and attitudes toward war, peace, and terrorists were compared. Results indicated that those children who had been exposed to shelling in the immediate vicinity showed evidence of increased valuing of the attribute of courage in their peers compared with children in areas that had not been shelled. Interestingly, there were no differences between the two groups in overt aggression toward terrorists, although there was some evidence of increased covert aggressive attitudes and increased patriotism among children in areas that had been shelled. Both groups equally valued peace. Children in areas that had been shelled did not show increased positive attitudes toward war compared with children from areas that had not been shelled. Exposed children appeared to demonstrate a stronger identification with the community, however. In another Israeli study, Ziv and Nebenhaus (1973) assessed more than 600 children to determine their wishes and feelings about peace during different periods of war intensity. Only one child expressed any felt hostile wishes toward the perceived aggressor, a finding that suggests that the phenomenon of "identification with the aggressor" was quite infrequent.

It seems possible that the outcome of war, both defeat and victory, shapes immediate perceptions of one's country and relative status in the world. Longer-term effects are less clear. Thus, the U.S. role in forging the international coalition in Operation Desert Storm, and the successful outcome, seemed to be related to a general sense of power and elation among children, youth, and adults, and few persons who witnessed these events would dispute their immediate effects on the U.S. emotional climate and national self-esteem. Yet, these positive effects were ephemeral and were quickly overtaken by subsequent events. President George Bush seemed "unbeatable" in opinion polls shortly after the war, but economic factors quickly took center stage in national attention during the presidential elections, resulting in his defeat.

Mediators of the Effects of War

Parental and Family Responses

Understandably, the preschool-age child living within the security of a constantly available and supporting family often mirrors the parental response to wartime stressors. When there is parental physical injury, significant parental emotional responses, premorbid parental psychopathology, or excessive intolerance of the child's tendency to regress behaviorally, an emotional contagion may occur that passes on, as in a "ripple effect," to the child (Bloch et al. 1956; McFarlane 1987; Newman 1976; Pynoos et al. 1987). Although these concepts are grounded in a substantial clinical and developmental literature, the actual extent to which parent-child emotional contagion occurs is unclear, and inferences about such factors are often drawn from selected clinical cases (e.g., children whose parents were in concentration camps [Bergman and Jucovy 1982; Epstein 1979; Sigal and Rakoff 1971]).

Although parental responses are likely to shape important adaptive and maladaptive outcomes in children, no evidence supports the notion that many adverse outcomes are explained by this phenomenon, particularly in view of the relatively remarkably positive outcomes in most children exposed to war events and processes. Likely, most parents respond quite appropriately during wartime conditions on behalf of their children. Inferences from clinical samples should not be applied to the broader populations exposed to these stressors.

Child-Specific Factors

Variables intrinsic to the individual child that are likely to affect ultimate outcomes in children exposed to wartime conditions include age, inborn coping style and capacity, cognitive level and other developmental factors, guilt, temperament, and preexisting psychopathology (Table 4–2). Some evidence suggests that a substantial proportion of children are able to call upon intrinsic coping capabilities during wartime crises and generate new levels of adaptation and coping. For example, during the 1967 Arab-Israeli War, as de Shalit (1970) reported, many children responded in a remarkable manner, often displaying high levels of self-sacrifice and desire to help the community. In this situation, children's fears often seemed less than one might have expected. One child said to his mother (a child psychiatrist), "At a time like this, each of us has a job to do. Mine is to go to school and be with my friends. We must not try to get out of our obligations." When war affects the home front, children (like adults) may prefer active roles (e.g., filling sandbags) to passive roles (e.g., sitting in shelters).

The opportunity to play an active role and to exert some control over one's individual responses to war stressors may have important eventual consequences on children's outcomes. Baker (1990) studied self-esteem, locus of control, and behavioral symptoms in 796 Gaza and West Bank children. The author

Table 4–2. Factors affecting children's adjustment to war events and processes

Family and parental support

Child-specific factors
  Age
  Coping style/locus of control
  Cognitive level
  Guilt
  Temperament
  Preexisting psychopathology

Social and community factors
  Social context and meaning
  Community support, cohesion, and leadership

found evidence of higher levels of positive self-esteem and locus of control since the inception of the Intifada, which allowed the children to more actively respond to the stresses of the Israeli occupation of that territory on the local residents. The ability to exert and develop an internal locus of control may be more characteristic of older children, and it may be the adaptive result of a response to stressors. Lifschitz (1975) found that adolescents who had lost fathers during the Six Day War or the Yom Kippur War tended to exercise a more internal locus of control and assert responsibility for their lives compared with control subjects.

Age and developmental factors may set important limits on children's and adolescents' capacity to respond adaptively to war crises. The young child lacks the cognitive capacities that are available to the adult. His or her theories of causality are egocentric, and he or she may be unable to talk about frightening experiences. Unable to transform internal conflicts and feelings into words, the child may express such feelings in action, play, or aggressive behaviors and/or activities. In contrast, the older child and adolescent may have a wider repertoire of adaptive responses and coping capabilities.

Possibly, younger children may be at increased risk for later consequences of war stress because of the increased preponderance of idiosyncratic and egocentric thought in this age group. Thus, a young child whose father is killed during wartime may wonder why the father was killed. He or she might wonder whether, for example, the father had failed somehow. Young children's tendency to attribute blame associated with their inner feelings is well described among clinical populations and may be an important contributing factor for some adverse outcomes. Interestingly, Freud and Burlingham (1943) suggested that very young children must be protected from war and violence, not because the horrors are strange and traumatic, but because the outer violent circumstances may parallel the children's inner experiences. Under such conditions, the normal processes of sublimation and repression are made much more difficult.

When considering the role of war stressors upon children and adolescents, one must keep in mind that the traumatic experiences of war may unmask latent psychopathology or, perhaps more commonly, may serve as a framing construct for more normal developmental fears. Thus, the child who at a given age may be quite normally afraid of certain animals or strangers may just as well become afraid of that country's enemies (e.g., the Iraqis for the U.S. child, the Israelis for the Palestinian child) and vice versa. In this sense, the war events may serve as metaphors, or "vehicles," for the child to express normal developmental anxieties.

Social and Community Contexts

Beyond the role that child and family characteristics may play in shaping children's reactions to war, the social context of specific war-related events is likely also an important mediator of eventual outcomes. One social contextual factor is the meaning of the war-related tensions within the community. For example, Ziv and Israeli (1973) suggested that Israeli children who were exposed to bombings may have been protected from further negative outcome by their "hero" status, because their situation was well known and met with great sympathy throughout the country. Conceivably, war-related stresses occurring during a war that was viewed by a significant proportion of the society as unjustified (e.g., the Vietnam War) could have quite different consequences from similar events occurring during a war that was widely regarded as justified and "moral" (e.g., Operation Desert Storm).

Other researchers of the effects of war on children have concluded that the presence of strong social and community supports may buffer the effects of adverse experiences upon children and adolescents. Lifschitz and colleagues (Lifschitz 1975; Lifschitz et al. 1977) noted that among children who had lost their father during the war, those who lived in kibbutzim fared better than those who lived in less cohesive supportive settings (e.g., the moshav or traditional environments). Among

children living in the 150 kibbutzim across Israel, it was noted
that the incidence of psychological disturbance following the
Yom Kippur War was no higher than that in the 2 years before
the outbreak of that war (Milgram 1982). Similar findings have
been noted for adults, which indicates that under high levels of
stress, a higher degree of social supports may buffer the effects
of stressful events (Zuckerman-Bareli 1979).

Ayalon (1983) has identified a number of community variables
that may mediate child and family responses to terrorist- and
war-induced stresses. First, the historical and cultural characteristics of the community, as well as its previous experience with
such traumas, may shape its reactions to subsequent traumas.
Second, community features such as leadership, community
cohesion, and communication can play an important role, particularly during and after the stressful situations. Third, the community's specific anticipatory responses to the possibility of the
occurrence of such traumatic events likely shape responses during and after the traumas. Last, it seems plausible that the community's specific responses after the traumatic situation may
further shape eventual outcomes.

Interventions and Treatment

Child-Specific Interventions

It is not totally clear what constitutes an ideal intervention for
children who have been affected by war-related acts. Some
authors (e.g., Ayalon 1983) have described a series of interventions including ventilation, abreaction, channeling of aggression, gradual in vivo exposure to feared situations, and
cognitive reappraisal. Shaw and Harris (1989) proposed a transitional psychosocial program to facilitate war-traumatized children's reorganization of their lives to enable them to once again
meet normal developmental expectations and to participate in
family and community. This program, which consists of an intensive residential program with high levels of staff involve-

ment, group activities, psychodrama, and psychiatric consultation, is currently being implemented in Mozambique (Shaw and Harris 1994). However, such interventions may be most useful for children whose traumatic experiences have entailed the separation and massive disruption of family and social ties, and would not apply to children of U.S. or multinational forces under the circumstances seen during Operation Desert Storm.

Child-focused interventions in clinical settings often entail 1) identifying and understanding the pattern of symptoms and dysfunction, 2) facilitating the child's expression of emotions, fears, and anxieties embedded in the symptom complex, and, ultimately, 3) enabling the child to express his or her interpretation and understanding of the traumatic situation (Table 4–3). Younger children with behavioral or emotional symptoms may be usefully given an opportunity to draw or play out their experiences, thus providing a forum for discussion. Older children and adolescents can be more directly encouraged to express and verbalize feelings, questions, and concerns so that they will not feel overwhelmed with feelings of guilt, shame, grief, and helplessness. Avenues must be made available for the expression of affects, conflicted feelings, confusing and muddled

Table 4–3. Interventions for children affected by war

Child-directed interventions
   Ventilation, abreaction, and in vivo exposure
   Transitional psychosocial residential program
   Group treatment

Family interventions
   Family therapy
   Keeping absent parent's place "open"

Community interventions
   School-based didactic/cognitive preparation program
   "Therapeutic teaching"
   Community consultation
   Emergency drills/rehearsal

impressions, and perceptions, which otherwise are too often quickly distorted in a search for egocentric explanations of causality. Although there are a number of therapeutic avenues by which one can address traumatized children and adolescents, a critical component employed in most settings is a psychosocial treatment designed to facilitate the child's assimilation and integration of the reality and meaning of the traumatic situation, in such a way that he or she will be able to progress with developmental and life's tasks.

Using less traditional clinical approaches, Lifschitz and colleagues (Lifschitz 1975; Lifschitz et al. 1977) noted that children who have lost their fathers benefit from identification with and pairing with "big brothers" or "big sisters." Other observers (Eloul 1982; Morawetz 1982) have noted that many children do not seem to be able or willing to cope directly or verbally with loss, but do like to be with other children who have experienced similar losses. Parents should know that such difficulties in coping do not constitute a lack of love for the lost one or shallowness on the children's part and do constitute a relatively common response.

Group intervention with child victims of war is a promising technique, with its provision of opportunities for clarification of cognitive distortions, normalization of the recovery process, and further assessment of psychiatric and psychological co-morbidity. However, one must be aware that children may suffer from a spectrum of emotional and behavioral problems that will require individualized, targeted interventions. Nonetheless, because there are many different contexts and great variations in children's responses to war situations, great care must be given and interventions developed in consideration of the child and family's ecological and cultural contexts.

Family Interventions

At the level of family interventions, traditional individually focused mental health concepts and approaches may need further restructuring. How does one treat families during times of crises without disrupting the social structure? If children's responses to war events are partly mediated through the effects on the broader family structure, interventions designed to assist the larger family group may be most effective. For families in which a parent is away because of war (either as a prisoner of war or as a result of more routine military combat duty), Frank and co-workers (1981) recommend that the absent parent's place be kept "open" during the time of separation to facilitate that parent's eventual reintegration into the family upon return. Many workers in the field recommend the use of frequent letters and tapes from the absent parent whenever possible, as well as the provision of ongoing support structures for the remaining parent (e.g., through the use of support groups), although we are unaware of systematic research evidence documenting the actual usefulness of such strategies.

Dremen and Cohen (1982) have recommended specific family therapy approaches as a strategy for dealing with children and adolescents who have been affected by war-related events. With this strategy they deemphasize the importance of individual psychopathology and concentrate instead on promoting family strengths, cohesion, and coping.

Community Interventions

Given the broad and far-reaching impact of war-related events and processes upon children and families, it seems likely that conventional mental health practices at the individual or even family level may not be possible during wartime because of the lack of available resources. In addition, it is possible that such individual- or family-specific interventions may be wasteful, ineffective, or even harmful. Traditional mental health concepts are often derived from Western thought and culture and may not be useful in other cultural contexts. Benyamini (1976) has recommended, as one method of choosing among treatment approaches, the consideration of community-level interventions for broad and potentially mild problems (e.g., school interventions), group-level interventions for more severe problems (e.g., family or group therapeutic approaches), and individual-level interventions (e.g., child and family therapeutic approaches) for the most severe war-related difficulties.

Community-level interventions draw upon the premise that the breakdown of social structure may be a critical factor in determining the overall impact of war upon children and families. Because the social structure provides the norms and context for interpreting and understanding traumatic events and circumstances, interventions at the level of these community structures may constitute a highly relevant, potentially effective vehicle for intervention. Benyamini (1976) described a school psychological emergency intervention after a terrorist attack. Similarly, Koubovi (1982) has advocated the use of "therapeutic teaching" of literature at the community and school level during war-related events and their aftermath. This approach involves selecting books with war-related themes and conducting classroom discussion. Koubovi suggested that such an approach promotes intellectualization, cognitive reappraisal, and reassurance of the likelihood of positive outcomes, while avoiding the unstructured and potentially harmful ventilation of feelings.

In Israel, some communities have prepared for the threat of war and terrorist attacks by systematic training and development. Such approaches are characterized by attack drills, allocation of roles and responsibilities to individual members, and the development and utilization of communications structures (Ayalon 1983). These approaches seem plausible, but as Ayalon (1983) has cautioned, an actual terrorist attack or war may be so traumatic that no amount of preparation through cognitive approaches can prepare one for the actual assault. Furthermore, it is possible that such rehearsals may increase children's anxieties and phobic responses and reinforce children's stereotyping of others as "the enemy." Nonetheless, promising systematic approaches have been developed to orient a community and its children to respond to emergency situations (e.g., COPE, or Community Oriented Preparation for Emergency, developed at the University of Haifa), but studies of the effectiveness of such interventions are needed.

Had massive casualties been sustained during Operation Desert Storm (as the Iraqi leaders were predicting), and had such casualties affected large stateside or Europe-based military communities, large-scale, community-directed consultation and interventions may have been clinically warranted. However, it should be noted that although a variety of child-, family-, and social system–level approaches have been developed and advocated, no research evidence exists documenting the superiority of one intervention over another. Benyamini's (1976) recommendations for interventions at three system levels (based upon the severity and breadth of the problem) are sensible, but implementation of this approach may not be possible under widespread and/or severe war-related conditions. Studies of combat stress reactions in the U.S. and Israeli military suggest that group- and social-level interventions may be more effective than individually focused interventions. In adult soldiers, traditional, individual, psychopathology-oriented psychotherapeutic interventions may lead to prolonged morbidity (Wise 1988). Although these adverse outcomes may be partly due to secondary gain resulting from ongoing morbidity in military soldiers, caution is warranted in the use of individual approaches without careful consideration of the broader context in which the traumas occurred and of the systems and cultures in which people must adapt after the resolution of the traumas.

Ethical and Political Issues

The recent events of Operations Desert Shield/Desert Storm have galvanized concerns among advocacy and professional groups that all efforts should be made to prevent the separation of mothers from their children during times of national mobilization and preparations for war. Interestingly, the same concern and recommendation was raised 40 years ago by Stoltz (1951), who noted that mothers should be the last source of manpower during wartime. In the instance of families with two active-duty parents, similar policy considerations may be warranted concerning whether to allow both parents to be mobilized and sent to a war area. Such recommendations deserve careful consideration, both with regard to the best interests of children and with regard to national security. A full consideration of these issues may warrant a special "blue-ribbon" panel of scientists, lawmakers, children's advocates, and military leaders to consider the scientific evidence for and against such a step, as well as to assess the potential impact of such a decision upon military families and national security.

Conclusions

Our review suggests that closer attention must be paid to the adequate assessment of children and families who have been affected by war. Although the traditional domain of psychopathology as a potential outcome remains relevant for research, additional studies assessing the impact of wartime conditions upon the values and attitudes of children and families are of great importance. A better understanding of why some children seem to acclimate to low to moderate levels of stress while others remain anxious or become dysfunctional is needed. Health care providers and community leaders must be aware of the range of factors that shape children's responses to war events and processes, and careful consideration of the optimal level of intervention for war-affected children and communities is necessary.

Consideration of the psychological and geographic proximity of the wartime stressors has provided useful clues to comprehending the magnitude of war-related effects under some circumstances. However, additional research is needed to increase our understanding of how similar events with similar psychological and geographic proximity exert dissimilar effects in some persons and some communities compared with others. Hopes have been raised for a "new world order," but the long and continuing history of international disorder indicates that these research agendas deserve ongoing highest priority.

References

Alcock AT: War strain on children. BMJ 1:124, 1941

Arroyo W, Eth S: Children traumatized by Central American warfare, in Post-Traumatic Stress Disorder in Children. Edited by Eth S, Pynoos RS. Washington, DC, American Psychiatric Press, 1985, pp 101–120

Ayalon A: Coping with terrorism, in Stress Reduction and Prevention. Edited by Meichenbaum D, Jaremko M. New York, Plenum, 1983, pp 293–339

Baker AM: The psychological impact of the Intifada on Palestinian children in the occupied West Bank and Gaza: an exploratory study. Am J Orthopsychiatry 60:496–505, 1990

Benyamini K: School psychological emergency intervention: proposals for guidelines based on recent Israeli experience. Mental Health and Society 3:22–32, 1976

Bergman MS, Jucovy ME: Generations of the Holocaust. New York, Basic Books, 1982

Bloch D, Silber E, Perry S: Some factors in the emotional reaction of children to disaster. Am J Psychiatry 113:416–422, 1956

Bodman F: War conditions and the mental health of the child. BMJ 2:486–488, 1941

Boulding E: Family adjustments to war separation and reunion. American Academy of Political and Social Science Annals 272:59–67, 1950

Chimienti G, Nasr JA, Khalifeh I: Children's reactions to war-related stress: affective symptoms and behavior problems. Soc Psychiatry Psychiatr Epidemiol 24:282–287, 1989

Cohen AA, Dotan J: Communication in the family as a function of stress during war and peace. Journal of Marriage and the Family 38:141–148, 1976

Cook PH: Evacuation problems in Britain. Transactions of the Kansas Academy of Sciences 44:343–345, 1941

de Shalit N: Children in war, in Children and Families in Israel: Some Mental Health Perspectives. Edited by Jarus A, Marcus J, Oren J, et al. New York, Gordon & Breach, 1970, pp 151–182

Dremen S, Cohen EC: Children of victims of terrorist activities: a family approach to dealing with tragedy. American Journal of Family Therapy 10:39–47, 1982

Dunsdon MI: Juvenile delinquency in war time: report from the British Child Guidance Clinic. Lancet 2:572–574, 1941

Elizur E, Kaffman M: Children's reaction following the death of the father: the first four years. Journal of the American Academy of Child Psychiatry 21:474–480, 1982

Elizur E, Kaffman M: Factors influencing the severity of childhood bereavement reactions. Am J Orthopsychiatry 53:668–676, 1983

Eloul J: A description of group work with war widows, in Stress and Anxiety, Vol 8. Edited by Spielberger CD, Sarason IG, Milgram NA. Washington, DC, Hemisphere, 1982, pp 207–212

Epstein H: Children of the Holocaust. New York, Putnam, 1979

Fee F: Responses to a behavioral questionnaire of a group of Belfast children, in A Society Under Stress: Children and Young People in Northern Ireland. Edited by Harbison J, Harbison J. Somerset, UK, Open Books, 1980, pp 31–42

Frank M, Shanfield SB, Evans HE: The in-and-out parent: strategies for managing reentry stress. Mil Med 146:846–849, 1981

Freud A, Burlingham DT: War and Children. New York, Medical War Books, Ernst Willard, 1943

Garmezy N: Children at risk: the search for antecedents of schizophrenia, Part II: ongoing research programs, issues, and intervention. Schizophr Bull 9:55–125, 1974

Garmezy N, Rutter M: Acute reactions to stress, in Child and Adolescent Psychiatry: Modern Approaches, 2nd Edition. Edited by Rutter M, Hersov L. Oxford, UK, Blackwell Scientific, 1985, pp 152–176

Hill R: Families Under Stress: Adjustment to the Crises of War Separation and Reunion. Westport, CT, Greenwood Press, 1949

Hillenbrand ED: Father absence in military families. The Family Coordinator 25:451–458, 1976

Koubovi D: Therapeutic teaching of literature during the war and its aftermath, in Stress and Anxiety, Vol 8. Edited by Spielberger CD, Sarason IG, Milgram NA. Washington, DC, Hemisphere, 1982, pp 345–350

Lifschitz M: Long-range effects of father's loss: the cognitive complexity of bereaved children and their school adjustment. Br J Med Psychol 49:187–197, 1975

Lifschitz M, Berman D, Galili A, et al: Bereaved children: the effects of mother's perception and social system organization on their short range adjustment. Journal of Child Psychiatry 16:272–284, 1977

McCubbin HI, Dahl BB: Prolonged family separation in the military: a longitudinal study, in Families in the Military System. Edited by McCubbin HI, Dahl BB, Hunter EJ. Beverly Hills, CA, Sage, 1976, pp 112–144

McFarlane AC: Posttraumatic phenomena in a longitudinal study of children following a natural disaster. J Am Acad Child Adolesc Psychiatry 26:764–769, 1987

McWhirter L: Northern Ireland: growing up with the "troubles," in Aggression in Global Perspective. Edited by Goldstein AP, Segall MH. New York, Pergamon, 1983, pp 367–400

Milgram NA: War related stress in Israeli children and youth, in Handbook of Stress: Theoretical and Clinical Aspects. Edited by Goldberger L, Breznitz S. New York, Free Press, 1982, pp 656–676

Morawetz A: The impact on adolescents of the death in war of an older sibling, in Stress and Anxiety, Vol 8. Edited by Spielberger CD, Sarason IG, Milgram NA. Washington, DC, Hemisphere, 1982, pp 267–274

Newman J: Children of disaster: clinical observations at Buffalo Creek. Am J Psychiatry 133:306–312, 1976

Nice DS: The androgynous wife and the military child, in Children of Military Families: A Part and Yet Apart. Edited by Hunter EJ, Nice DS. Washington, DC, U.S. Government Printing Office, 1978, pp 25–37

Pynoos RS, Frederick C, Nader K, et al: Life threat and post-traumatic stress in school age children. Arch Gen Psychiatry 44:1057–1063, 1987

Rofé Y, Lewin I: The effect of war environment on dreams and sleep habits, in Stress and Anxiety, Vol 8. Edited by Spielberger CD, Sarason IG, Milgram NA. Washington, DC, Hemisphere, 1982, pp 67–79

Saigh P: Affective and behavioral parameters of traumatized and non-traumatized adolescents. Paper presented to the annual meeting of the Society for Traumatic Stress Studies, Washington, DC, October 1991

Shaw J, Harris J: A prevention-intervention program for children of war in Mozambique. Paper presented to the annual meeting of the American Academy of Child and Adolescent Psychiatry, New York, October 1989

Shaw J, Harris J: Children of war and children at war: child victims of terrorism in Mozambique, in Individual and Community Responses to Trauma and Disaster: The Structure of Human Chaos. Edited by Ursano RJ, McCaughey BG, Fullerton CS. Cambridge, UK, Cambridge University Press, 1994, pp 287–305

Sigal JJ, Rakoff V: Concentration camp survival: a pilot study of the effects on the second generation. Canadian Psychiatric Association Journal 6:393–397, 1971

Stoltz L: The effect of mobilization and war on children. Social Casework 32:143–149, 1951

Wise MG: Adjustment disorders and impulse disorders not otherwise classified, in The American Psychiatric Press Textbook of Psychiatry. Edited by Talbott JA, Hales RE, Yudofsky SC. Washington, DC, American Psychiatric Press, 1988, pp 605–620

Ziv A, Israeli R: Effects of bombardment on the manifest anxiety level of children living in kibbutzim. J Consult Clin Psychol 40:287–291, 1973

Ziv A, Nebenhaus S: Frequency of wishes for peace of children during different periods of war intensity. Israeli Journal of Behavioral Sciences 19:423–427, 1973

Ziv A, Kruglanski AW, Shulman S: Children's psychological reactions to wartime stress. J Pers Soc Psychol 30:24–30, 1974

Zuckerman-Bareli C: Effects of border tension on residents of an Israeli town. Journal of Human Stress 5:29–40, 1979

5 Chemical and Biological Weapons: Silent Agents of Terror

Carol S. Fullerton, Ph.D.
George T. Brandt, M.D.
Robert J. Ursano, M.D.

> Late in the afternoon in the Spring of 1915 French troops near the city of Ypres experienced a new type of warfare. A strange opaque cloud of greenish-yellow fumes drifted towards them. Soldiers fell down in terrible agony, gasping for breath and terror and panic spread throughout the ranks. In the chaos, soldiers ran in all directions, wild with confusion. Greenish-gray clouds descended, moved across the countryside and destroyed everything in its path. The soldiers, coughing and heaving, were unable to speak. Others were blinded. Hundreds of soldiers died in the gas-soaked trenches. It was demonic and unconscionable. (Joy 1988)

War is one of the most complex of the human-made disaster environments. The psychiatric symptomatology of war is manifold and varies across individuals and across different types of war trauma (Green et al. 1990; Laufer et al. 1985; Rundell et al. 1989). In the present world climate, the possibility of chemical and biological warfare (CBW) persists and causes great concern. The behavioral and

111

psychological responses that might affect health and performance in a context in which use of CBW is a possibility or CBW has actually been introduced (referred henceforth in this chapter as the *CBW environment*), however, are not well understood.

Recently, in the Persian Gulf War, the world was reminded that the use of chemical and biological agents in combat is a realistic concern (Ursano et al. 1992). Although the missiles used in the Persian Gulf War were equipped only with conventional warheads, the threat of CBW was a chronic stressor. The terror and fear of chemical and biological weapons caused panic that resulted in psychological stress casualties. After a SCUD missile explosion in Tel Aviv, Israel, 60 individuals sought emergency care, thinking they had been exposed to chemical and biological warfare agents. No exposure had occurred, but the terror of these weapons had led them to an erroneous belief. Bleich and colleagues (1992) examined 773 individuals taken to the emergency room at 12 Israeli hospitals following the SCUD missile attacks. Forty-three percent were diagnosed as psychological casualties. Twenty-seven percent had mistakenly injected themselves with atropine. We can expect that when CBW is actually used, the numbers of stress casualties will be high.

Chemical and biological weapons have profound effects as agents of terror. Although the tools used to terrorize vary, their effects are similar. Terrorism disrupts common beliefs and habits; safety, security, and predictability are destroyed, and uncertainty and fear emerge in their stead. Chemical and biological weapons are especially well suited to be agents of terror: no sight, smell, or sound effectively defines their presence. Thus, the entire environment becomes potentially life threatening, and individuals' physical and emotional energies are taxed by constant vigilance and apprehension in this state of continuous threat.

The psychological trauma of chemical weapons is based on their capacity to contaminate and insidiously destroy an individual's sense of security and trust in the environment (Fullerton and Ursano 1990). Behavioral and psychological responses to

CBW can put individuals and groups at increased risk. The stress of CBW is compounded by wearing protective gear and living and working in protective shelters. In the CBW environment, running while in protective gear, removing a protective mask, experiencing panic while in the confines of a chemical protection shelter or interpersonal withdrawal—all can increase the individual's chance of becoming a casualty (Fullerton and Ursano 1990).

To better understand the psychological mechanisms associated with CBW and the resulting acute and chronic stress reactions, we examine in this chapter 1) the history of CBW, 2) the biological mechanisms of action in toxic agents, 3) the psychological responses to CBW, 4) protection in CBW, and 5) issues in modern-day CBW (i.e., the Persian Gulf War, medical care in CBW, and chemical stockpiles).

History of Chemical and Biological Warfare

The Hague Convention

The Hague Convention, an international meeting convened in 1899 to limit the horrors of war, was an important marker in the history of CBW (for review of CBW history, see Joy 1988). Although chemical and biological weapons (or in the vernacular of the time, poison gases) were not new, the controversial moral questions about CBW had not been raised in an official forum before The Hague Convention. Were shells with asphyxiating gases inhumane or unnecessarily cruel? The Hague agreement to outlaw chemical warfare was superseded as World War I became the testing ground for gas as a weapon of war and the development of effective protection. The Hague Convention became a worldwide symbol for the moral dilemma posed by CBW. Much of this controversy, far from being settled at The Hague Convention, has continued to this day.

World War I

Chemical and biological warfare in World War I began with the German introduction of portable flamethrowers (see Joy 1988). However, there were a number of problems with flamethrowers: they only lasted a minute or two, had a tendency to blow up and kill the operator, and were easy to combat by shooting the operator.

In warfare, the goal of chemical and biological weapons is to degrade the enemy unit's effectiveness, deny territory, and decrease command and control. Historically, military units have been fairly resistant to these effects. Complete breakdown of units only occurred twice in World War I. In April 1915, two elite French Divisions panicked and became disorganized after being attacked with chlorine gas. The Germans released approximately 150 tons of chlorine from 6,000 cylinders. They achieved immediate tactical success. They hit 15,000 troops, leaving approximately 800 soldiers dead and another 3,000 incapacitated. Although the German military command was not ready for follow-up and did not trust the weapon, this marked the beginning of the race between weapon protection and development.

By September 1915, the British were moving chlorine cylinders to the front lines. The Levin Projector, a weapon that could throw shells or bombs, was used to propel cylinders containing 1.5 gallons of either chlorine or phosgene. The Germans introduced smoke mixed with gas to make an impending heavy attack look lighter; then, when the opposition could not clearly gauge the extent of the attack, a heavy attack was launched. In January 1917, the Germans activated the last chemical attack against the French, near the village of Persons in the Champagne sector. The gas (chlorine mixed with either phosgene or chloropicrin and with smoke) was released in high concentrations. It spread to the back of the combat line, where the soldiers were without protection.

In April 1917, the United States entered the war relatively unprepared for CBW. At that time, the U.S. had no established principles for implementation of and defense against CBW;

troops were not trained and were without chemical protective equipment. As a result, the U.S. Bureau of Mines initiated research and development, primarily at universities, on chemical agents. A leading scientist, Yandall Henderson of Yale University, internationally known for his work in respiratory physiology, became the principal consultant to the medical aspects of the program. The Signal Corps was tasked with making the gas alarms, the Ordnance Corps with making the weapons and ammunition, and the Corps of Engineers with providing troops with the chemical weapons and training them in their use. The Army Medical Department was directed to manufacture protective equipment and to provide troops with training in their use. The Medical Department performed physiological studies on the energy costs and pulmonary function of people wearing masks. They also conducted controlled gas exposure studies by exposing volunteers to gas and then testing the efficacy of various masks.

Dichlorethyl sulfide (mustard gas) was introduced in the summer of 1917 and marked a new era in chemical warfare. Mustard gas had the ability to penetrate ordinary fabric and leather and attack the entire skin surface. In addition, mustard gas was persistent. Burns and temporary blindness occurred in large numbers. Mustard gas could remove large numbers of troops from the lines as short-term casualties. If inhaled, mustard gas could be lethal. In July, the Germans used mustard gas against British troops at Ypres. Delivered by artillery shells, the mustard attack resulted in 20,000 casualties. The troops were often unaware they had been gassed until an hour after the attack, when there was marked inflammation of their eyes (Gilchrist 1928; Gilchrist and Matz 1933). The mustard gas caused severe vomiting and erythema of the skin. (The first cases were diagnosed as scarlet fever.) Later, casualties suffered severe blistering of the skin, especially where the uniform had been contaminated. Upon arrival at the clearing stations, the gassed men were virtually blind and were led by an orderly in a line with each man holding on to the one in front.

By late 1917, the chemical attacks delivered by cylinder were replaced by shell attacks called "gas surprise fire." The Germans used phosgene or similar agents in green-cross shells. First, they fired nonlethal blue-cross shells containing arsenic compounds to force the opposition to remove their gas masks (the removal of the masks prompted by the tearing and discomfort caused by the shells). The green-cross shells were then fired on the unprotected soldiers. By 1918, approximately 25% of all artillery fire was made up of chemical rounds. These new weapons were produced in the thousands of tons by both sides. For good or for ill, this new weapon had come to stay.

In World War I, the United States had about 250,000 casualties (for review, see Joy 1988). Of those, 13% were killed in action, and 87% were wounded. Approximately 225,000 soldiers needed medical care, and of those, 30% were gas casualties. Gas is an effective weapon—it wounds but does not kill. Mustard gas was the most effective. The British suffered approximately 20,000 casualties from lung irritants and about 160,000 from mustard gas. From a logistics, personnel, and engineering support perspective, days lost per case because of hospitalization constitute an enormous burden on the command. Again, gas proved to be an effective weapon. It disables by imposing a major logistic and medical burden, but it does not primarily kill. Approximately 95% of the people wounded by chemicals survived. The death rate was around 4%. In the Russian Army it was somewhat higher (about 11%) because they were late in producing even very primitive masks. Interestingly, this general low lethality and high morbidity rate in World War I led many people to see the chemical weapon as holding great promise for the future of war.

The U.S. military paid attention to CBW agents and trained its troops in the interwar years in both simulated and real chemical environments. After the war ended, work at the Edgewood Medical Research Laboratories in the U.S. continued (Vedder 1925). New gas masks were developed. Masks for the U.S. Navy had high eyepoint lenses so that naval officers could use binoculars. Researchers also experimented with masks with speaker diaphragms, because it was difficult to hear through a mask. Early on, the people at Edgewood developed oilcloth and rubber uniforms for protection from mustard gas (Vedder 1925). Later, they developed resin and chloramide uniforms. Smoke and gas delivery systems were added to weapons such as the tank and the airplane.

World War II

During World War II, the use of chemical agents was minimal (for review, see Joy 1988). Chemical attacks were successful in two major unprotected populations during World War II (i.e., the Italians and the Japanese used these weapons against the Ethiopians and the Chinese, respectively). Hitler was not in favor of chemical and biological weapons because of his personal experience in the trenches in World War I and the mistaken belief that the Allies had the capability to make nerve agents. This belief, however, kept the Germans from using their vastly superior capability. In the initial hours of the invasion at Normandy, there was panic and fear that the Germans would use chemical weapons to defend the beachheads.

Edward Vedder (1925) was in charge of the medical laboratory at Edgewood at the time. His group produced new mask cannisters that could filter smoke as well as the standard respiratory agents. They reported clinical cases and animal work on the agents as well as experimental work in humans and attempts at new treatment. In 1925, he published a superb text that contained excellent data on the pathology and physiology of the various chemical agents (particularly mustard gas) and on the time course of the lesions. Although the book has largely been forgotten, much of it is germane today. On the front inside cover of the book is a picture of a soldier horribly wounded by shrapnel. Vedder argued that if this is the result of a humane weapon, then the chemical weapons, by comparison, are much more humane. Again, we see the theme expressed by some at that time that gas is more humane than bullets.

The Bari disaster, a disaster involving a cargo of gas that occurred in 1943 in Bari, Italy, heightened awareness of the

dangers of mustard gas (D. M. Saunders, unpublished manuscript, 1994). The USS *John Harvey,* an American ship in the
harbor, had a highly classified load of 2,000 100-pound mustard
bombs. When the Germans hit the Bari harbor in a surprise
bombing raid, fire on the USS *John Harvey* caused a mustard-
laden smoke that spread into the city, producing eye inflammation, choking, pulmonary signs and symptoms, and burns. The
mustard gas mixed with the oil from the damaged tankers and
rapidly spread throughout the Bari harbor. In the chaos that followed the raid, no one "remembered" that the USS *John Harvey*
had such a deadly cargo. The garlic smell of mustard was
masked by oil, gas, and smoke fumes. Many men who were covered in mustard-contaminated oil were left wrapped in blan-
kets for 12 to 24 hours. They later developed severe burns,
particularly of the eyes. The most severe cases had swallowed
the oil-mustard mixture and developed severe internal (gastrointestinal tract) burns. The first mustard death occurred just
hours after the raid. Of the 617 known mustard casualties, approximately 83 died.

Biology of Chemical and Biological Weapons

> *Toxin* is the Greek word for bow. Historically, arrow
> wounds became septic. With no germ theory at hand, the
> bow and arrow were viewed as poisons since poisons were
> understood. Thus, the bow and arrow became a poisoning
> weapon. (Joy 1988)

Toxic Agents and Their Mechanisms of Action

Nerve gases, although chemically related to some pesticides,
are far more toxic and act much faster. Nerve gases can enter
the body both through the lungs or by absorption through the
skin. Lethal doses of nerve gases can be as little as 0.4 to 1 mg,
with exposures by respiratory inhalation and skin absorption

(Meselson and Robinson 1980). Nerve gases poison through binding acetylcholinesterase, an enzyme necessary in the metabolism of the neurotransmitter acetylcholine. After this enzyme is inactivated, the neurotransmitter quickly increases, giving cholinergic effects: muscle tension, perspiration, diarrhea, hyperventillation, shaking and tremors, irritability, urination, and pounding heart (Martin and Manning 1990). These symptoms are difficult to distinguish from expected physiological responses to combat. A sufficient dose of nerve agent, if it goes unchecked, quickly leads to exhaustion of the muscles, then paralysis, and finally death from asphyxiation. Long-term neurological and psychiatric disorders can develop after high levels of exposure.

When nerve gases are used on the battlefield, soldiers can self-administer antidotes; however, the antidotes themselves are potentially debilitating if used incorrectly. Soldiers are instructed about the signs and symptoms of early chemical exposure to nerve agents and told to take the antidote at the onset of these symptoms. However, these symptoms are virtually indistinguishable, even by a physician, from the normal psychophysiological responses to combat. In addition, they are also difficult to distinguish from the early signs and symptoms of heat stress, which one would expect to be present in a large percentage of troops who are dressed in mission oriented protective posture (MOPP) suits.

Sarin and soman were first produced in Germany in 1938 and 1944, respectively. The modern-day chemical weapons of war are often nerve gases. There are three main nerve agents: GB, or sarin; GD, or soman; and VX. Biological agents such as anthrax spores and botulina toxin are somewhat less toxic than nerve agents. They are more frightening in other ways. These agents are undetectable until an epidemic of unusual illness presents. The agents may persist in the environment for years. The anthrax spore can be aerosolized, infect the lungs, and lead to an overwhelming pneumonia and death. Because of the thick glucopolysaccharide coat on this bacterium, white blood cells cannot recognize the bacterium to effectively fight off an infection. In addition, it is difficult to create an adequate vaccination to this coating on the bacterium. Exposure to the botulina toxin can result in flaccid paralysis and death.

Mustard Gas

Mustard gas was introduced in the summer of 1917 and was the first agent to be used in artillery shells. This gas has a mechanism of action far superior to those of the poison gases in use at that time. Mustard gas is a persistent agent and has remained active up to 30 years in concrete. Mustard gas has effects at a low dose and is not very noticeable. In addition to being a lung agent, it is a potent skin agent. Mustard gas is heavier than air and therefore settles on the ground and remains dangerous for days and even weeks. The effect is analogous to that of land mines. Mustard is toxic through direct contact, causing chemical burns to the skin. It penetrates regular clothing and attacks the skin. It is lipid soluble and is 80% to 90% absorbed through the skin, resulting in systemic toxicity (Heully and Gruninger 1956). Mustard is even more lethal when inhaled, causing severe chemical burns to the lungs.

In World War I, mustard gas made everyday living for the soldier in a combat zone extremely difficult. Areas previously safe were no longer so. The air the soldier breathed and the objects he touched became potential weapons. How could he know when his area was contaminated? How could a soldier eat, drink, sleep, perform bodily functions, use his weapon, or give and receive commands when such uncertainty existed?

Medically, the volatility and low-dose capability of mustard gas required the medics to segregate the mustard patients and establish specialized evacuation systems and equipment. Such specialized systems were necessary because mustard gas contaminated everything it came in contact with. Skin burns were treated in a variety of ways. First, the patients were washed down by corpsmen who themselves wore protective clothing. The burns were initially treated with grease, which only enhanced infection. Later, sodium hypochlorate was used as a constantly running solution and was also administered by soaking the skin. Patients who died from mustard gas inhalation showed gross destruction of the tracheobronchial tree. These lesions were much worse to treat than those induced by phosgene or chlorine. In terms of eye problems, acute conjunctivitis was induced by mustard gas. Immediate eye irrigation was the treatment. Most of the eye cases cleared up in several weeks. During the resolution stage of mustard-related acute conjunctivitis, patients were photophobic for a considerable period.

Psychology of Chemical and Biological Weapons

Expecting the Unexpected: A Project to Study the Psychological Effects of Chemical and Biological Warfare

> When he heard the drums beat at Waterloo in 1915, Sir Charles Bell, a surgeon, thought to himself with fearful expectation, that the nature of the wounds of those who may be brought to him should have occupied his mind earlier. (Joy 1988)

Several years before the Persian Gulf War, a project to examine the behavioral and psychological responses to CBW was undertaken (Ursano and Fullerton 1988a, 1988b, 1988c, 1988d, 1988e, 1988f). In the mid-1980s, a multidisciplinary group of national and international scientists, brought together by Ursano and colleagues, was formed to investigate the psychological, behavioral, cognitive, and physiological responses to the CBW environment. Up to that time, the psychological and behavioral aspects of CBW had not been well conceptualized. The group took an innovative approach to learning about a stressful environment that is hard to study. They examined analogous environments that share some of the characteristics of the CBW environment (e.g., toxic contaminations, contained environments, and isolated group and individual functioning). This work underscores the value of looking across high-stress situations to add to our knowledge of human behavior in extreme environments. Such events include naturally occurring and human-made conditions characterized by the presence of high stress, which are not reproducible in the laboratory. These conditions are present in natural disasters, man-made disasters, accidents, and prisoner-of-war and hostage situations, as well as other experiences such as military training exercises.

Ursano and colleagues held a series of scientific meetings. Experts from around the world presented historical and current research and discussed the human factors involved in a world that must plan ahead for the possibility of CBW. The group examined a broad range of stressors (e.g., handling of dead bodies, coping with isolation and deprivation, the fear and restricted life of prisoners of war and hostages). The findings and implications of these investigations (see Ursano and Fullerton 1988a, 1988b, 1988c, 1988d, 1988e, 1988f) have application to the broad spectrum of research on human behavior in high-stress environments and the complex interface among personality, stress, and environmental factors.

Toxins and Terror

> Stories that use terror to frighten often show nothing that is actually grotesque. Rather, each person is invited to recall their most frightening fantasy and to relive their worst nightmare. (Stephen King 1981)

Those who have experienced a trauma or disaster are familiar with terror—in themselves, in their family and friends, in rescue workers, or even in the community at large, as after Chernobyl (Fullerton 1988), the San Francisco and Armenian earthquakes,

Hurricanes Hugo and Andrew, and the recent devastating floods in the U.S. Midwest. Breslau and Davis (1991) estimated the lifetime prevalence of exposure to traumatic events as 39.1% in a random sample of 1,007 young adults from a large health maintenance organization in Detroit, Michigan. Norris (1992) estimated that 6% to 7% of the U.S. population are exposed to a disaster or trauma each year—ranging from motor vehicle accidents and crime to hurricanes and tornados. In a representative sample of women over the age of 18 in the U.S., Kilpatrick and Resnick (1993) found that 68.9% had been exposed to a traumatic event sometime in their life.

To understand the psychological responses to and recovery from trauma agents, of which CBW is one, it is important to understand the terror response (Holloway and Fullerton 1994). The role of terror can be seen in everyday life through our literature and films. Horror films threaten our view that the world is safe but nonetheless reassure us of conventional outcomes. Many individuals voluntarily expose themselves to terror by going to horror movies and reading terrifying novels. They often achieve a sense of mastery and control by watching films of terror (Terr 1989). Vicarious exposure to terror may help us deny actual terrors—we can watch a horror movie from a distance and not be destroyed. According to Terr (1989), the fear is loss of control; knowing is controlling. The imagination creates its own terrifying fantasy. Stephen King (1981) divides tales of terror into two groups: those that result from an intended act or conscious decision to do evil, and those that are caused by nature, for example, a lightning strike. It is interesting to note that actual traumatic events can be divided into the same two groups: human-induced trauma such as terrorism and rape, and natural disasters such as floods and earthquakes.

Recently, the world was reminded that terror is also induced in both individuals and groups by weapons, such as those used in CBW. These weapons cause shock, horror, helplessness, and panic. As mentioned earlier, 60 individuals in Tel Aviv sought emergency care after a SCUD missile explosion, thinking they had been exposed to chemical and biological warfare agents.

Soldiers in Saudi Arabia reportedly slept in their protective masks and gear for both protection and psychological comfort. The psychological trauma of chemical and biological weapons is based on these agents' capacity to induce terror, to contaminate and insidiously destroy an individual's sense of security and trust in the environment (Fullerton and Ursano 1990). CBW increases the risk of behavioral and psychological disturbances in combat (Fullerton and Ursano 1988, 1990; Newhouse 1987; Rundell et al. 1989; Ursano and Fullerton 1988a, 1988b, 1988c, 1988d, 1988e, 1988f).

People respond to the unknown with fear. Panic may be induced by trying to deal with a situation for which one is untrained, unprepared, and unprotected. Chemical and biological weapons are regarded as inherently insidious and, therefore, terror inducing. There have been instances of wars in which dead corpses full of plague were thrown over city walls because they frightened people (Joy 1988). Some of the terror of CBW is the result of the uncanny, seemingly new and unnatural characteristics of killing and incapacitating without damaging. In World War I, lethal gas was new, so there was the fear of the unknown as well as the panic of a situation that one is not trained or prepared for or protected from. CBW can be invisible or almost invisible and can have delayed effects that show up hours or even days later. The anticipation of CBW attack can result in performance degradation, psychologically induced physical symptoms, and reporting to a medical station.

One of the most significant features of CBW is surprise. Although this is not new or unique to CBW, surprise is important in any military conflict. However, it plays a particularly important role in CBW. Unlike conventional weapons of war, CBW agents do not destroy or blow up buildings; nor do they leave mutilated, grotesquely torn apart, bloody victims. Their mechanism is to create the chronic stress of uncertainty and surprise and of the burden of operating in protective gear (see below). Chemical and biological weapons kill and incapacitate without disrupting the terrain or destroying structures, as does conventional warfare. They persist in the environment, continuing to kill and incapacitate, and thus deny certain areas and positions to the enemy and make the entire field of combat feel unsafe, with no haven for rest and respite.

The Burden of Protection

To know how a gas mask feels, it has been said that all one needs to do is to seize one's nose with a pair of fire tongs, bury his/her face in a hot feather pillow, take a gas pipe between the teeth and breathe through it while performing routine functions. It may be safe, but it is not sane! (Joy 1988)

The first protective mask was developed by the Germans. It was made of leather and had pads inside soaked in bicarbonate and sodium hypochlorate with some charcoal layers. The French developed a form-fitting Tissot mask that was similar to the German mask. The early American mask was designed with a nose clip and an internal mouthpiece. The English began by using veil respirators. To use these masks, soldiers would put a gauze over their mouth and then wrap the veil around to hold it in place. The English rapidly moved to a flannel hood in which the whole flannel bag was soaked in glycerin and hydrochloride and then donned over the head. Horses were the prime movers in World War I and also had to be protected from chemicals. Artillerymen, quartermasters, and transport people were directed to mask their horses before masking themselves.

In 1916, the British developed a box respirator with a hose to connect the mask to a canister of protective chemicals and filters. The Germans developed respirators with the canister in front on the mask. Soldiers carried the unit in a can on their belt.

The protective suits, used in conjunction with the mask respirators, greatly hampered performance. The chemical protective gear was difficult to don and wear, causing people to tire quickly and experience heat stress. As a result of the difficulties with the protective devices, protection was not always in place. Thus, the element of surprise became crucial.

A wide range of methods of delivery were tried during World War I in efforts to surprise the enemy with something new and for which they were unprepared. Attack in the dark became best for a surprise attack. In 1916, the Germans employed a random attack pattern to catch the enemy without respirators. By 1918, the properly worn masks were very effective and were approximately 99% efficient. If one had on this type of mask, it worked. The biggest problem was vision. In fact, there are many accounts of artillerymen taking the mask off because they could not read the gunsight.

Current empirical and observational studies indicate that when chemical protective gear is worn, performance is seriously degraded by a number of factors, including psychological responses, heat stress, manual dexterity problems, and communication difficulty (for review, see Taylor and Orlansky 1993). Findings suggest that training in protective clothing decreases difficulties if heat stress is not a factor. Communication and even recognition of others in the group while wearing the protective mask are difficult and sometimes seem not worth the effort unless absolutely necessary, resulting in withdrawal and isolation (Fullerton and Ursano 1990; Taylor and Orlansky 1993). The suits induce considerable heat stress, reduce dexterity, restrict respiration, and limit communication, thereby diminishing the effectiveness of military units.

Modern chemical protective gear works well against nerve agents. However, this gear can be overcome with very high concentrations. Wearing a mask in a high-concentration chemical environment for a long period causes the absorbent surface to become saturated. Chemical protective gear is still difficult to don and wear. During the Persian Gulf War, the Iraqis used the threat of chemical weapons against the Israeli civilian population. Difficulty with the masks increased the anxiety and had serious health consequences (e.g., an increase in the rates of myocardial infarction during the missile attacks) (Hiss and Arensburg 1992).

Modern-Day Chemical and Biological Warfare

The Persian Gulf War

Although biochemical warfare is not known to have been used during the Persian Gulf War, some small areas of contamination have been reported by other countries, presumably because of leakage or wreckage of Iraqi armament. The Iraqis had used chemical weapons frequently and effectively in the 8-year Iran-Iraq War. Chemical weapons, particularly mustard gas, were a standard part of the Iraqi doctrine of war.

Exposure to mass casualties can be expected in CBW. Fortunately, this was not the case in Operation Desert Storm. However, anticipation in and of itself is a source of stress. McCarroll and colleagues (1993a, 1993b; Ursano and McCarroll 1994) examined the anticipated stress of working with the dead of Operation Desert Storm. McCarroll et al. (1993b) studied 386 individuals who would handle remains (mortuary workers) and 87 who would perform tasks other than working with the remains. The mortuary workers reported higher levels of distress than the others. Interestingly, the nonvolunteer mortuary workers had higher levels of distress than did the volunteers. Experienced mortuary workers reported fewer intrusive and avoidant symptoms than did the inexperienced workers. Those at highest risk for distress were the inexperienced nonvolunteer mortuary workers. The study has important implications for the selection, training, and supervision of, and the need for aftercare of, those individuals anticipating working with the dead. Further, those who recovered war dead during Operation Desert Storm reported greater intrusive and avoidant symptoms than those who did not (McCarroll et al. 1993a). If there had been mass casualties as a result of CBW, these symptoms would have been much more pervasive.

Fear of CBW was prominent in troops immediately before the beginning of hostilities. Vaitkus and Martin (1992) surveyed

1,400 ground troops in the days before the January 15th deadline for Saddam Hussein to withdraw from Kuwait. In addition to assessing anxiety among these troops, the investigators inquired about what the soldiers perceived to be most stressful. Fear of Iraqi use of chemical and biological weapons was the highest rated of all stressors, even higher than the fear of having a buddy killed.

Aboard the USNS *Comfort,* the hospital ship deployed to the Persian Gulf, the anxious uneasiness associated with training in gas masks was observed. The crew feared that Iraqi stores of anthrax spores could be aerosolized by agricultural sprayers mounted on small boats and sprayed onto their ship. There was not an adequate supply of antibiotics for prophylaxes aboard. The spores were rumored to be able to kill all inhabitants of the ship and make it uninhabitable for decades (Dinneen et al. 1994).

The Iraqis used the threat of chemical agents against the Israeli civilian population in the Persian Gulf War. The SCUD missile attacks had a dramatic terrorizing effect on the civilian population. Fear and a heightened state of arousal were prominent in this population. We all can recall the images of panic-stricken television news journalists rushing to put on gas masks while describing the SCUD missles streaking toward them. The calm of the night was shattered by the shrill pitch of sirens. Although the SCUD missiles carried conventional warheads, there was the ongoing threat of chemical attack.

Data collected from the emergency rooms of 12 Israeli hospitals and the Medical Corps of the Israel Defense Forces after each SCUD missile attack indicated that 43% of the 773 casualties evacuated to hospitals were psychological casualties (Bleich et al. 1992). Twenty-seven percent of the total casualties had mistakenly injected themselves with atropine. There was also an increase in death from suffocations and myocardial infarction (Bleich et al. 1992; Hiss and Arensburg 1992). The gas masks distributed to the Israeli population had two component parts: the mask itself and a filter canister. The canister was attached to the mask at the time of use. The canister was sealed with a plastic plug. If the mask was put on before the canister was "un-plugged," air could not flow. This error, brought on by fear, led to several individuals being suffocated (Hiss and Arensburg 1992). The added stress of anxiety may explain the increase in rates of myocardial infarction during the missile attacks.

After return home from the Persian Gulf War, approximately 60 to 79 soldiers from the 123rd ARCOM complained of symptoms and problems they felt might have been related to their deployment during Operation Desert Storm (DeFraites et al. 1992). The symptoms included fatigue, intestinal pains, headache, joint pain, eye sensitivity to light, unexplained fever, ache in the gums or teeth, repeated unexplained memory loss, sweats, anxious distrust, disorientation, rash, cough, phobia, anger and mood swings, and insomnia and nightmares. The common beliefs about the cause of the symptoms were exposure to radiation (both microwave and nuclear), toxins (from pesticide-laced fish, SCUD fragments, petrochemical residuals, etc.), biological agents (anthrax vaccine or whatever substance[s] was administered to them through the immunization process), and endemic disease (e.g., leishmaniasis). Concerns were also raised by the soldiers about whether during their deployment they may have been exposed to something from which they might become ill in the future (e.g., long latency for virus, malignancy) or that might be passed along to their offspring (Agent Orange and human immunodeficiency virus were mentioned as examples). None of the soldiers had sustained battle-related injuries.

The fears of contamination from CBW or other toxins continue today. Beginning with the group of soldiers in Indiana (see DeFraites et al. 1992), the fear of occult contamination in the war has grown to now include thousands of individuals who have contacted the Veterans Administration (VA). Although the underlying cause(s) of these symptoms is unknown, they are unlikely to represent posttraumatic stress disorder. However, the large number of people who have contacted the VA reflects, in part, the powerful effects of fear of contamination and toxic exposure.

Medical Care

Little is known about the psychological effects of providing medical care in the CBW environment. Knowledge of the predictors of vulnerability and of the mediators of the stress of CBW has important implications for health care delivery in CBW. Medical care must be given in a confined chemically protected shelter such as the Survivable Collective Protection System—Medical (SCPS-M). The chemical protective gear limits one's ability to obtain information about a casualty's injury, slowing triage of casualties and the delivery of emergency care (Xenakis et al. 1985). Communications among staff, between staff and patients, and with the outside world become laborious and difficult. Feelings of isolation are common because communication is limited. This can often affect the level of perceived support. Social supports are important buffers of war stress (Solomon et al. 1986, 1987), particularly through effects on group cohesion (Spiegel 1944).

In a preliminary investigation of a health care delivery team in a simulated CBW environment (Fullerton and Ursano 1988, 1990, 1994; Fullerton et al. 1992; Ursano and Fullerton 1990), simulated casualties ("patients") were processed through the decontamination and medical care procedures in a protected shelter (SCPS-M) used for the delivery of medical care in the CBW environment. The study examined the best predictors of 1) psychological symptoms after the exercise (depression, anxiety, and global symptoms), 2) perceived social support (cohesion) during the exercise, 3) fatigue during the exercise, and 4) active training (Table 5–1). The major findings of this portion of the study can be summarized as follows:

1. Anticipatory stress (i.e., pre-exercise anxiety) made a substantial contribution to psychological outcome. Lower state anxiety before the exercise predicted less depression and less global psychological symptomatology postexercise. State anxiety explained 8% of the variance in depression and 21% of the variance in global psychological symptomatology.

Table 5–1.   Important predictors of psychological responses to the chemical and biological warfare environment

Anticipatory anxiety

Perceived social support from family

Perceived social support during experiences that involve high levels of stress

Active training

Fatigue

2. Perceived social support predicted both depression and anxiety after the exercise. Higher perceived social support from family predicted lower depression (4% of the variance); higher perceived social support from friends predicted lower anxiety. It is important to recall that during war, including the Persian Gulf War, the availability of mail, telephones, newspapers, and television influences the perception of friend and family support (Dinneen et al. 1994). The effect of information both as a stressor and as a stress buffer may have operated in part through the alteration of perceived social supports.

3. Individuals with greater active training reported less anxiety postexercise. Active training is an important component of preparation for military and rescue groups involved in high-stress environments. Stress inoculation, confidence in one's own performance, and increased skills in social relatedness during high-stress events are control components of active training, in contrast to the cognitive knowledge learned in seminars and lectures. Greater active training and greater perceived social support from friends at baseline also predicted higher social support during the exercise, a measure of unit cohesion. Active training, rather than passive training (e.g., watching videotapes, classes, reading), was a better predictor of perceived social supports during the exercise. Active training, in contrast to passive training, may directly increase interpersonal contact among the group as well as foster greater levels of task-

specific confidence and self-esteem, both of which may also contribute to the formation of social supports.

4. Lower reported social support during the exercise was correlated with higher anxiety before the exercise, although state anxiety was an insignificant predictor when other variables were considered in the stepwise regression analysis. Whether those who are more anxious are less likely to seek support or are less likely to be offered help (or to recognize it) is unclear. Highly anxious individuals may be at increased risk in high-stress environments both because of their anxiety and because of the effects of that anxiety on social support during the event.

5. Fatigue is often described by those in combat and in other disaster environments as having a substantial effect on performance and psychological health. It can be modified by rest and respite. Our fatigue measure had been used in studies of other high-stress environments and was correlated with performance demands (Harris et al. 1971; Hartman et al. 1974; Storm and Gray 1978). The multiple regression analyses indicated that 36% of the variance in fatigue could be explained by perceived social support during the exercise (22%) and perceived social support from family (14%). Interestingly, individuals reporting high social support during the exercise were less fatigued, whereas those reporting high family social support were more fatigued. Perceived social supports during the exercise may have been related to instrumental support received during the exercise that could decrease physical exertion. The relationship between family support and fatigue, however, is counterintuitive. Fatigue was measured at the end of the exercise, before individuals were to return home. Our fatigue measure may have identified a general "nostalgia" or homesickness. Alternatively, those with high family support may have been in poorer physical condition and therefore more fatigued. This seems unlikely, however, because all participants were generally subject to the same height and weight standards and aerobic testing.

Understanding how health care teams respond to the CBW environment and other high-stress environments is important in improving care for individuals and groups exposed to such trauma. (See Table 5–2 for summary of behavioral and psychological responses during CBW exercises.) Overall, the exploratory study whose findings were described above identified state anxiety, perceived social support from family and friends, and active training as predictors of psychological outcome, even after trait and pre-exercise psychological variables had been considered. These variables are important because interventions directed at them may improve psychological health in a CBW environment.

In another part of this study, behavioral responses that might have indicated health or performance problems were identified. Behavioral and psychological casualties were defined as those individuals exhibiting responses that indicated psychiatric disease or disrupted performance, or whose behavior placed the individual or group at increased risk, such as breaking the protection requirements that in a real CBW environment would lead to potential contamination and death. We observed 14 cases of such behavioral and psychological casualties involving a total of 18 individuals: 3 staff and 15 patients (Table 5–3). Cases 1 to 13 each involved 1 individual, and case 14 involved 5 individuals.

These behavioral and psychological casualties involved claustrophobia, difficulty with the protective mask, overheating, feelings related to having failed, overdedication to the group, alcohol use, failure to recognize danger, and anxiety. The most common responses were claustrophobia (cases 6–10, 11, 13), difficulty with the protective mask (cases 3, 6–10), and overheating (cases 1, 3, 5, 11). These difficulties were all the result of performing in the chemical protective gear within the protective shelter. Clearly, individuals and leaders must be alert to the warning signs of overheating and intervene immediately. Proper hydration maintained on timed schedules can help reduce this risk and decrease dependence on the individual's subjective assessment. Overdedication to the group (cases 1, 3, 14–18) may

Table 5–2.   Behavioral and psychological responses during chemical and biological warfare (CBW) training exercises

1. Overall, state anxiety, perceived social support from family and friends, and active training stand out as predictors of psychological outcome, even after trait and pre-exercise psychological variables are considered.
2. Understanding the mechanisms of social support during high-stress events is important in designing programs for fostering disaster-specific social supports.
3. Fatigue is an important measure of overall performance in long-duration combat and disaster events and potentially a predictor of psychological outcome.
4. Understanding how health care teams respond to the CBW environment and other high-stress environments is important to improvement of care for individuals and groups exposed to such trauma. Interventions directed at state anxiety and active training may offer mechanisms to decrease the psychological distress of the high-stress environment.
5. Claustrophobia is common in the confines of the protective mask and chemical shelter and may result in panic responses.
6. Protective masks present problems, among which are difficulty in breathing, hyperventilation, fatigue, sweating, claustrophobia, and, potentially, malfunctioning of the drinking apparatus. These problems may result in panic and removal of masks, especially in patients who are waiting for medical treatment.
7. Overheating is common when one is working in the protective gear within the chemical shelter. Individuals and commanders must be alert to the warning signs of overheating and intervene immediately.
8. Feelings of having failed, including embarrassment, disappointment, and anger, are expectable in the high-stress CBW environment. These feelings may interfere with the accurate assessment of physical or emotional limitations and may be expressed through anger and annoyance at leaders.
9. Overdedication to the group may interfere with an individual's or supervisor's accurate assessment of physical limitations.
10. Group behaviors can arise that adversely affect performance in the CBW environment (e.g., when one member could not access fluid, all refused fluid).
11. The use of alcohol is of substantial concern in the CBW environment because of the risk of dehydration.
12. Failure to recognize the danger of certain behaviors can result in contamination in the CBW environment.

Table 5–3.   Behavioral and psychological responses during chemical and biological warfare exercises

Response	n	Case number(s)[a]	Subject role
Claustrophobia	7	6–10	Patients
		11	Patient
		13	Patient
Difficulty with mask	6	3	Staff
		6–10	Patients
Overheating	4	1	Staff
		3	Staff
		5	Patient
		11	Patient
Feelings of failure	4	4	Patient
		5	Patient
		11	Patient
		13	Patient
Overdedication to the group	7	1	Staff
		3	Staff
		14–18	Patients
Dehydration and overheating secondary to alcohol use	2	1	Staff
		5	Patient
Failure to recognize danger	1	2	Staff

Source.   Fullerton and Ursano 1994.
[a]Some cases appear in more than one response category.

interfere with the recognition of physical limits, causing inaccurate assessment of one's physiological limits and/or denial of individual limitations.

Chemical Stockpile: How Safe Is Safe?

The Geneva Protocol of 1925 prohibited the use of poison gas and other chemical weapons in war. Some nations accepted the agreement as absolute. Others viewed it as a no-first-use agreement, having formally reserved the right to retaliate if the protocol was violated. As a result, nations stockpiled chemical weapons in defense of CBW. Chemical agents are thought to be stable for years and, if stored properly, can remain toxic for years. Media articles and reports about poison gas stockpiles, often targeting issues of safety, continue to evoke concerns and in some cases terror and fear in civilian populations. Questions about accidental contamination remain at the center of much of the current controversy.

Congress ordered the destruction of all existing U.S. stockpiles of poison gas weapons by 1997. However, individual states can outlaw burning in the state, forcing the transportation of the weapons to other sites from the eight current sites. The risk may be increased because of difficulties moving old munitions, which may be deteriorating and may not be stable. The affected states opposed the railroad shipment of munitions. The problem remains unanswered.

Safe disposal of poison gases is problematic (for a review, see Smith 1989). Ocean dumping was used after World War II by Britain and in the 1970s by the United States. Such dumping is now prohibited. Chemical neutralization was used to destroy more than 20,000 chemical bombs in the mid-1970s in Colorado. However, this method takes a great deal of time and does not eliminate all the poison. It also results in 2 pounds of hazardous waste per pound of nerve agent. Incineration was tested by the U.S. Army in 1988 near Salt Lake City, Utah. Although this method was reported to be safe after 8 years of testing and after construction and use of a $67 million facility, the controversy continues (Smith 1989). On occasion, aberrant ideas for the disposal of chemical agents (e.g., radiation, nuclear blasts, dumping munitions into active volcanoes) have sparked debate and created intense opposition.

Isolated incidents of the discovery of buried toxic munitions have caused fear and apprehension. On March 9, 1956, the discovery of an old mustard shell by children playing in a field resulted in a disaster that spread to those who helped the children. Three children were playing with an old artillery shell in the woods near Verdan, France. The shell exploded, giving only light fragmentation wounds to the children. The two children nearest the explosion were dowsed with a clear, slightly yellowish substance that was difficult to discern from the blood, oil, earth, and tar covering the children. These two children died 3 and 4 hours after their exposure with a frothy pulmonary edema and burns all over their bodies. The third child did not catch the full explosion. She had a difficult course over the next 10 days, with altered mental status, pulmonary compromise with a purulent bronchitis, and burns. She was treated supportively with fluids and antibiotics and recovered well. Twelve other individuals who treated or came in contact with the children developed symptoms of mild to moderate mustard gas exposure. Ocular and skin lesions were most prominent in these individuals, in addition to some purulent bronchitis.

In January 1993, artillery shells from World War I that were thought to contain mustard gas were unearthed during construction of new homes in an affluent suburban Washington, D.C., community. Controlled excavation exposed a total of 15 artillery shells. Documents confirmed that the homes were on the site of a World War I munitions depot.

Conclusions

Chemical and biological warfare increases the stress of the combat environment primarily through the induction of terror and burdens of protection from contamination. Exposure to unseen, fear-inducing agents, the necessity to work in contained environments, and the fears and problems of contamination are stressful aspects of the battlefield or of a threatened civilian population in a CBW environment. For troops, the ability to sustain oneself in small group operations with little contact with the outside is critical to the operation of contained protected environments. Risk perception is an important aspect of the stress of the CBW experience and influences leaders and troops as well as civilians. The ways in which threats are perceived and the experience of risk are always mediated through group values and culture. The psychological, behavioral, and physical effects of performance in the face of such fear require further study. Anticipatory anxiety, social support from family and friends, cohesion, active training, and fatigue stand out as predictors of psychological outcome because interventions can be expected to affect these variables. The management of and level of exposure to the media's portrayal of risk can affect an entire nation's feelings of threat.

References

Bleich A, Daycian A, Koslowsky M, et al: Psychiatric implications of missile attacks on a civilian population: Israeli lessons from the Persian Gulf War. JAMA 268:613–615, 1992

Breslau M, Davis GC: Traumatic events and posttraumatic stress disorder in an urban population of young adults. Arch Gen Psychiatry 48:216–222, 1991

DeFraites RF, Wanat ER, Norwood AE, et al: Investigation of a Suspected Outbreak of an Unknown Disease Among Veterans of Operation Desert Shield/Storm. Washington, DC, Walter Reed Army Institute of Research, 1992

Dinneen MP, Pentzein RJ, Mateczun JM: Stress and coping with the trauma of war in the Persian Gulf: the hospital ship USNS Comfort, in Individual and Community Responses to Trauma and Disaster: The Structure of Human Chaos. Edited by Ursano RJ, McCaughey BG, Fullerton CS. Cambridge, UK, Cambridge University Press, 1994, pp 306–329

Fullerton CS: Treating the Chernobyl victims: individual and group response of the UCLA medical team, in Groups and Organizations in War, Disasters and Trauma. Edited by Ursano RJ, Fullerton CS. Bethesda, MD, Uniformed Services University of the Health Sciences, 1988, pp 99–106

Fullerton CS, Ursano RJ: Behavioral and psychological response to toxic exposure, in Individual Response to Disaster (DTIC: A203310). Edited by Ursano RJ, Fullerton CS. Bethesda, MD, Uniformed Services University of the Health Sciences, 1988, pp 113–128

Fullerton CS, Ursano RJ: Behavioral and psychological responses to toxic exposure. Mil Med 155:54–59, 1990

Fullerton CS, Ursano RJ: The chemical and biological warfare environment: psychological responses of a health care delivery team. Mil Med 59:524–528, 1994

Fullerton CS, Ursano RJ, Kao T, et al: The chemical and biological warfare environment: psychological responses and social support in a high stress environment. Journal of Applied Social Psychology 22:1608–1623, 1992

Gilchrist HL: A Comparative Study of World War Casualties From Gas and Other Weapons. Edgewood, MD, Edgewood Arsenal, Chemical Warfare School, 1928

Gilchrist HL, Matz PB: The Residual Effects of Warfare Gases. Washington, DC, U.S. Government Printing Office, 1933

Green BL, Grace MC, Lindy JD, et al: Risk factors for PTSD and other diagnoses in a general sample of Vietnam veterans. Am J Psychiatry 147:729–733, 1990

Harris DA, Pegram GV, Hartman BO: Performance and fatigue in experimental double-crew transport missions. Aerospace Medicine 42:980–986, 1971

Hartman BO, Hale HB, Harris DA, et al: Psychobiologic aspects of double-crew long-duration missions in C-5 aircraft. Aerospace Medicine 45:1149–1154, 1974

Heully F, Gruninger M: Collective intoxication caused by the explosion of a mustard gas shell. Annales de Medecine Legale 36:195–205, 1956

Hiss J, Arensburg B: Suffocation from misuse of gas masks during the Gulf War. BMJ 304:92, 1992

Holloway HC, Fullerton CS: The psychology of terror, in Individual and Community Responses to Trauma and Disaster: The Structure of Human Chaos. Edited by Ursano RJ, McCaughey BG, Fullerton CS. Cambridge, UK, Cambridge University Press, 1994, pp 31–45

Joy RJT: The history of medical defense against chemical warfare, in Individual and Group Behavior in Toxic and Contained Environments (DTIC: 203267). Edited by Ursano RJ, CS Fullerton. Bethesda, MD, Uniformed Services University of the Health Sciences, 1988, pp 3–17

Kilpatrick DG, Resnick HS: Posttraumatic stress disorder associated with exposure to criminal victimization in clinical and community populations, in Posttraumatic Stress Disorder: DSM-IV and Beyond. Edited by Davidson JRT, Foa EB. Washington, DC, American Psychiatric Press, 1993, pp 113–143

King S: Danse Macabre. London, Futura, 1981

Laufer RS, Brett E, Gallops MS: Dimensions of posttraumatic stress disorder among Vietnam veterans. J Nerv Ment Dis 173: 538–545, 1985

Martin JA, Manning FJ: Psychiatric casualties in future combat, in Wartime Medical Services. Second International Conference, Stockholm, Sweden, 25–29 June 1990: Proceedings. Edited by Lundeberg JE, Otto U, Rybeck B. Stockholm, FOA, 1990, pp 310–314

McCarroll E, Ursano RJ, Fullerton CS: Symptoms of posttraumatic stress disorder following recovery of war dead. Am J Psychiatry 150:1875–1877, 1993a

McCarroll E, Ursano RJ, Fullerton CS, et al: Traumatic stress of a wartime mortuary: anticipation of exposure to mass death. J Nerv Ment Dis 181:545–551, 1993b

Meselson M, Robinson JP: Chemical warfare and chemical disarmament. Sci Am 242(4):38–47, 1980

Newhouse P: Neuropsychiatric aspects of chemical warfare, in Contemporary Studies in Combat Psychiatry. Edited by Belenky G. New York, Greenwood Press, 1987, pp 185–202

Norris FH: Epidemiology of trauma: frequency and impact of different potentially traumatic events on different demographic groups. J Consult Clin Psychol 60:409–418, 1992

Rundell JR, Ursano RJ, Holloway HC, et al: Psychiatric responses to trauma. Hosp Community Psychiatry 40:68–74, 1989

Smith RJ: Army poison gas stockpile raises worries in Kentucky. The Washington Post, January 22, 1989, A1

Solomon Z, Mikulincer M, Hobfoll SE: Effects of social support and battle intensity on loneliness and breakdown during combat. J Pers Soc Psychol 51 (6, suppl):1269–1276, 1986

Solomon Z, Mikulincer M, Hobfoll SE: Objective versus subjective measurement of stress and social support: combat-related reactions. J Consult Clin Psychol 55:577–585, 1987

Spiegel HX: Psychiatric observations in the Tunisian campaign. Am J Orthopsychiatry 14:381–385, 1944

Storm WF, Gray SF: Minuteman missile crew fatigue and 24-hour alerts. USAF School of Aerospace Medicine Technical Report, SAM-TR-78-19. Brooks Air Force Base, Texas, 1978

Taylor HL, Orlansky J: The effects of wearing protective chemical warfare combat clothing on human performance. Aviat Space Environ Med 64(3):A1–A41, 1993

Terr LC: Terror writing by the formerly terrified: a look at Stephen King. Psychoanal Study Child 44:369–390, 1989

Ursano RJ, Fullerton CS: Exposure to death, disasters and bodies (DTIC: A203163). Bethesda, MD, Uniformed Services University of the Health Sciences, 1988a

Ursano RJ, Fullerton CS: Groups and organizations in war, disasters and trauma (DTIC: A203161). Bethesda, MD, Uniformed Services University of the Health Sciences, 1988b

Ursano RJ, Fullerton CS: Individual and group behavior in toxic and contained environments (DTIC: 203267). Bethesda, MD, Uniformed Services University of the Health Sciences, 1988c

Ursano RJ, Fullerton CS: Individual response to disaster (DTIC: A203310). Bethesda, MD, Uniformed Services University of the Health Sciences, 1988d

Ursano RJ, Fullerton CS: Performance and operations in toxic environments (DTIC: A203162). Bethesda, MD, Uniformed Services University of the Health Sciences, 1988e

Ursano RJ, Fullerton CS: Training for the psychological and behavioral effects of the CBW environment (DTIC: 203680). Bethesda, MD, Uniformed Services University of the Health Sciences, 1988f

Ursano RJ, Fullerton CS: Cognitive and behavioral responses to trauma. Journal of Applied Social Psychology 20:1766–1775, 1990

Ursano RJ, McCarroll JE: Exposure to traumatic death: the nature of the stressor, in Individual and Community Responses to Trauma and Disaster: The Structure of Human Chaos. Edited by Ursano RJ, McCaughey BG, Fullerton CS. Cambridge, UK, Cambridge University Press, 1994, pp 46–71

Ursano RJ, Fullerton CS, McCarroll JE, et al: Stress and Coping With War Support Providers and Casualties of Operation Desert Shield/Storm (DTIC: A256195). Bethesda, MD, Uniformed Services University of the Health Sciences, 1992

Vaitkus MA, Martin JA: Correlates of anxiety and depression among U.S. soldiers awaiting combat in the Gulf War. Paper presented to the World Congress of the International Traumatic Stress Society, Amsterdam, 1992

Vedder EB: The Medical Aspects of Chemical Warfare. Baltimore, MD, Williams & Wilkins, 1925

Xenakis SN, Brooks FR, Balsom PM: A triage and emergency treatment model for combat medics on the chemical battlefield. Mil Med 150:411–415, 1985

6 The Threat and Fear of Missile Attack: Israelis in the Gulf War

Arieh Y. Shalev, M.D.
Zahava Solomon, Ph.D.

From the time of Iraq's invasion of Kuwait in August 1990, war in the Middle East was imminent. It was not clear, however, whether Israel would be involved directly. Numerous "experts" appeared in the media and made a wide variety of predictions. The Iraqi threat to use chemical and biological warfare against civilians was voiced repeatedly. Shocking pictures of the nerve gas used by Iraq in its war with Iran made the threat all the more terrifying and believable.

In October, gas masks were distributed to the entire population of Israel, implying an admission on the part of the government and the Army that the threat of chemical warfare was real. Life went on as usual. As the Allied forces' January 15 ultimatum approached, instructions for self-protection against chemical warfare were provided by the military. Sealed rooms were to be prepared in every apartment, office, and public place; people were told to stock up on food, drinking water, and medications. Films were shown on television explaining what people were to do in case of emergency.

Tension rose sharply as January 15 approached and the threat of war filled the air. On January 16, all educational institutions were shut down to avoid the risk of large gatherings. When the Allied forces' attack began, all residents of Israel were instructed to remain at home, within reach of their gas masks and their sealed rooms. This situation continued for 4 days, during which the Iraqi missile attacks on Israel commenced. From January 16 to February 28, there were 18 different attacks in which 39 missiles were fired. Most landed in the densely populated central region of Israel. The missiles caused extensive destruction of property, bodily injury, and some loss of life. The reality of the threat was brought home daily by on-the-spot television coverage of the mounds of rubble that were once dwellings and by interviews with the survivors who had lost their homes and all their possessions in a flash.

During this period, some adults returned to work, but the schools remained closed. The country gradually adjusted to what became known as a state of "emergency routine." This meant return to work and gradual reopening of some schools, but places of entertainment remained closed, and it was forbidden to meet in large groups after dark.

A new lifestyle developed. In the morning, life went on as if conditions were nearly normal. From early afternoon on, there was a large outpouring of cars from the central region to outlying areas. In the evenings, most people retired to their homes, close to their sealed rooms and gas masks, and readied themselves for night, when the missiles would fall. At night, a voluntary curfew took effect.

There was a stirring of social and political debate over a number of issues: whether Israel should continue to endure the missile attacks without retaliation; whether it was justified to keep the entire labor force at home; whether the protective devices provided by the government were really effective; whether people were better off going to sealed rooms when the sirens sounded, as was being recommended by the authorities, or to bomb shelters that would provide better protection against conventional missiles but would be less safe in the case of chemical warfare. Many families in the areas that were hit by missiles abandoned their homes in search of safer areas. This response to attack aroused further debate over whether those who left were smart survivors or were abandoning the battlefield in the midst of a war.

The Gulf War provided a natural laboratory for the study of stress. In this war, the entire population of Israel was exposed to an anticipated and relatively long-lived period of threat. The conditions precipitated by this unfortunate situation were the basis for numerous investigations. According to our estimation, more than 50 independent studies were carried out that assessed the effects of the crisis on groups that were at high risk for stress-related illnesses, such as children, Holocaust survivors, and persons with mental illness, as well as on large representative samples of the population. In this chapter we present some of the main findings from these studies and focus our attention on reactions of both adults and children in the community at large.

Psychological Reactions of the Adult Population

Morale

In a study conducted by the Israeli Institute of Applied Social Research (Levy 1991), investigators examined public morale during the Gulf War in the context of data on morale in Israel that had been collected on a regular basis over the previous 15 years. As operationalized in this study, public morale consisted of three components: personal ability to adjust, mood, and general assessment of the state of Israel.

Of the three dimensions of morale, the only one that seems to have been at all undermined by the Gulf War was people's views of their ability to adjust. Fewer than 80% of the respondents (70% in Haifa and Tel Aviv, where missiles landed) reported that they adjusted well, in comparison with a usual pattern of 80% to 90% endorsing ability to adjust in peacetime.

This decrease in perceived ability to adjust may have reflected a transient sense of personal vulnerability; a large proportion of the population who were under direct threat, by their own admission, adjusted well to the war's stresses.

Improvement was actually seen in the other two dimensions over the years preceding the war. A somewhat higher proportion of respondents reported better mood than they had had over most of the preceding 15 years. Dr. Levy, who conducted this study, pointed out that there is a precedent for external difficulties leading to an improvement in mood among Israelis (Levy 1991). People's appraisal of the country's situation was also better than it had been for most of the preceding 15 years.

One of the interesting findings that emerged from this study is that public morale, when all three of its aspects are taken as a whole, was higher during the Gulf War than during certain periods of peace. Interestingly, the lowest level of morale was charted not during wartime but during the peacetime years of 1980 to 1981, when the economy was in deep recession. This finding suggests that mundane economic strains may have a more detrimental effect on citizens' morale than the life threat of missile attacks.

The picture of personal vulnerability among part of the public, along with the positive mood and positive assessment of the country's situation, is consistent with findings from other studies, as will be reported below. All of the studies show a mixed reaction: people displayed signs of distress on the one hand, and control and a sense of proportion on the other.

Sleep

Sleep disturbances are recognized as a common response to stress. Lavie and colleagues (1991) examined sleep disturbances during the war by employing both a telephone survey and assessment via actigraphic monitoring. In the telephone survey, 28% of those queried complained of difficulties falling asleep and/or midsleep awakenings. Compared with reports obtained in a previous study of Israeli industrial workers, the overall rate of sleep disturbance reported during the war was only slightly higher than that recorded during peacetime (28% vs. 22%, respectively). On the other hand, about four times as many people reported both types of sleep disturbances during the Gulf War as compared with before the war (13.5% vs. 3.4%, respectively). Also of interest was the finding that sleep problems were more prevalent among residents of the areas that sustained missile attacks than among those who lived in other areas. (The prevalence of sleep problems reached 36.5% in Tel Aviv and 39.1% in Haifa, two areas that sustained missile attacks, compared with the national average prevalence of 28% mentioned above.) Results of the actigraphic monitoring, on the other hand, showed that in contrast to the increase in complaints of insomnia, overall objective measures of sleep were only minimally affected during the war in general. The time it took to fall asleep and the duration and efficiency of sleep were no different from the quality of sleep of the same persons recorded in 1987. The researchers pointed out that many persons who experienced insomnia simply misperceived their sleep quality and that they suffered only from "fear of sleep." This fear was provoked by worry that they would sleep through the missle attack alarm or that, even if they did hear it, they would be too slow to protect themselves. These findings suggest that even if people were uneasy and felt that they slept poorly, the objective measure did not reveal abnormal patterns of sleep that would indicate major and obtrusive distress.

Fear and Anxiety

As with objective measures of sleep, which showed relative equilibrium from peacetime to wartime, fear and anxiety have been shown in two studies to be relatively consistent between peacetime and wartime (Ben-Zur and Zeidner 1991; Gal 1992). Yet, these studies also demonstrated a process of habituation with time. Both studies found that although subjects reported more fear, anxiety, and distress at the beginning of the war, the fear and distress, as reported by respondents, decreased somewhat with the number of days elapsed since the start of the war.

The most comprehensive of these studies was undertaken by the Department of Behavioral Sciences of the Israel Defense Forces (IDF) (Carmeli et al. 1992). The study consisted of 23 surveys of the general population carried out over a 7-month period beginning in August 1990 and ending at the end of February 1991. Data were gathered via nationwide telephone surveys of random samples consisting of 8,000 subjects. We present here only selected findings of this comprehensive study. These findings clearly demonstrate the nature and extent of a process of gradual habituation to the crisis as the war progressed.

Perception of the threat was assessed by the following question: How likely is a conventional and/or chemical attack on Israel in the near future? For the better part of the war, a considerable proportion of the public continued to expect missile attacks. As the war progressed, there was a decrease in expectations of both conventional and chemical attacks. Yet, the overall decline notwithstanding, the expectancies fluctuated with the actual missile attacks, rising sharply right after each attack and then subsiding a day or two later.

With regard to apprehension, two diverse trends coexisted: emotional accommodation and persistent nervousness. As the war progressed, the public's emotional reactions to the war decreased in intensity, as was evident in two ways. First, as the war progressed, gradually fewer people reported feeling strong fear during the interval between attacks. Second, fewer people reported experiencing strong fear during the attacks. In February, fewer people endorsed greater apprehension about the consequences of a possible conventional attack than in January, and fewer reported strong concern with the security situation. The researchers referred to the overall downward trend as "habituation" and the decline in the percentage of people who responded intensely to each missile attack as "mini habituation." They observed a dual process of habituation and mini habituation.

The other trend, that of persistent nervousness and of remaining on edge, was evident, for example, in the substantial amount of apprehension about chemical attacks that persisted throughout the war. It was also seen in the increase of fear associated with every reminder of the danger, actual or symbolic.

The public's behavioral responses were assessed in two ways: somatic symptoms in the sealed, chemically protected room and coping. Anxiety, as measured by the severity of somatic symptoms in the sealed room, was intense early on but increasingly decreased in intensity, reflecting a process of accommodation. Bodily symptoms such as burning sensations, tears, breathing difficulties, and so forth were reported by 38% of the respondents on January 18, at the start of the war, yet by only about 20% in the third week of the war. Similarly, in January, when asked to rate their coping, 73% of the respondents answered that they were coping well, whereas by the last week of February 90% reported that they were coping well. For most of the public the sense of mastery improved steadily during the course of the war. Again, it seems that people learned to cope with the threat and to live adaptively while continuing to experience relatively high levels of fear.

In summary, the findings of the IDF Department of Behavioral Sciences study point to two simultaneous responses. On the one hand, the population responded to the war in a well-disciplined, self-controlled manner. Most people kept their anxieties under control, followed the emergency instructions, and maintained their sense of mastery under the attack. Somatic and behavioral disturbances were relatively rare. Moreover, as the war progressed, anxiety levels declined and a sense of mastery increased. On the other hand, signs of nervousness and apprehension continued unabated.

Psychological Casualties

Although, overall, most people responded adaptively during the Gulf War, this war, like all other wars, inevitably had its share of physical and psychological casualties. Israel's succession of frequent wars has created a structure enabling real-time assessment of wartime medical and psychological needs. The Gulf War was no exception. During the war, psychological casualties were not only treated but also monitored and documented. The IDF Medical Corps collected data on emergency admission to all 12 major hospitals throughout the country during the first 8 hours after each missile attack. Data were collected both for actual missile attacks and for alarms (Bleich et al. 1992; Krsenty et al. 1991). These data indicate that although 39 missiles fell, almost all of them on residential areas, relatively few people were killed or injured. Around three-quarters of the direct casualties were physical injuries, and just fewer than one-quarter of casualties were from acute psychological reactions. Out of 1,059 war-related hospital emergency room admissions, 234 were for injuries resulting from the explosion of the missiles. Only two of these casualties died of their wounds. The overwhelming majority of the injured (221) suffered mild injuries, 10 were classified as having suffered moderate wounds, and only one person, a 3-year-old girl, was severely injured.

In addition to the injuries resulting from the missile explosions, 825 indirect casualties related to the warning sirens were admitted to the emergency rooms nationwide. Injuries in these subjects stemmed to one degree or another from the fear aroused by the alert signals rather than from actual exposure to the missiles. The indirect casualties of the war included 11 deaths: 7 from suffocation due to faulty use of the gas masks, and 4 due to heart attack. In fact, more people died from the results of fear than from actual exposure to the missiles. Forty people suffered physical injuries while rushing to safety shelters after hearing the warning siren, and a further 230 patients were admitted after needlessly injecting themselves with atropine (the nerve gas antidote that was distributed to all residents of Israel before the outbreak of the war). During this time, an astonishing 544 patients were admitted to hospital emergency wards throughout the country with symptoms of acute psychological distress. Most of these admissions for acute stress or un-justified atropine injection followed the first missile attack. The numbers dropped sharply afterward. The public was quite dis-tressed after the first missiles landed in a densely inhabited area. Uncertainty and fear about the use of chemical weapons were much more prevalent following the first attacks than later on.

These findings indicate that extreme fear reactions were sometimes fatal. Although these reactions occurred frequently following the first missile attack, over time, the public adjusted and learned to cope, resulting in fewer hospital referrals. These data on treated populations are consistent with the findings from studies of the general public (i.e., an untreated popula-tion). Both sets of data demonstrate intense reactive distress and habituation with time.

Children's Responses to the War

Children are thought to experience considerable distress dur-ing wartime, but there is uncertainty about the extent of these effects because few empirical studies have been conducted. De-spite the fact that millions of children around the globe have been exposed to the horrors of war, and although there have been many studies of war-induced stress, very few of these stud-ies have focused on children. Even in Israel, which has known many wars, direct research on the impact of war on children has been limited and has focused primarily on terrorist attacks and flare-ups along the northern border (Milgram 1982). This pau-city of studies is perhaps not surprising. Wartime is a difficult and most inappropriate time to conduct research. Both sub-jects and researchers are inevitably engrossed in their own survival, so the feasibility of conducting a systematic study is greatly diminished. This is particularly true for children facing adversity; these children are protected by adults, who often de-cline to let them participate in psychological research.

In a crisis such as war, it is considered imperative that the education of the young continue and that children occupy themselves with familiar educational and recreational routines. This rule rests on the assumption that children tolerate crisis situations best when there is minimal dislocation from familiar surroundings, peers, authority figures, and the customary routines of daily living. The school system is regarded not only as a peacetime institution that should continue to function during war, but also as a wartime provider of mental health services to the children themselves and, through the children, to their families (Milgram 1993).

In stark contrast to these conceptions, however, Israeli schools and kindergartens were closed for almost the entire duration of the Gulf War. Moreover, after the first 4 days of the war, adults were required to return to work. Many children thus not only lacked the benefit of a consistent school environment and the support of teachers and friends, but were also denied the support of their parents for extended periods.

However, there was, in contrast to other wars, a considerable amount of research on the psychological adjustment of Israeli children during the Gulf War. Here, we present only three examples of these studies, which we believe are representative of many others. The first study examined changes in the prevalence of common emotional and behavioral problems in children; the second study looked at anxiety levels of children and their parents; the last study focused on coping in the sealed room and war-related posttraumatic stress disorder (PTSD).

Behavioral Problems

Ronen and Rahav (1991) compared the frequency of common behavioral problems in children before and during the war. Participating in the study were 316 second-graders and sixth-graders in a Tel Aviv school. These children had been assessed by their teachers 2 months before the war, as part of another project, and were reexamined during the third week of the war, a day after the schools reopened.

The main findings indicate that a significant increase in most behavior problems had occurred during the war as compared with the period before the war. Problems that increased included bed-wetting, nightmares, and headaches. Age appeared to be an important factor in the children's behavioral problems. Each of the problem behaviors was reported more often in the second-graders than in the sixth-graders. That is, the younger children were at higher risk for emotional problems during the war than were the older children.

The researchers also examined whether changes in the number of problems were related to the number of prewar problems. Results showed that in both age groups children with an above-average level of prewar behavioral problems displayed a greater increase in problems during the war than did children with fewer behavioral problems before the war. This trend was particularly evident in the second-graders.

Anxiety

Michael Rosenbaum and Tammie Ronen (1991), of Tel Aviv University, examined anxiety levels in children and parents. Respondents were asked to rate their own anxiety and the anxiety level of the other two members of the family during three general periods of the day (i.e., morning, evening, and night) and during three other specific times (i.e., upon hearing the alarm, being in the sealed room, and immediately after being released from the sealed room). In the fifth week of the war they were asked to rate current levels of anxiety and also, retrospectively, what the levels had been in the first week of the war.

The study sample consisted of 112 children: 52 boys and 60 girls from the fifth and sixth grades of a large public school in a suburb of Tel Aviv, and their parents. The major findings were as follows:

1. All subjects—parents as well as children—reported higher anxiety at week 1 than at week 5 of the war.
2. Both parents and children reported greater anxiety at night, when the danger was greater, than during the day.

3. On the whole, the mothers' self-reported anxiety was higher than that of the children.
4. The children's self-reported anxiety was similar to that of their fathers during the day but was higher than their fathers' at night and when the alarms sounded.
5. In general, there was a moderate degree of correspondence between the children's self-reports and the parents' perceptions of their children, particularly with regard to the sealed room, when families were together and could observe one another's responses. The mothers, however, tended to view their children as being more anxious than did the fathers.

PTSD and Coping

In a study that one of the present authors conducted with a group of colleagues (Schwarzwald et al. 1993), the efficacy of different types of coping behaviors and the rates of PTSD were assessed. PTSD is a psychiatric syndrome that belongs to the category of anxiety disorders, as defined by DSM-IV (American Psychiatric Association 1994). PTSD may follow exposure to any type of extreme or traumatic stress and is characterized by symptoms of intrusion, avoidance, and hyperarousal.

In this study, 5th-, 7th-, and 10th-graders were administered questionnaires in their schools 1 month after the end of the war, and their teachers were also asked to report on changes in the social and scholastic functioning of each child. Two-thirds of the schools were in the suburbs of Tel Aviv, which sustained missile attacks, and the remainder were in the nearby city of Netanya, where no missiles fell during the war.

Although three-quarters of the children (75.8%) reported feeling tense in the sealed room, all of the other highly endorsed emotional responses in the sealed room had a positive orientation. Examples of such responses were "I felt sure that everything would be OK" (80%), "I felt relaxed" (78.2%), and "I acted as if everything was the same as usual" (74.2%). In contrast, infrequently endorsed items were mostly negative, such as "I cried" (17.4%) and "I thought I would go crazy" (17.8%).

Certain coping behaviors in the sealed room were reported by almost everyone. Examples of these coping behaviors were information seeking from the radio and television (96.6%) and talking to others in the sealed room (90.6%). Another set of commonly shared activities can be categorized as monitoring and assisting others. These activities included checking to see whether everyone was OK (89.8%), helping others (89.8%), calming others (85.4%), and checking gas masks (82.6%). A third set of shared responses involved wishful thinking; examples of these responses were wishing for a miracle (88.5%), wishing the missile alert were a false alarm (82.2%), and wishing that the missiles would fall elsewhere (81.2%). The findings showed that a month after the war, nearly 25% of the Tel Aviv children displayed a constellation of symptoms consistent with a DSM-III-R (American Psychiatric Association 1987) diagnosis of PTSD, compared with 13% of the children in Netanya—that is, almost double.

In this study the investigators also found a significant effect of age: the younger children endorsed more symptoms and qualified for PTSD diagnoses more often than did the older children. Nearly one-third (33%) of the 5th-graders were eligible for PTSD diagnosis, compared with 14% of the 7th-graders and 9% of the 10th-graders. In other words, the rates of PTSD among the 5th-graders were more than twice as much as those among the 7th- and 10th-graders. Furthermore, as in many other studies conducted in Israel during the Gulf War, in this study the investigators found that girls were more vulnerable than boys. Girls endorsed significantly more stress symptoms than did boys. Interestingly, teachers did not display a high degree of sensitivity to their students' distress: they reported a deterioration in academic functioning in only 24% of the children who were eligible for a PTSD diagnosis; impairment in social functioning was reported by teachers for only 11% of the children who had received the diagnosis of PTSD.

Children who were more active in the sealed room, more involved in checking protective devices, and more attentive to others were found to report more stress reactions in the long run. In contrast, children who used more avoidance and distraction fared better in the long run. Older adolescents were more likely to embrace a pattern of effective coping than were their younger counterparts. Taken together with the finding that emotional reactions in the sealed room were primarily positive in nature, this finding suggests that denial of the threat was a very common and very beneficial strategy that contributed to children's well-being.

Although in this section we have presented the findings of only three studies, they are representative of results found in many other studies as well. In summary, the first finding that these studies have in common is that, on the whole, the large majority of children responded adaptively to the stresses of war, even when the danger of a missile attack was very close to home. Although a certain percentage of children responded with exacerbation of prewar problems, with anxiety, or even with PTSD, most of the children did not display signs of psychopathology.

Although the studies discussed in this section were all conducted either during or shortly after the war, and data from long-term follow-ups are not yet available, it does appear that the overall pattern of findings reflects a tendency toward habituation of stress responses. That is, the most severe reactions were observed at the start of the war, and the frequency and severity of these reactions dropped sharply over time. Like adults, children got used to the threat very quickly and were less affected with repeated exposure.

The Professional Community at Work

As in many disaster areas, therapists and patients during the Gulf War were under the same threat. Therefore, the treatment could not be conducted with the same professional perspective as it usually is. Moreover, issues of diagnosis, outcome, and treatment strategies were unclear. Therapists found it difficult to correctly diagnose, reliably predict the outcome, and accurately treat the patients seen during the war. The diagnostic category of acute stress disorder is mainly descriptive, and very little is known about its face—and prospective—validity. PTSD diagnoses could not be made on cases seen during the war because of the short duration of the symptoms. Moreover, anticipatory anxiety and insomnia, and not intrusion, numbing, and avoidance, were salient features of the clinical picture, and many instances of these features were self-limited. Finally, no data are available on the long-term effects of treatment, and contrasting statements may be found regarding treatment modalities such as pharmacotherapy, hypnotherapy, and so forth.

Despite these shortcomings, mental health professionals were often called to intervene in states of emergency and, of course, among the evacuees. Several hot-line services were made available to the public, and many mental health providers at mental health services provided telephone consultations to their patients, who, during the first days of the war, could not travel. Psychologists and psychiatrists who followed their patients reported frequent reactivation of PTSD in previously traumatized subjects.

Mental health professionals in all hospitals were part of readiness programs that were designed to decontaminate and treat victims of chemical attacks. They trained with the hospital's personnel in diagnosis and triage of chemical casualties and participated in emergency shifts. Psychologists and psychiatrists also participated in numerous programs in the media, in which they were called to provide information regarding stress reactions and to help the audience understand the nature of their responses to help delineate excessive from normal responses.

Conclusions

War is not a novelty in Israel. The Gulf War, however, presented the Israeli population with a new scenario that entailed absence of concrete military conflict, forced passivity, extremely serious and unprovoked threat directed at the civilian population, and stress endured within families.

We have limited our discussion to the public at large. Yet, although the war entailed considerable stress and disruption for the entire population, there were certain segments that were at particularly high risk for psychological distress. Holocaust survivors (Solomon and Prager 1992) and traumatized war veterans (Kaplan et al. 1992) were reminded of their earlier ordeal and thus were most vulnerable to reactivation of their trauma. New immigrants, singles living on their own who lacked the support of kin and friends, persons with mental illness, and individuals suffering from physical diseases such as cardiac problems—all were more vulnerable during the Gulf War. Although these individuals were in fact at higher risk and as groups did display more distress than the general public, on the whole, their responses were also quite contained (Solomon, in press).

When considering the data presented above, one must remember that the circumstances of the Gulf War in Israel were indeed unique. This was a limited war in that it entailed only relatively few casualties and the physical damage was contained. Furthermore, the military authorities were able to alert the public in advance to the upcoming bombardment, thus enabling people to take cover in sealed rooms and to put on protective gear in time. The public was provided with continuous real-time, reliable information regarding areas hit and the extent of damage, thus strengthening their individual sense of control. These circumstances are probably implicated in the relatively calm and restrained psychological reactions and habituation to reported distress over time. Therefore, caution should be exercised when generalizing from the current findings and extrapolating them to other military conflicts involving civilians.

Finally, it seems to us that the increased recent interest in PTSD should be extended also to the issue of acute traumatic reactions (characterized, in part, as acute stress disorder in DSM-IV [American Psychiatric Association 1994]). Increasing our knowledge with regard to the course of acute stress reactions and developing appropriate and effective treatment modalities should be of major concern to researchers and therapists alike.

References

American Psychiatric Association: Diagnostic and Statistical Manual of Mental Disorders, 3rd Edition, Revised. Washington, DC, American Psychiatric Association, 1987

American Psychiatric Association: Diagnostic and Statistical Manual of Mental Disorders, 4th Edition. Washington, DC, American Psychiatric Association, 1994

Ben-Zur H, Zeidner M: Anxiety and bodily symptoms under threat of missile attack: the Israeli scene. Anxiety Research 4:35–44, 1991

Bleich A, Dycian A, Koslovsky M, et al: Psychiatric implications of missile attacks on civilian population. JAMA 268:613–615, 1992

Carmeli A, Mevorach L, Leiberman N, et al: The Gulf War: Home Front in a Test of Crisis, Final Report. Tel Aviv, Department of Behavioral Sciences, Israel Defense Forces, 1992

Gal R: Stress Reactions in Israel to the Missile Attacks During the Gulf War. Zichron Ya'acov, Israel Institute of Military Studies, 1992

Kaplan Z, Kron S, Lichtenberg P, et al: Military mental health in the Gulf War: the experience of the central clinic of the IDF. Isr J Psychiatry Relat Sci 29:7–13, 1992

Krsenty E, Shemer J, Alshech I, et al: Medical aspects of the Iraqi missile attacks on Israel. Isr J Med Sci 27:603–607, 1991

Lavie P, Carmeli A, Mevorach L, et al: Sleeping under the threat of the Scud: war-related environmental insomnia. Isr J Med Sci 27:681–686, 1991

Levy S: Morale during the Gulf War. Lecture presented at the Israeli Institute for Military Studies, Zichron Ya'acov, June 1991

Milgram NA: War-related stress in Israeli children and youth, in Handbook of Stress: Theoretical and Clinical Aspects. Edited by Goldberg L, Breznitz S. New York, Free Press, 1982, pp 656–676

Milgram NA: Stress and coping in Israel during the Gulf War. Journal of Social Issues 49:103–123, 1993

Ronen T, Rahav G: Children's behavior problems during the Gulf War. Paper presented at the Israeli Ministry of Education Conference on Stress Reactions of Children in the Gulf War, Ramat Gan, Israel, 1991

Rosenbaum M, Ronen T: How did Israeli children and their parents cope with the threat of daily attack by Scud missiles during the Gulf War? Paper presented at the Israeli Ministry of Education Conference on Stress Reactions of Children in the Gulf War, Ramat Gan, Israel, 1991

Schwarzwald J, Weisenberg M, Waysman M, et al: Stress reactions of school-age children to the bombardment by Scud missiles. J Abnorm Psychol 102:404–410, 1993

Solomon Z: Coping With War-Induced Stress: The Gulf War and the Israeli Response. New York, Plenum (in press)

Solomon Z, Prager E: Elderly Israeli Holocaust survivors during the Persian Gulf War: a study of psychological distress. Am J Psychiatry 52:1707–1710, 1992

Part III
Preparation for the War

7

Those Left Behind: Military Families

Ann E. Norwood, M.D.
Carol S. Fullerton, Ph.D.
Karen P. Hagen, R.N.

Families are important to the well-being and effectiveness of military personnel, both in peacetime and in times of war. Families provide support critical to the military member's performance and to his or her readiness and ability to carry out the military's mission. During the Persian Gulf War, in particular, receiving information from home and knowing that family members were safe was of utmost importance to those serving in the Gulf (Dinneen et al. 1994).

In this chapter, after a brief review of the health effects of family support, we present a general overview of the changing needs of military families and of efforts to support these families during the Persian Gulf War. In subsequent sections we examine in greater detail the experiences of two subgroups of military families who were felt to be especially stressed by the war: military families living in Europe and reserve and National Guard families here at home. We conclude the chapter with a discussion of the role of support programs for military families during the war and an example of one such program.

Family Support and Coping: Physical and Mental Health Effects

Familial support, particularly in the spouse/significant other relationship, is an important aspect of coping with many types of stress. A substantial amount of research has documented the health effects of receiving social support from families and friends (for reviews, see S. Cohen and Wills 1985; House et al. 1988). However, providing support to family members can be stressful for the support provider, particularly following traumatic events (Fullerton et al. 1993; Shumaker and Brownell 1984; S. D. Solomon et al. 1987; Taylor 1990) and in times of war (Z. Solomon et al. 1993). Wives of combat veterans may be distressed as a result of psychiatric and physical health problems experienced by their husbands (see Kulka et al. 1988; Rosenheck 1986; Z. Solomon et al. 1991). Z. Solomon and colleagues (1991) found increased somatic complaints and psychiatric distress among the wives of veterans with combat stress reactions and posttraumatic stress disorder (PTSD). The wives' stress was associated with the increased responsibility secondary to the husband's illness and with identification with the husband's symptoms. Interestingly, Solomon et al. found that the degree of expressiveness in the marital relationship was associated with the wives' mental health.

Now and Then: The Changing Face of the Military

Just as the Persian Gulf War highlighted changes in the technology of fighting wars, it also focused attention on changes in the composition of the military and the military family. An estimated 3.5% of the United States population are either in the military or a member of the immediate family of a servicemember. If one includes past military members and their families, roughly one-third of the U.S. population have or have had an affiliation with the military (Black 1993). Since the Revolutionary War, the American military family has been sculpted by many forces: the pool of individuals from which the military has drawn, cultural trends, advances in technology, and economic pressures, to name just a few. Despite the changes in the military family, however, many themes about life in a military family have remained the same.

Then

Camp Followers

During the Revolutionary War, most families stayed behind while their sons, brothers, and fathers left home to fight. However, as many as 20,000 women did not stay at home, but instead accompanied the soldiers as they marched from battle to battle. Many of these "camp followers" were laundresses authorized by the Continental Congress to support the soldiers. These women and their children received a camp follower's stipend of half-ration for the women and quarter-ration for each child (Alt and Stone 1991). While many laundresses were wives of senior enlisted personnel, some others were prostitutes; indeed, the origin of the term "shacking up" has been attributed to the practice of soldiers living with prostitutes in shacks outside of camp (Little 1971). Officers' wives, too, accompanied their husbands, Martha Washington being one of the more prominent among them.

Women served important roles during the Revolutionary War, beginning a long tradition of American women's contributions to war efforts. As they would again in the wars that followed, women at that time carried out a host of support roles: nursing the wounded, cleaning and mending clothes, foraging for supplies, and cooking. Women were also exposed to combat and the attendant horror of warfare, some receiving congressional pensions for their service. Life for Revolutionary War–era women accompanying their husbands was marked by deprivation and hardship; one colonel's wife was noted to have become so depressed in this environment that she committed suicide (Alt and Stone 1991).

In the Revolutionary War era, just as today, the conflict between military duty and family created tension. This dilemma of dual obligation was apparent to General Knox, who was forced to leave his wife, Lucy, to her own devices when he heard that the British fleet had sailed into New York Harbor. Although he was aware of the "distress and anxiety Lucy had [with] the city in an uproar, the alarm guns firing, the troops repairing to their posts, and everything in the height of battle," he reported to his command post because "my country calls loudest" (Alt and Stone 1991, p. 10).

The camp-following families of the Revolutionary War represent the experience of the minority of soldiers' families. Then, as now, it was far more common that women and children remained back home.

Changes in the Military and in Military Families

Military families did not exist in substantial numbers until the 20th century, when it became more acceptable for military members to be married and there was a larger standing military force. Originally, the military was composed predominantly of volunteers called up from the colonies. Because there were concerns that a large standing army would threaten the fledgling democracy, the Continental Congress discharged virtually all troops following the Revolutionary War; 25 men were assigned to Fort Pitt and 55 men were asked to stay on at West Point (Alt and Stone 1991).

The size of this standing army gradually increased in response to contingencies created by the growth of the nation, such as the westward expansion. Until relatively recently, most men who were recruited to serve in the Army were single; at times, Army regulations specifically prohibited married men from enlisting. As late as the 20th century, enlisted men and noncommissioned officers (NCOs) were required to obtain their commander's permission to marry. Until the early 1900s, officers tended to postpone marriage until they were in their 30s (Goldman 1976).

As the numbers of military families grew, Congress and the military were compelled to address the needs of these families. By the mid-1800s, Army regulations acknowledged the need to provide basic services to the families of officers and NCOs. The most profound changes in recognizing military families and their needs have come about since World War II. World War II witnessed the conscription of millions of married men. In response to the hardships created by the loss of husbands and fathers, the Army Emergency Relief Society was established to provide financial assistance for needy families. In the years following World War II, increasing attention was focused on issues affecting military families, such as housing problems and children's schooling (Albano 1994).

While the vast numbers of military families during wartime captured bureaucratic interest, so did the peacetime need to maintain a fighting force of experienced servicemembers. For example, difficulties in retention of soldiers in active-duty positions following the Korean War prompted the initiation of the first studies to examine the family's impact on decisions relating to continuing in the military and choosing it as a career. The next major impetus for military family research was the shift after the Vietnam War to an all-volunteer force in the 1970s. It was recognized that the servicemember family's satisfaction with military life contributed heavily to the member's decision to make the military a career versus returning to civilian life.

Another change in composition of military families resulted from the retention and inclusion of female servicemembers with children; it was only in 1975 that the policy allowing women to be involuntarily discharged for pregnancy and parenthood was dropped (Albano 1994). The new phenomenon of women being allowed to serve in the military in addition to being wives and mothers has created a "new" military family.

Because of, in large part, these changes in the composition of the military and the military family, the 1970s and 1980s were

watershed decades for the military family. Military family support programs were initiated, and research on the military
family was supported. In 1979, the Air Force issued a directive
that recognized the family's contribution to military readiness.
In 1983, the Army Chief of Staff issued a document that laid out
an administrative structure to improve the quality of military
family life.

Now

During Desert Storm, it was possible to observe how well the
major changes in policies related to military families that occurred following the Vietnam conflict generalized to times of
war. It is helpful to compare the demographics of the military
during the Vietnam War and during the Gulf War. Changes in
the population and the end of the draft have had a profound
effect on the demographics of the military and the structure of
the military family (Table 7–1). The composition of the military
has become increasingly diverse. On average, military members
are better educated and more likely to be married and have
children than their counterparts of the 1960s and 1970s
(Department of Defense 1992). In Vietnam, 16% of those in-
country were married with children, whereas in the Gulf War,
almost 60% were married with children (Department of Defense 1992). In addition, the uniformed personnel of the 1990s

Table 7–1.   Changes in the military since the Vietnam War era

All-volunteer force
More women in the military
More dual-career military couples
More married servicemembers
More servicemembers with children
More military wives working out of the home
Higher education level
Wider range of occupational specialities for military women

are an all-volunteer force, in contrast to the large number of draftees during the Vietnam War.

Like her counterparts in the civilian community, the military wife has also changed. Today's military wife or significant other is likely to work outside the home and to be less active in traditional volunteer activities. In fact, women whose husbands are in the military in many cases are themselves members of the military.

Women now constitute approximately 10% of all Americans serving in uniform and hold a much wider range of occupational specialities than in the past. During the Gulf War, approximately 5,700 dual-career military couples were deployed. Further, the large influx of military women has created a large number of "military husbands" (i.e., civilian husbands with active-duty wives), a population that has not been well studied. The past decades have also brought a dramatic increase in the number of single-parent families.

Family Life in the Military

Issues Specific to the Military Family

In addition to facing many of the same issues that civilian families face, military families also are confronted by challenges specific to military life (Ridenour 1984; Ursano and Holloway 1985) (Table 7–2). The military family must contend with a broad spectrum of issues. For example, similar to spouses of police officers, military spouses must contend with anxiety and worry over the possibility of death or injury to their mates, but in the case of military spouses, this worry is also compounded by lengthy separations and frequent moves. Segal (1986) has characterized the military as a "greedy institution," citing the military as unusual in the pattern of demands it places on its members and their families. One routine part of military life that places many of these special demands is deployment.

Table 7–2.   Aspects specific to military life

Frequent separations and reunions
Regular geographic relocations
"The mission must come first"
Regimentation and conformity of military service
Early retirement relative to civilian counterparts
Threat of death or injury during training and deployment
Threat of capture during deployment
Structured and hierarchically organized social systems
Separation from the nonmilitary community

Stress of Family Separation Due to Deployment

Deployment entails family separation. Family separation consists of three stages: anticipation before the deployment, separation during the deployment, and reunion after the deployment (Table 7–3). Each of these stages is associated with a specific set of stressors, and how the family copes is affected by the circumstances occurring during that period. The frequency of past separations, the length of the present separation, and the timing of the present separation (whether it occurs during peacetime or during a period of war) influence the experience of a deployment by a military family. The family's experience is affected by the role and gender of the parent left behind as well as the coping skills and past separation experiences of this parent. The child's experience of the separation will be affected, in part, by his or her developmental stage and by familial conflicts and attachments (Blount 1992).

Anticipation phase.   The anticipation phase usually begins 6 to 8 weeks before deployment. This phase is often characterized by conflicting desires and emotions—the need to feel close to one's partner and yet to begin to distance oneself in order to prepare for the upcoming loss. Generally, wives report that they begin the separation process earlier than their deploying husbands (Amen et al. 1988). This can lead to anger and hurt as

Table 7–3.   Stress of family separation due to deployment

Stage 1: Anticipation

- *Expectation of separation* (6–8 weeks before deployment)
  Feelings: denial, fear, anger, resentment, hurt
  Activities: financial planning, making car repairs, making home repairs
- *Emotional withdrawal* (1 week before deployment)
  Feelings: confusion, ambivalence, anger, pulling away
  Activities: talking, sharing, fighting, planning reunion

Stage 2: Separation

- *Emotional confusion* (1–6 weeks after departure)
  Feelings: sense of abandonment, loss, emptiness, pain, disorganization
  Activities and reactions: crying, loss of sleep, loss of appetite, keeping busy
- *Adjustment* (most of deployment)
  Feelings: hope, confidence, calmness, less anger, loneliness
  Activities: establishing routine, establishing communications, promoting self-growth
- *Expectation of reunion* (6–8 weeks before homecoming)
  Feelings: apprehension, excitement, high expectations, worry, fear
  Activities: planning homecoming, cleaning, dieting

Stage 3: Reunion

- *Honeymoon* (1 day until first argument)
  Feelings: euphoria, blur of excitement
  Activities: talking, reestablishing intimacy, readjusting
- *Readjustment* (6–8 weeks after return)
  Feelings: uncomfortableness, role confusion, satisfaction
  Activities: renegotiating relationships, redefining roles, settling in

---

Source.   Adapted from U.S. Navy: "The Stages of Deployment," in *Navy Family Deployment Guide* (Norfolk Gen, 7000/1 1/87, 0199-LF-007-0000). Norfolk, VA, Navy Family Services Center, 1987.

the husbands detect the wives pulling away. Other common feelings include denial that the deployment will take place and resentment.

Numerous activities must be accomplished before the active-duty member departs. Often, the military member works long hours preparing for the deployment. This diminishes the time at home for taking care of automobile and house repairs, making sure finances are in order, and having the discussions that are necessary to keep the home functioning smoothly during the member's absence.

Separation phase.   The extended absence of a spouse creates new stressors and opportunities for the individual left behind. Responsibilities and decisions related to managing the household that normally are shared must now reside with the husband or wife remaining at home. If there are children in the family, the parent left behind temporarily becomes a "single" parent. He or she must assume all the responsibilities of caring for the children while the other parent is away. During the deployment, the stay-behind spouse often experiences emotional confusion that can last for several months. The initial experience of the separation is frequently characterized by feelings of abandonment, loss, pain, and disorganization. Frequently, the spouse will report mild and transient depressive symptoms of tearfulness and loss of sleep or appetite. Generally, these feelings subside as the family settles into a new routine. Often, the spouse at home will develop greater confidence as he or she negotiates the activities of daily life as a temporarily "single" person or parent. Ideally, the couple stay abreast of each other's experiences through phone calls and frequent letters.

As the deployment nears an end, expectations about reunion begin to build. There is a sense of excitement about being reunited but also apprehension about how the individuals will have changed. Often, there are last-minute diets, decisions over what to wear, house cleaning, and a flurry of other activities centered on welcoming the spouse home.

Reunion phase. When the couple is reunited after the deployment, the reunion phase begins. As with other hoped-for events, expectations are often very high. The reality of reunion often does not live up to these fantasies. Reunion begins with a "honeymoon" phase that lasts until the first major argument. As the couple reestablishes intimacy, there are commonly feelings of euphoria and excitement. However, after the blush of the initial excitement wears off, the couple must wrestle with a period of readjustment typically for 6 to 8 weeks. This process is characterized by intermittent discomfort as the relationship is renegotiated and roles are redefined.

The Military Family in Times of War

Research on Stressors of War and the Family

In addition to the stress related to separation, a host of additional stressors on military families are invoked by war. Research on military families coping with the effects of war not only has proved beneficial to the military but also has advanced our understanding of families under stress. Lavee and Ben-David (1993) have summarized the enormous impact on family stress theory spawned by research attempts on families' reactions to war. They cite the strong influence that World War II had on Reuben Hill's (1949) development of the ABCX model to explain a family's crisis in response to a stressor event. They also note that studies on coping in families of prisoners of war and those of military personnel missing in action (Boss 1977, 1980; Nice et al. 1981) led to McCubbin and Patterson's (1983) formulation of the double ABCX model of family postcrisis adaptation and adjustment, in addition to Boss's (1977) development of the boundary ambiguity concept in family stress theory.

War-related military family research has generally focused on three issues: the effects of father/son absence on the family, the family's concerns about the soldier's safety, and the effects of postdeployment reunion on the family (Lavee and Ben-David 1993). Special subpopulations of military families have been studied, namely, families of prisoners of war and families in which a father is missing in action (Hunter 1986; McCubbin et al. 1975). The impact of the father's death or injury on his family has also been the subject of investigation. More recently, studies of the effect of a soldier's PTSD or combat stress reaction on families and spouses have been initiated (Rosenheck 1986; Z. Solomon 1988). The changing demographics of the military suggest that future researchers will need to address the impact of the death and injury of mothers on children and husbands as well.

Family Experiences in Operation Just Cause

Some of the stressors experienced by families when loved ones are in combat were evident during and in the aftermath of Operation Just Cause. Families of elite Army units deployed to Panama during Operation Just Cause expressed anger at the secrecy involved in not revealing information about the soldiers' mission (Scurfield and Tice 1992). They also described feeling angry and confused about the perception that their soldier/spouse gave the military higher priority than the family. Fears were expressed that their spouse would be psychologically scarred by his or her experience in Panama as they believed had happened to Vietnam War veterans. The family members reported heavy consumption of news about the war; interestingly, they felt the news exacerbated their anxiety and depression. Some spouses had nightmares that their spouse would be maimed or killed, and others employed the defense of denial, not entertaining any thoughts of possible harm to their spouse. Many reported that they feared going to a military mental health facility because it might hurt their spouse's career or anger him or her.

Upon the return of the soldiers from Operation Just Cause,

clinicians noted additional themes. Many voiced anger that the returning veterans received all the attention and support, while the sacrifices endured by the veterans' families were not acknowledged. Some families were also concerned and perplexed by the symptoms displayed by some of the servicemembers: isolation, moodiness, disrupted sleep, and detachment (Scurfield and Tice 1992).

The Persian Gulf War and American Military Families

Because reserve elements were activated during Operation Desert Shield/Storm, the impact of the Persian Gulf War was experienced not only by families who were full-time members of military communities but also by reserve and National Guard families embedded in civilian communities throughout the country. Although many of these organizations had family support groups, these groups were hampered by geographical distance. Moreover, some segments of the reserves may have been at higher risk. Families of personnel assigned as Individual Mobilization Augmentees (IMAs) may have been especially vulnerable to a perceived lack of support. Because these individuals are not assigned to specific reserve units, they are not automatically a part of any support or outreach program (Pehrson and Thornley 1993).

Ninety percent of military families are headed by women in the event of a war. Although women have been posited to be more likely than men to respond in a supportive manner during times of stress (Kessler and McLeod 1985), women also may experience strong social supports as burdensome. This seems to be especially true after a traumatic event (S. D. Solomon et al. 1987). Wives also may be heavy consumers of news on trauma. A. A. Cohen and Dotan (1976) found that during the 1973 Arab–Israeli War, there was more intensive use of both interpersonal and mass communication by women. Exposure to such news may be stressful in itself.

Single-parent households may be especially vulnerable to the stress of deployment. During the Gulf War, special concerns were raised about the effects of war on children left by their primary caretaker either through the deployment of both active-duty parents or the single parent. During Operations Desert Shield/Storm, approximately 22,895 single parents (including reservists) deployed, and it is estimated that 32,048 children were affected by the deployment of their single parents (Department of Defense 1992). Joint service marriages in which both parents deployed (both active and reserve elements) were estimated to involve 5,706 couples and 4,656 children. Additionally, with the increased role of women in the military, the phenomenon of women deploying to war and leaving husbands home to care for families occurred on a broader scale than ever before. Little is known about the effects of deployment on those families in which fathers assumed both parental roles.

During the Gulf War, advances in communications presented new opportunities and dilemmas for servicemembers and their families. CNN broadcasts brought the war into living rooms in "real time." This round-the-clock reporting created a new set of stressors for Americans, who were bombarded by scenes reflecting the horror of war. The new technology has created a powerful stressor, the effects of which have not yet been well studied.

There may be populations who are especially vulnerable to adverse effects from viewing and reading the news of war. Safran (1993) has written of the need to observe the ways in which patients' reactions to stressful media events like the Persian Gulf War resemble their reactions to more directly experienced stressors. Psychiatric patients across a variety of inpatient and outpatient settings experienced worsening of their conditions apparently as a result of media accounts of the Gulf War (Safran 1993). Another population at risk are children—regardless of proximity to the war—who are exposed to media coverage. Viewing explicit televison images of mutilation increased the severity of Kuwaiti children's posttraumatic stress reactions (Nader et al. 1993). Still another population at risk for adverse effects from viewing extensive media coverage may be persons who have friends or loved ones "in harm's way."

Preliminary data suggest that persons who had loved ones in the Gulf saturated themselves with news. In his description of a support group formed to help individuals and families in dealing with the Gulf War, Wadsworth (1993) noted the group theme of members' "'lives being on hold'" and being "'addicted to the news' in their hunger for information and loyalty to their loved ones" (p. 68).

The "hunger for news" was observed in other populations as well. In the course of studying the effects of Hurricane Hugo, Kaniasty and Norris (1991) assessed the impact of the Gulf War on residents in four southeastern cities. Among other items, their study measured traumatic stress, relationship of the respondents to persons in the Gulf, and use of news. More than half (52%) of their sample of 833 knew at least one person serving in the Gulf, including 15% who had an immediate family member in Southwest Asia. They found that those with greater ties to the war experienced more symptoms that resembled those associated with posttraumatic stress, even after prior symptoms (which contributed very strongly to levels of traumatic stress symptoms) were controlled for. News seeking was assessed based on the frequency of following war news through television/radio, newspapers, and discussion with other people. Older age, married status, more education, and close ties to the war (e.g., having deployed relative) were associated with use of multiple media for news about the war. Interestingly, this study found that weariness of hearing about the war was more prominent among women, blacks, single persons, persons of higher occupational prestige, and persons with more psychological symptoms before the war.

The availability of telephones allowed an immediacy of communication not experienced in past wars. This increased immediacy created problems, such as when informal information and rumors were disseminated before updates were given through official channels, as often happened. Additionally, family support center workers noted instances of monthly phone bills in excess of $1000 (*Military Family*, July 1991), a crippling amount for an enlisted servicemember who earns on the order of $1500 per month.

The use of "real time" television and telephone also carried implications for casualty notification. For example, when the SCUD missile struck the warehouse in Dhahran, Saudi Arabia, television news and phone calls back to the States added considerably to the apprehension and anxiety of families and friends of individuals in the affected units. Live television coverage increases the pressure to rapidly identify casualties, which can lead to a greater possibility of misinformation being given.

Support for Military Families During the Persian Gulf War

In the Gulf War, as in previous wars, both peer-led self-help and professionally facilitated support groups were used to help spouses deal with the dilemmas posed by separation due to deployment. Group support can be helpful during peacetime as a means of sharing coping strategies and educating spouses new to the installation or to the service about the variety of services available at the particular locale. During wartime, support groups take on a new primacy, offering emotional support in addition to information. During the Gulf War, support groups were made available throughout the country to family members and friends of deployed servicemembers. In addition to military-sponsored groups, civilian agencies and individuals also offered their services, frequently without remuneration.

A Psychiatric Hospital–Sponsored Support Group

Wadsworth (1993) described his work as leader of one such group that was sponsored by a psychiatric hospital and open to the general public at no cost. The weekly meetings began approximately 1 week after the initiation of the air war. The group was composed of 10 Caucasian women, all of whom had a relative or close friend either already in the Gulf theater or slated to deploy there. Several observations made by Wadsworth are important for leaders of future support groups during war.

Serendipitously, the hospital administrator who attended the first group meeting to welcome members was a Vietnam War veteran. In this first meeting, the group members availed themselves of his consultation to discuss military issues. His sharing of information and reassurance that U.S. forces were well prepared had a reassuring effect. The unplanned success of his consultation suggests the benefits of periodic consultation from "experts" to support groups.

Several themes emerged over the course of the 15-week series of meetings. A sense of cohesion and mutual understanding with fellow group members developed that was in contrast to the frustration and disappointment caused by responses of the general community. The members had felt that they were either receiving hollow reassurance from or being avoided by the general community. The group also discussed their struggle with loyalty. They were concerned about how much time they should center their thoughts on their loved ones or on watching the news versus taking part in diversionary activities to help them cope. Existential themes were prominent in the discussion of strong emotions among the family members in the face of possible death in the Gulf. Group members contacted each other outside the group and kept apprised of absences from group. These actions seemed to facilitate the cohesion of the group.

After the cessation of hostilities, the group's focus shifted to the issues of reunion with loved ones. Their concerns echoed those expressed by families in previous wars: wondering how their loved ones would be changed by the experiences of war and how they could best talk about these issues in a supportive manner.

The group leader's level of activity in guiding the group varied considerably. The higher the group's distress, the more active a role he played. In turn, the group's distress correlated highly with developments in the war. The group was most upset when the beginning of the ground war was imminent. This group leader's report of his experiences suggests that support group leaders need to be flexible and attuned to shifting requirements in activity levels.

A Family Support Program Implemented by a Psychiatric Army Reserve Unit

Members of a psychiatric Army reserve unit based in Minnesota has described their unit's implementation of a family support program (Rabb et al. 1993). In the predeployment phase, discussions of stress management were offered as part of servicemembers' in-processing before moving on to their mobilization site. A children's support group was held to give children (ages 5 to 15 years) a chance to share their feelings and concerns. Individual, family, and command consultations were also offered during this phase.

During the deployment phase of the Gulf War, the psychiatric detachment created a stress management team that visited family assistance centers and met with families of mobilized servicemembers. The team was proactive in using telephone outreach to assess how family members were handling the separation. Recommendations and referrals were provided for family members who were in need of further assistance.

Reunification education included education on the normal reactions and adaptations to reunion, tips for improving the transition, enhancement of communication skills, and other practical advice. Although a formal assessment of the effects of the psychiatric unit's intervention was not made, many participants voiced their appreciation for the services.

Military-Sponsored Programs for Active-Duty Servicemembers

Each branch of the armed forces has its own structure for providing family support. Generally, the most basic level of support is the unit (i.e., company level for the Army, the ship for the

Navy, etc.). Support at this level usually includes the unit's chaplain, the servicemembers left behind whose duties include assisting families (referred to as the "rear detachment" in the Army), and family support groups (Amen et al. 1988). In units with successful family support programs, activities include pre-deployment and reunion briefings for family members, social functions, telephone trees, and newsletters.

At the community level (base or post) there are many formal support systems available to assist families. Army Community Service, the chaplains' Family Life Center, and mental health services are organizations typically available to assist the family. They often provide courses on child rearing, stress management, anger control, and communications skills. Each service also has publications to assist military members and their families in coping successfully with separation and the other stressors of military life.

Family support programs such as those mentioned above played a key role in helping military families cope with the stressors of deployment to the Persian Gulf. Each service has its version of a family support structure, named differently from those of the other services—for example, in the Army the support structure is referred to as the "chain of concern," a variation of the military member's structure, the "chain of command." Although medical units train for wartime mobilization, combat concerns are not predominant themes of day-to-day experience for most hospital personnel—in contrast, for example, to submariners or infantrymen. Moreover, when medical personnel leave their duty stations for another mission, the peacetime mission must still be carried out: other health care providers must take the places of those who deploy so that provision of care for the ill can be continued. Deployment, then, raises special challenges for hospital staff members and their families. An in-depth discussion of the experiences of a family support program created to provide assistance for staff and families of the National Naval Medical Center (NNMC) in Bethesda, Maryland, is presented below. This first-hand account by one of the authors (K.H.) illustrates the activation of a family support plan during Operation Desert Storm, highlighting the successes and lessons learned.

National Naval Medical Center Family Support Program During the Persian Gulf War

The NNMC is a major teaching hospital for the Navy and is familiar to most readers as the hospital where the president or members of Congress, often, are treated. Many military health care providers assigned to the NNMC are also designated to be staff for the hospital ship the USNS *Comfort*. Deployment of the USNS *Comfort* or her sister ship, the USNS *Mercy,* requires intensive staffing. Both essentially are floating medical centers. Although it is customary for physicians, nurses, and other military health care providers to be assigned temporarily to other duty stations, this usually occurs on an individual basis. With the decision to send the USNS *Comfort* to the Persian Gulf, hospital personnel from the NNMC were deployed en masse. Setting up a support system for the families of the *Comfort* personnel presented a great challenge. The NNMC focused on four primary issues in order to improve family and staff support: 1) expanding the ombudsman program, 2) creating the *Comfort* support office, 3) establishing a command family support team, and 4) creating a regional subcouncil to incorporate other military organizations in the immediate area.

Structure of the Program

Navy Family Ombudsman Program.   The Navy Family Ombudsman Program is normally the primary family support unit within any naval command. The ombudsman is a family member volunteer appointed by the commanding officer to act as the liaison between the command and the families. There is an open-door policy with the commanding officer, the executive officer (second-in-command), the command master chief (the senior enlisted member of the command), and the ombudsman.

Having completed an extensive training program, the ombudsman is on call 24 hours a day to meet the needs of the families.

Within 3 days of the initial notice of the mass deployment to staff the hospital ship *Comfort,* coverage of the ombudsman office was expanded. To meet the extra demands created by the war, four additional ombudsman were trained, bringing the total to six. Experienced Navy spouses and ombudsmen voluntarily staffed the office, working throughout the week. At other times the office was open as indicated by the events in the Gulf.

Information about deployments and the ombudsman program was distributed at every opportunity. Within the first few days, the ombudsman office received more than 2,000 calls, prompting the command to increase the number of telephone lines into the office from two to four, including a long-distance phone line. One volunteer with extensive personal experience in deployments was always available to answer questions. Ombudsmen from other commands also helped staff the office and rotated 24-hour call. As the deployment wore on, the ombudsmen played an increasingly central role in providing support to families, who used the services provided extensively. The office received more than 63,000 calls during the deployment, in addition to hundreds of walk-in visits.

Comfort **support office.** When the deployment of the hospital ship was announced, the Comfort support office (CSO) was created. The office had two, and sometimes three, active-duty Navy staff and served as the military point of contact for all deployed staff, including those not assigned to the *Comfort* (some hospital personnel were sent to other assignments to provide coverage). The CSO handled official message traffic and other military issues and played a key role in providing official information that helped minimize rumors and other misinformation.

Preparing for the mass deployment of hospital personnel represented a significant logistical challenge. Staff from many departments in the hospital worked around the clock to ensure a smooth departure of the deploying staff. An important part of preparing personnel for departure was assuring them that their families would be provided for during their deployment and, as was a common worry, in the event of their death. To facilitate preparation for deployment, the command ran "one-stop shopping" locations for deploying staff. In one room, deploying staff could go to a booth staffed by personnel experts to ensure that their pay was distributed the way they wanted and that their personnel records were current; a booth for the legal staff to address the need for wills, powers of attorney, and other special needs; a booth for immunizations; a booth to ensure that identification cards and Geneva Convention cards (cards identifying their holders as medical personnel and noncombatants) were in order; and a booth to handle sundry needs, such as dental record updates.

One of the key objectives of family support leaders before deployment was obtaining information about the families left behind. There simply were not enough staff available to ensure that the ombudsmen would receive copies of each updated form that gave information about family members. Rather than relying on official paperwork, which can be outdated, the CSO obtained voluntary next-of-kin sheets from departing servicemembers. These family information sheets included names, mailing addresses, and telephone numbers of the primary and secondary next of kin, names and birthdates of children, and space for the servicemember to add any special concerns. The information was computerized at the CSO and the sheets given to the ombudsmen. These sheets were kept in a locked cabinet and used only for official command purposes, by the ombudsmen. They were kept current, including telephone numbers at which the spouse could be reached during a trip or following a move back home to be with parents. These sheets were the single most important part of the family support program. Without them, or the computerized backup, it would not have been possible to contact the families quickly for any reason.

Obtaining accurate information about deployed friends and loved ones is a major concern for those left behind. A toll-free 24-hour message machine was maintained in the CSO. Each week there was a new recorded message from the ship and a short space to leave a message after listening. It was not uncommon to hear messages from a concerned wife who had not heard anything from her husband, asking for verification that he was still alive and well. One testimonial to the success of the outreach program was a call from the wife of a sailor who was augmented to the USNS *Comfort* from the Australian Navy!

A reserve liaison office was created to assist with both deploying reserve staff and reservists who were augmenting the staff at the NNMC. The reserve liaison office also assisted families of reserve staff assigned to Bethesda. Deployed reservists' families were added to the ombudsman rosters for support.

Command family support team. The command family support team (CFST) was established to coordinate support and identify problem areas. This team was made up of key representatives from the various elements within the command, who worked with families: command master chief; the spouses of the hospital commander, deputy commander, commander of the USNS *Comfort,* and the *Comfort*'s command master chief; an ombudsman representative from the subcouncil; chaplain; representatives from the Social Services Department (social worker), Navy–Marine Corps Relief Society, and American Red Cross; representatives from Psychiatry, Psychology, and Pediatrics services; and representatives from the reserve liaison office and the CSO.

The CFST usually met weekly. Its charter was to observe trends, identify needs, and recommend the appropriate action for family support to the command. The broad composition of the team enabled the sharing of information about the military members and families from a variety of sources and perspectives in a forum that was confidential. Information was synthesized, and a comprehensive plan of coordinated support was instituted. An important task of this group was the identification of distressed family members who required more in-depth assistance. Because of the unified efforts of this team, the family support program was immensely effective.

NNMC Area Ombudsman Subcouncil. To enhance medical/dental family support within the entire Washington, D.C., region after the initial deployment and the large demand for assistance was proven, the NNMC Area Ombudsman Subcouncil was established. It comprised ombudsman from other military organizations in the immediate area, as well as from outlying medical units from the region. The subcouncil provided broad access to families.

Family Support Activities

Meetings. The ombudsmen and the CFST participated in all predeployment briefings, informing deploying personnel that support services would be available to their families and that the services would be provided in a confidential manner, except where prohibited by law (e.g., in cases of child abuse). The ombudsmen planned and staffed weekly support meetings for children as well as adults. The support meetings were held on weekends to maximize attendance. Early meetings centered on practical issues of general interest. For example, the first meeting offered was "Care and Feeding of Your Children," followed by a meeting on a topic such as "Care and Feeding of Your Car." Special programs were offered for adolescents, who later developed their own consistent support group. A Christmas party was held in October, complete with video opportunities and pictures with Santa. One wife used a photograph taken at this event for the family's annual Christmas card, writing friends that her husband was not home to see his baby's first Christmas but that the Navy was taking good care of her.

The changing composition of the military was reflected by the fact that many of the staff deployed to the *Comfort* were women who had left behind husbands and children. However, despite the formation of a male spouse support group, few male spouses attended the support meetings. Several did call the office on a regular basis to stay abreast of the issues that concerned them.

Support groups.   Regular family meetings were supplemented with support groups for distressed individuals. Counseling staff assisted members of the CFST in running these groups. Individuals who were undergoing professional psychotherapy often tended to dominate the group discussion time, and volunteer facilitators needed special training in how to manage this situation.

Newsletters.   Monthly newsletters were sent to family members, both to those in the local area and to those living away from the metropolitan region. The newsletters contained useful telephone numbers, informational articles about deployment in general, and specific information about current events. The newsletter was a tremendous tool and source of comfort to those far away, especially for parents who had no emotional preparation for potential deployments. It also served to control rumors and to educate families about Navy procedure. For example, information was provided on what the families could expect in the unlikely event that the USNS *Comfort* or another unit sustained damage.

Rumor control.   Because the war was covered in "real time," all the time, the family support program played an important role in managing the anxieties of the families about their loved ones. News reports were sometimes inaccurate and frequently sensationalized. The CSO and the ombudsmen received many calls asking for verification of what was really going on. Many family members reported that knowing they could call for accurate information was a major source of comfort. One of the important pieces of advice provided was that it was helpful to turn off the radio and television once in a while.

Publications.   During the war, military and civilian organizations worked feverishly to distribute publications aimed at helping servicemembers and their families prepare for the stressors associated with deployment. In addition to pamphlets already in existence, new brochures were developed for the specifics of the Gulf War. Many of these publications were excellent, offering practical and helpful suggestions for spouses and children.

Educational programs for schools. In response to a specific problem and complaints that schools were not being understanding of some student's emotional needs, special presentations were made to the schools in the local area. These talks were aimed at increasing the teachers' and counselors' awareness of the military child's special needs. They also served to inform them about the military support networks available to assist the families. The schools were most responsive, with a few schools even developing their own parent-student-teacher support groups.

Telephone tree.[1] Attempts to create a telephone tree were generally unsuccessful due to privacy act considerations and time limitations. There literally were families in every state of the union, and there were insufficient resources to dedicate to the acquisition of the appropriate release-of-information forms and the organization of the lists.

Family notification. One of the painful tasks for the CFST was planning a response in the event of a mass casualty. It was felt that if a disaster were to befall the USNS *Comfort,* it would probably be of such magnitude that it would also impact many other ships and shore units at the same time. It was anticipated that the Navy's special units designed to respond to such crises, SPRINT teams, already busy, would be overwhelmed and unable to assist every group in need. In addition, the CFST projected

---

[1]A *telephone tree* is a network used to disseminate information rapidly among groups of people. Essentially, it is a roster of individuals and their phone numbers organized in a cascade. When leadership wants speedy and concise communication, it notifies a few individuals designated as primary callers, who, in turn, contact specified secondary callers on the list. The persons on the second tier then contact persons on the third tier and pass on the information, and so forth, until everyone on the list has received the information.

that in the event of a mass casualty, the NNMC would be lower in priority for assistance than other facilities and commands due to its already available medical and professional resources. For these reasons, a mass casualty plan for support of the families was created. Communication was established with the Casualty Affairs Office coordinator, specifying who, by position and not name, would do exactly what job and where. A specific location was designated for the families to assemble and wait. Various methods for "breaking the bad news" were discussed. Plans were developed, with rooms designated to be used for private counseling, provision of child care and food, and so forth. Provisional arrangements were made with the phone company that in the event of a disaster, several additional phone lines would be installed for computer terminal needs and a bank of pay phones. Plans were also developed in cooperation with local hotels for special discounted accommodations if needed. Firm plans were in place to both assist the media and control media access to the families, if they chose not to grant an interview. Families were advised that if anything did happen, they would get a call from the ombudsman, with a statement prepared and approved by the command, telling them as much as possible about what really happened and what their next step should be, whether it was to stay in place or to go to the designated area.

Reunion

When word was sent out that the USNS *Comfort* would be returning to port, the ombudsmen were able to contact more than 80% of the families to inform them when their loved one was expected home. There were mandatory reunion briefings on every Navy ship, including the USNS *Comfort.* At the NNMC, reunion briefings for family members were held; because of the short notice, however, these briefings were poorly attended but were much appreciated by those who came.

Major portions of the *Comfort*'s medical staff flew home while the ship was en route. They were met at Andrews Air Force Base and brought by bus to the NNMC. When they got off the bus, it was with a 2-week leave chit in their hands, and, for most, families were waiting inside the main lobby, ready to celebrate the safe return. Despite the uncertainty surrounding exactly when the staff would return, parents and spouses from across the country came to welcome their loved ones home. The USNS *Comfort* arrived in Baltimore, Maryland, a short time later to a large welcoming reception.

The CSO closed when the USNS *Comfort* returned. Some of their "lessons learned" were consolidated as contingency plans. The CFST continued to meet in order to monitor the "pulse" of the command. The ombudsman office gradually wound down, with fewer calls and walk-ins. By the middle of May 1991, the extra telephone lines were removed, and it was back to business as usual.

Lessons Learned

Following Operations Desert Storm/Shield, the Department of Defense sponsored joint service family support outreach teams to travel to 24 sites throughout the world to assess the effectiveness of the family support centers during the war. The teams used town meetings, interviews, and family focus groups to solicit perceptions of what had worked well and what should be improved.

Families felt that the most important aid was accurate information. Family members who had pursued information through family centers, rear detachments, support groups, and other organized support services reported that they coped relatively well with the stresses of war. Conversely, family members who did not use these formal information resources were more likely to have been buffeted by rumors and misinformation, and reported more anxiety and distress.

Getting reliable information was a challenge during the war. There were significant problems with the mail. Many units compensated for the mail problems somewhat by providing regular communication back to the rear detachments via fax, phone, or message. This information was passed on to the families through phone trees, newsletters, or recorded messages.

Although each single parent is required to have a family care plan that outlines provisions for child care in the event of deployment or other absences, many units found that many servicemembers' plans were outdated or flawed. A uniform and comprehensive instruction is needed to ameliorate some of the problems that arose during Desert Storm mobilization. Preparing families in case of deployment is clearly important. Family readiness is a key responsibility of each servicemember. Monitoring the currency of wills, the family care plan, family member ID cards, and other documents is important and clearly critical when servicemembers deploy, leaving their families behind. Predeployment and mobilization briefings for family members are clearly helpful. These are envisioned to be comprehensive, addressing benefit issues, resources available to families, and other information, as well as providing details about the deployment. These briefings will also prepare families for problems that have been experienced in past deployments (e.g., mail delays, financial consequences of relying too heavily on phone calls). It is important that in major training exercises, the family support systems also be exercised. As was noted earlier in the chapter, units in which family support systems were already in place were more successful than those in which the support groups were developed only after the initiation of Operation Desert Shield.

There are many excellent publications for health care professionals who work with military families and for military families themselves. The Office of the Assistant Secretary of Defense for Force Management and Personnel has established a clearinghouse for information about military families. The military Family Resource Center maintains a resource collection that contains model programs and training curricula for development of support programs. It also contains a research collection of journal articles, popular magazine articles, and other materials relating to military family life. The address of the Family Resource Center is as follows:

Military Family Resource Center
Ballston Centre Tower Three, Suite 903
4015 Wilson Boulevard
Arlington, VA 22203-5190
Telephone: (703) 696-5806/5807
Fax: (703) 696-1703

Conclusions

Since the Vietnam War, there have been numerous changes in today's military: there are more women holding a wider variety of jobs, the draft has been replaced by an all-volunteer force, and single-parent households are more common. As a result of these changing demographics, the military family of today differs from that of the Vietnam War era. Research is needed to maximize the ability of today's military families to adapt to the stressors of military life. In view of the changes in demographics in the past three decades, research should focus on increasing our understanding of the "new" military families and their adjustment patterns; single-parent households, dual-career military couples, and the impact of mother absence on families are all areas meriting study.

In an era of cost containment, it must be remembered that families play an important role in readiness. Resources are needed to ensure that family support programs are functional in all units. Training of key family members, unit representatives, and mental health professionals in issues pertaining to family support is important to both the active and the reserve forces. To ensure that information is up-to-date, family support programs need to be tested in conjunction with training exercises for the active-duty member. For example, when an Army National Guard unit activates for its yearly training, a telephone tree for family members could be activated to provide details about the training. Increasingly, the reserve forces will be relied upon to round out active-duty members in future operations. The special challenges associated with reserve units must be addressed.

References

Albano S: Military recognition of family concerns: Revolutionary War to 1993. Armed Forces & Society 20:283–302, 1994

Alt BS, Stone BD: Campfollowing: A History of the Military Wife. New York, Praeger, 1991

Amen DG, Merves E, Jellen L, et al: Minimizing the impact of deployment separation on military children: stages, current preventive efforts, and system recommendations. Mil Med 153:441–446, 1988

Black WG: Military-induced family separation: a stress reduction intervention. Social Work 38:273–280, 1993

Blount BW, Curry A: Family separations in the military. Mil Med 157(2):76–80, 1992

Boss PG: A clarification of the concept of psychological father absence in families experiencing ambiguity of boundary. Journal of Marriage and the Family 39:141–151, 1977

Boss PG: Normative family stress: family boundary changes across the life span. Family Relations 29:445–450, 1980

Cohen AA, Dotan J: Communication in the family as a function of stress during war and peace. Journal of Marriage and the Family 38:141–148, 1976

Cohen S, Wills TA: Stress, social support, and the buffering hypothesis. Psychol Bull 98:310–357, 1985

Department of Defense: DoD report on Title III of the Persian Gulf Conflict and Supplemental Authorization and Personnel Benefits Act of 1991 (Public Law 102-25, Title III, Part B, Section 315). Washington, DC, U.S. Department of Defense, Office of Family Policy, Support, and Services, 1992

Dinneen MP, Pentzein RJ, Mateczun JM: Stress and coping with the trauma of war in the Persian Gulf: the hospital ship USNS Comfort, in Individual and Community Responses to Trauma and Disaster: The Structure of Human Chaos. Edited by Ursano RJ, McCaughey BG, Fullerton CS. Cambridge, UK, Cambridge University Press, 1994, pp 306–329

Fullerton CS, Wright KM, Ursano RJ, et al: Social support for disaster workers after a mass-casualty disaster: effects on the support provider. Nordisk Psykiatrisk Tidsskrift 47:315–324, 1993

Goldman NL: Trends in family patterns of U.S. military personnel during the 20th century, in The Social Psychology of Military Service. Edited by Goldman NL, Segal DR. Beverly Hills, CA, Sage, 1976, pp 119–149

Hill R: Families Under Stress. New York, Harper & Row, 1949

House JS, Landis KR, Umberson D: Social relationships and health. Science 241:540–545, 1988

Hunter EJ: Families of prisoners of war held in Vietnam: a seven-year study. Evaluation and Program Planning 9:243–251, 1986

Kaniasty K, Norris FH: Some psychological consequences of the Persian Gulf War on the American people: an empirical study. Contemporary Social Psychology 15:121–126, 1991 [correction Contemporary Social Psychology 16:10, 1992]

Kessler RC, McLeod JD: Social support and mental health in community samples, in Social Support and Health. Edited by Cohen S, Syme SL. New York, Academic Press, 1985, pp 219–240

Kulka RA, Schlenger WE, Fairbank JA, et al: Contractual Report of Findings From the National Vietnam Veterans Readjustment Study. Research Triangle Park, NC, Research Triangle Institute, 1988

Lavee Y, Ben-David A: Families under war: stresses and strains of Israeli families during the Gulf War. Journal of Traumatic Stress 6:239–254, 1993

Little RW: The military family, in Handbook of Military Institutions. Edited by Little RW. Beverly Hills, CA, Sage, 1971, pp 247–270

McCubbin HI, Patterson JM: The family stress process: the double ABCX model of adjustment and adaptation, in Social Stress and the Family. Edited by McCubbin HI, Sussman M, Patterson J. New York, Haworth Press, 1983, pp 7–37

McCubbin HI, Hunter EJ, Dahl BB: Residuals of war: families of prisoners of war and servicemen missing in action. Journal of Social Issues 31(4):95–109, 1975

Military Family, July 1991, pp 1, 8 [published by the Military Family Resource Center]

Nader K, Pynoos RS, Fairbanks LA, et al: A preliminary study of PTSD and grief among the children of Kuwait following the Gulf crisis. Br J Clin Psychol 32:407–416, 1993

Nice DS, McDonald B, McMillian T: The families of U.S. Navy prisoners of war from Vietnam five years after reunion. Journal of Marriage and the Family 43:431–437, 1981

Pehrson KL, Thornley N: Helping the helpers: family support for social workers mobilized during Desert Storm/Shield. Mil Med 158:441–445, 1993

Rabb DD, Baumer RJ, Wieseler NA: Counseling Army reservists and their families during Operation Desert Shield/Storm. Community Ment Health J 29:441–447, 1993

Ridenour RI: The military, service families and the therapist, in The Military Family. Edited by Kaslow FW, Ridenour RI. New York, Guilford, 1984, pp 1–17

Rosenheck R: The impact of posttraumatic stress disorder of World War II on the next generation. J Nerv Ment Dis 174:319–327, 1986

Safran RD: Assessing stressors experienced through news media. Percept Mot Skills 76:293–294, 1993

Scurfield RM, Tice SN: Interventions with medical and psychiatric evacuees and their families: from Vietnam through the Gulf War. Mil Med 157:88–97, 1992

Segal MW: The military and the family as greedy institutions. Armed Forces & Society 13:9–38, 1986

Shumaker SA, Brownell A: Toward a theory of social support: closing conceptual gaps. Journal of Social Issues 40:11–36, 1984

Solomon SD, Smith EM, Robins LN, et al: Social involvement as a mediator of disaster-inducted stress. Journal of Applied Social Psychology 17:1097–1112, 1987

Solomon Z: The effect of combat-related posttraumatic stress disorder on the family. Psychiatry 51:323–329, 1988

Solomon Z, Waysman M, Avitzur E, et al: Psychiatric symptomatology among wives of soldiers following combat stress reaction: the role of the social network and marital relations. Anxiety Research 4:213–223, 1991

Solomon Z, Laor N, Weiler D, et al: The psychological impact of the Gulf War: a study of acute stress in Israeli evacuees. Arch Gen Psychiatry 50:320–321, 1993

Taylor SE: Health psychology: the science and the field. Am Psychol 45:40–50, 1990

Ursano RJ, Holloway HC: Military psychiatry, in Comprehensive Textbook of Psychiatry/IV, 4th Edition. Edited by Kaplan HI, Sadock BJ. Baltimore, MD, Williams & Wilkins, 1985, pp 1900–1909

Wadsworth RD: A Persian Gulf War support group: process, viability, and flexibility. Int J Group Psychother 43:63–76, 1993

8   From Citizen to Soldier: Mobilization of Reservists

Christine M. Dunning, Ph.D.

Each war contains unique elements and issues that distinguish it from other conflicts and fosters continued debate and discussion. This is also true of Desert Storm. The mobilization and deployment of a significant fighting force comprising reserve and National Guard members raised problems and issues that the military had never before needed to consider. The psychological and financial impact of military service on individual reserve and guard soldiers was not the primary concern of Command, whose major responsibility was to field a fighting force. Soldiers were expected to "give all" for country and to put aside the demands of civilian life in order to honor their military obligations. As the military continues to shift more of its assets from the active forces into the reserve and the National Guard, the effects of activating "civilian" soldiers on those servicemembers, their families, and their communities will have an impact on larger numbers of Americans. In this chapter I discuss the special challenges confronting reserve and National Guard members and their families. Lessons learned from the Persian Gulf War can better prepare reserve and National Guard servicemembers and their families for future deployments and can inform future policy.

Issues Related to the Expanded Role of the Reserve

Historically, the maxim held that "if the military had wanted you to have a family, it would have issued you one." That this maxim no longer applied by the time of the Persian Gulf War was evidenced by the deployment of a large reserve contingent to support the Persian Gulf conflict. As never before, the military was held accountable by society for the hardship and injury military service visited upon the personal life of "civilian" soldiers who had been called up for duty. Soldiers' issues were debated in the media, in Congress, and in schools, work sites, and homes across the United States. The stress of military duty in wartime, especially among part-time volunteer forces, was no longer perceived soley as the soldier's responsibility, but rather as a shared responsibility with society.

The logistical and combat issues related to fielding a reserve force must be examined so that society can better support the reserve/guard soldier. Indeed, it is society's obligation to support those who have assumed the hardship of combat duty on its behalf. Understanding the stress associated with reserve/guard combat service is important because future fighting forces will increasingly rely on this resource.

The call-up and mobilization of substantial numbers of reserve and National Guard troops to support and augment active-duty forces in the Persian Gulf precipitated considerable national discussion. Not only did policy analysts debate the readiness of reserve forces, they also expressed concern about the lives and well-being of these soldier citizens. The extensive use of reserve soldiers for whom the military was a secondary occupation engendered public comment about the impact of activation on the affected troops and their families.

Public attention focused on issues of the physical, psychological, psychosocial, and psychosomatic consequences of combat on military members, their families, and their primary employers. The public learned the danger inherent in combat encompassed more than physical threat. War stressors also included family disruption, financial difficulties, and the logistical problems associated with juggling modern family and employment commitments with military obligation. The nation as a whole recognized the importance of attending to the psychological welfare of deployed soldiers and of their families and others left behind. Considerable public debate centered around military policies that created situations contrary to prevailing societal values. These policies included sending women into harm's way, especially mothers of infants and small children. This was more apparent in reserve forces, many of which never expected to be activated.

The Decision to Activate the Reserve Force

When Iraq invaded Kuwait on August 2, 1990, it highlighted the impact of the reduction-in-force (i.e., drawdown) on military strength. The active military was deployed to the Persian Gulf by August 7, 1990. For the first time since the Vietnam War, the reserve military was alerted that mobilization was possible. On August 10, 1990, the Forces Command (FORSCOM) first indicated that presidential call-up was likely. Reserve troops had not played a major role in battle since World War II, except for a brief call-up during the Berlin crisis. Although reservists had only been nominally involved in Vietnam, many present reservists had served as active-duty personnel in that war (Summers 1992).

The military's reserve component—the Army and Air National Guard and the Army, Navy, Air Force, Marine Corps, and Coast Guard Reserves, along with the Reserve Officer Training Corps (ROTC)—comprises a mix of combat-experienced and non–combat-experienced soldiers. By 1990, 58% of the total strength of the United States Army, 31% of the Air Force, 29% of the Navy and the Marine Corps, and 32% of the Coast Guard consisted of reserves (Summers 1992). These soldiers represented the vast majority of support elements necessary to conduct war: heavy equipment maintenance, water resupply, hospital services, supply and transportation, refueling, evacuation support, and construction units. Despite the political consequences, President Bush had no choice but to activate a call-up of reserves to augment the active military for Operation Desert Shield.

The president is authorized, under the provisions in Title 10 of the U.S. Code, to call up 200,000 selected reserve members to active duty (Engelage 1991). Such a call-up can occur without a declaration of war or national emergency. Within 3 weeks of the Iraqi invasion, President Bush considered a call-up of the reserves. Exercising Section 673b, the president implemented a slow, rolling call-up instead of using other options such as accepting volunteers or invoking a "total force" mobilization (National Defense Research Institute 1992). The reserve and National Guard forces who were mobilized in support of Desert Shield and who ultimately served in Desert Storm represented the first use of this authority since World War II.

In the days following August 10, 1990, various military units received the initial alert for mobilization to implement the incremental, rolling call-up. Coast Guard personnel were included in the alert, as were the National Guard and reserve servicemembers. Selection was based on the unit's capability to perform mobilization and wartime missions and focused on personnel and equipment readiness and training status.

Between August 1990 and March 1991, approximately 227,000 reservists and guard members, including college students enrolled in ROTC, were called up. An additional 10,700 volunteered for service. A total of 1,819,000 servicemembers were available had the reserves been totally mobilized (Hiro 1992; National Defense Research Institute 1992; National Secretary for Defense Reserve Affairs 1991).

Roughly half of the activated reservists and guards (106,000) were deployed to the Persian Gulf or overseas (primarily to Germany) to backfill for overseas active-duty personnel deployed to the Gulf (National Secretary for Defense Reserve Affairs 1991). The remaining 54% of the activated reservists were assigned to various duty stations in the U.S. to augment or replace active military strength or to assist in the mobilization effort. Summers (1992) reported that a total of 143,211 Army, 34,693 Air Force, 30,548 Marine Corps, 19,119 Navy, and 990 Coast Guard reservists, representing states all across the nation, were deployed in the Desert Storm area of operation. Most were organized into 798 reserve units under the direction of the active military.

The Stress of Call-Up

Operations Desert Shield/Storm have been referred to as a "media war." Like the rest of the population, reservists and guard members followed media reports in order to gauge the likelihood of military intervention in the Gulf. These reports were an important source of information because most reservists, living in some cases hours away from their unit's base, did not have direct and continuing contact with command. Most reported spending the days, weeks, and even months following August 10th watching CNN and perusing newspaper reports for the most reliable information (Mowlana et al. 1992). It is not surprising, then, that reservists and their families reported becoming "addicted to the news" in their hunger for information (Wadsworth 1993).

> A 32-year-old reservist expressed frustration about the lack of formal communication from his command. His distance from the base (2 hours driving time) and from the closest fellow reservists contributed to a sense of living in limbo, not knowing whether or not to make serious preparations to leave. This lack of ready access to the base and a potential reserve community support system contributed to this reservist's feelings of isolation and unimportance. These feelings were heightened by the reservist's perception that there was a unit "in-group" that had received better information, whereas he felt "left out of the loop" and relied on rumors. A therapeutic intervention was created for this reservist by which he could be assisted in formulating a plan to actively pursue information. This was accomplished

through the establishment of an informal fan-out telephone chain for unit members to maintain contact, pass
information, and manage rumor.

Unlike in previous wars, our modern society does not field
troops composed of male soldiers who are the major wage earn-
ers supporting, in large part, stay-at-home wives. Today's soldiers are male and female, and either may be the major or equal
contributor to the finances of the family. When called up, reservists and guard members usually lost civilian incomes, with the
military pay being in no way comparable in amount. In a report
by the National Secretary for Defense Reserve Affairs (1991), the
finding was presented that half of the reservists interviewed experienced a drop in income because of activation. Some reservists were paid full or partial pay by their civilian employers while
on active duty, but this was far from universal. Additionally, most
all of the reservists interviewed complained that they did not
receive timely military pay while on active status. The pressure
of reduced income, burdening some already financially precari-
ous family circumstances, was a major source of concern expressed to the Department of Defense (National Secretary for
Defense Reserve Affairs 1991).

Whereas in the past a stay-at-home spouse could return to
work to supplement military pay to maintain the same family
economic level, in Desert Storm many male military personnel
already had working spouses, so augmentation was not an option. The female soldier faced the reduction of income contribution (military pay being generally less than civilian salary) to
family support because of military service. This had an impact
whether the female reservist was a single parent or part of a couple. When the reservist made payment of child support, the reduction in pay or change in military disbursement as a source of
income also caused stress, especially for the custodial parent.

In addition, deployment added additional strains to family
budgets as family services usually performed by the soldiers
(male or female) now had to be contracted (e.g., child care,
lawn maintenance, snow removal) This was especially apparent

in single-parent and in dual-reserve families (when both parents were mobilized), whether the soldier-parent(s) had to make paid arrangements for care of the children and household. It was not unusual for private practitioners, consultants, and service providers to supplement their income with the stability of reserve or National Guard employment. For many, reserve or National Guard service was seen as a side job, not a career. For others, reserve service was an obligation for costs incurred pursuing higher education. To lose or receive reduced civilian pay and to subsist on the heretofore supplemental pay of reserve duty placed some reservists in financial jeopardy. The financial stress of the loss of primary income and subsistence on supplemental income was frequently cited as the greatest stressor by reservists' families.

The values associated with society, family, and country had changed dramatically since the last major call-up of reservists in World War II. Some experienced conflict over interrupting a perceived primary obligation to family, business, or client, in order to fulfill their legal obligation and patriotic duty. Discomfort was magnified by an erosion in confidence in the government because of such events as Watergate, the Vietnam conflict, and the present state of the economy.

Families, too, experience the stressors associated with war, and these stressors often are particularly unfamiliar to, and thus possibly have an even greater impact on, families of reserve members. Historically, the soldier's family's role in military support was to "keep the home fires burning." Active-duty military families with 24-hour contact with military life afforded by living on base or in a military community understand this obligation and accept it as a way of life. Inconveniences caused by deployment are accepted and dealt with through greater support and accommodation. Yet, research has found that stress reactions surfaced in traditional enlisted/career military family members who experienced separation in the Gulf War (Wexler and McGrath 1991). Separation is much harder when the family does not perceive itself as being a part of the military and does not have support from other military families in close proximity.

Some families of reserve and guard personnel had not seriously considered that their family member would be exposed to the dangers of war. The level of concern and consideration paid to military families during Desert Storm reflected the changes in active-duty and reserve demographics.

Few studies exist regarding the impact of military conflict on wives and children of servicemen (Wexler and McGrath 1991). Even less is found to describe what happens to military dependents when family members who are female spouse or parent, or are caregivers of adult dependents or self-supporting relatives, are called up for conflict. Nearly all of the few studies that do exist focus on the physical and emotional stress symptoms experienced by active-duty military families when the male head of the family is deployed to war (Ursano et al. 1989). The families of female soldiers and reservists on active duty have not been studied in depth to date.

Wives of active-duty military personnel have reported anxiety, loneliness, anger, sadness, and worry as reactions to separation (Wexler and McGrath 1991). They also have reported physical symptoms of headaches, eating disturbances, insomnia, nervousness, distractibility, and difficulty concentrating. During the Persian Gulf War, a support group of family members of deployed active-duty soldiers expressed feelings of helplessness, hopelessness, and overwhelming stress (Wadsworth 1993). Common themes were the wish for control and predictability of the environment, and the anxiety aroused by events outside of their control.

One would expect that reserve and guard families would experience similar reactions. Indeed, it might be hypothesized that reserve and guard families would suffer more serious reactions because of the lack of a military social support system. For individuals not living in a military community, it was more difficult to locate peers who were experiencing similar challenges. On the other hand, it is possible that reserve families found a haven from stress through denial of the military role—a haven not available to active-duty families, who are faced daily with reminders of the military.

A wife of a reservist who had continued in the military after service in Vietnam reported conflict over the pressure to attend reservist family support groups. In her husband's absence during the Persian Gulf War, she assumed additional family duties and had to make ends meet on her husband's military pay, which was less than his work wages. As the spouse of a commanding officer, she was expected to participate in the support of other families. She thought of her role in relation to her husband's role as a spouse, father, and insurance agent. She resisted becoming involved in any group that, in her mind, made her a part of the military. She sought individual counseling to alleviate her stress, rather than join a group, which reminded her of the source of her stress, the military. Her therapist assisted her in accepting her new responsibilities, providing her with the time and space to accept a role thrust upon her almost overnight.

Call-up presented logistical problems of small and large proportions. The uncertainty and stress of deploying for Desert Storm stemmed from a range of decisions and responsibilities, from the more mundane, such as deciding what to pack in three duffel bags or less, to the extremely crucial, such as finding a home for one's children. The short duration between call-up and mobilization created what might appear to be minor, yet stressful, situations such as not having the chance to say good-bye in person to one's parents, family, co-workers, and friends. Some individuals faced larger issues of arranging legal and financial matters.

Reservists were dissatisfied and distressed by the short amount of advance notice received before activation. In many cases, the reservists had not anticipated the call-up. Uncertainty about the length of the call-up period added to the stress level experienced by called-up reservists, who heard rumors that the duration would be anywhere from 90 to 360 days (National Secretary for Defense Reserve Affairs 1991). In November 1990, under the authority of Executive Order No. 12727, the Secretary of Defense extended the initial 90-day activation period for reservists to 180 days (National Secretary for Defense Reserve Affairs 1991).

Not knowing their deployment destination was another source of stress for many reservists and guard members. For many, basic decisions about what to take and how to settle affairs were affected by their destination: would they be sent to the Gulf, or to Germany, or would they stay stateside? Some units were only partially activated, leaving those left behind to worry about when their call-up might occur.

Despite the lessons learned in Vietnam about the benefits of stability and group cohesion on coping with the stress of battle, deployment resulted in the break up of some reserve units and the dispersal of members to other locations. Many reservists also had the perception that maintaining unit integrity did not seem as high a priority for reservist and guard units as it was for active-duty units assigned to the Gulf. Solidarity and cohesion for these "orphan" reservists were established through work and close living conditions in their new units. Some members reported that they were assigned to jobs for which they had not been trained before arrival at their mobilization station, which further added to their stress level (National Secretary for Defense Reserve Affairs 1991). New workmates, new bunkmates, and new tasks further heightened the already stressful environment in which some reservists entered war.

Lack of time to prepare and plan was particularly troublesome for custodial parents, students in school, business owners, and self-employed individuals. A significant number of reservists came from private practice (medical personnel), from the post office, and from protective service agencies (police and fire). Many reservists and National Guard members experienced worry over obligations that could not be settled or remanded to the care of another in the period between notice and report. Although reservists were familiar with their statutory responsibility to be able to mobilize and deploy within 72 hours, the short time period between initial notification and reporting to duty (generally ranging from 2 to 9 days) was generally regarded as being inadequate. Although a 72-hour deadline may have been feasible in the past, new features of today's society make it more difficult to achieve: loss of extended families, single parenting, single adults maintaining independent households, female military membership, and private entrepreneurship. Issues such as dealing with leases, pets, contractual obligations, and so forth are more common today than during the 1940s, when the statute was created.

> A 34-year-old National Guard member sought counseling to assist her in deciding whether to seek a hardship discharge because of the strain that active duty would place on her responsibility to care for her elderly mother and on her already tenuous finances, and because of her concern that there would be no one left behind to "take care of things." She was torn between her responsibilities to her "civilian" work group, which would be overburdened by her absence, and her military unit, which would be "a man short" and might perceive her negatively if she rejected her "obligation." Because the likelihood of a hardship discharge was small, the guard member was assisted in diminishing the impact of her deployment. She was helped to research options for coverage of her family and family responsibilities and was supported in managing the stress of her situation until mobilization occurred.

Almost all reservists reported problems with winding up personal and occupational affairs before reporting for duty. When called up for duty, the 19-year-old soldier of yesteryear had only to make out a short will to dispose of his few assets and perhaps to visit home on leave before shipping out. The reservist of Desert Storm faced more complex and complicated settlement problems. For single reservists, homes and apartments had to be closed and arrangements made for security of possessions. Pet and plant care had to be arranged, without knowing whether permanent or long-term solutions were best. Agreements with landlords and roommates concerning obligations in the reservist's absence had to be negotiated. Mail had to be diverted to a responsible party. Deliveries had to be stopped and automobile storage arranged. In some cases homes had to be winterized in expectation of a long deployment over the ensuing winter months. Crime and violence in our contemporary society added to the fears that home and possessions were at risk in the reservist's absence.

Although family care plans are required to be updated yearly, many reservists had not made realistic arrangements, never having expected the type of deployment necessitated by Desert Storm. In rare situations in which family care problems could not be resolved, hardship discharges were issued. Receiving such a discharge may have resulted in feelings of guilt over letting down the unit or stress in having one's military career ended abruptly and unexpectedly.

Care arrangements for children and other dependents were especially difficult to make given the short period between notification and reporting to duty. In some cases, children could be enrolled in traditional child care facilities such as day or family care to cover the time the remaining parent was at work. For these parents, the selection of the right agency was quite stressful. In cases in which either the parent from a single-parent household or both parents deployed, the traditional workday (6 A.M. to 6 P.M.) child or family care facilities had to be supplemented with family, friends, paid strangers, or governmental agencies as interim caregivers, creating an even more stressful situation. Sometimes this required moving children hundreds of miles from home, school, and friends.

> A single-parent reservist sought assistance from a counselor because of the extreme anxiety and stress she was experiencing. She was trying to find a good placement option for her child because of her unit's deployment for Desert Shield. Although the reservist had developed a care plan, it involved sending her son to her mother, who lived in another state. The reservist had faced the realization that the plan, although fine theoretically, was not practicable. Her mother was neither physically nor emotionally prepared to accept the responsibility for a 13-year-old boy. The dilemma of providing care for her child was overwhelming for the reservist. She was assisted in constructing a plan that would place her son with another local reservist family in foster

care. This arrangement resolved many issues related to sending her son out of state, including her not wanting to overly burden her mother, as well as the financial cost, and allowed her to feel that she was still maintaining "custody" and control in a parental role. Her separation anxiety was lessened because she felt the foster family was especially attuned to her son's issues surrounding her deployment and therefore could provide the support necessary to assist him emotionally.

Parents of both sexes reported feeling as if they had abandoned their children; in some cases this was the perception of the children as well! Although the school, family, and friends may have rallied to support the child of an active-duty parent in resolving the separation anxiety resulting from parental deployment (or even the feeling associated with siblings' and friends' being sent to the Gulf), reservists did not have a comparable support system. Reports of difficulties in school, regression in skills, conflicts with peers, and displays of grief over the loss of the parent(s) further added to the parents' stress (Hobfoll et al. 1991).

A school social worker sought advice to assist in the implementation of a support group for children whose parents or siblings were being mobilized in support of Desert Shield. She felt that the worry and anxiety expressed to the teachers by affected students interfered with school performance. She thought the school should assist children in adapting to their circumstances. The social worker was quite resourceful, gaining assistance and materials from the National Guard's Office of Soldier Support and the American Psychological Association as well as other sources. Adapting school intervention plans developed by the National Institute of Mental Health for disaster situations, the social worker developed an age-appropriate support program for children and their caregivers affected by the Persian Gulf War.

Even when arrangements were not hastily made and were generally adequate, the public debate engendered by sending "mommy off to war" (accompanied in the press with pictures of a crying mother in uniform holding an infant while saying good-bye) exacerbated the feelings of guilt felt by many mothers who reported to military duty (Kater et al. 1992). Much was made in the media about women sacrificing the pleasures and responsibilities of nurturing their babies and the resultant harm that might be caused to the developing child. Among reservists, this guilt and its accompanying worries were felt to varying degrees by parents of both sexes. Because the majority of reservists were mobilized before the Christmas holiday, the distress was compounded by missing this traditional time of family togetherness. Although fathers in the armed forces have often missed out on the hallmarks of their children's lives, being absent for birthdays, special events, and stages of growth and development, in this war, some mothers, too, missed their babies' first steps, words, and teeth—all in the service of their country. Public sentiment of condemnation or disapproval of these female soldiers added to the pain already experienced by these parents.

> Although not seeking counsel for the anxiety she felt at leaving her 7-month-old daughter when mobilized in support of Desert Storm, a doctor experienced numerous physical stress symptoms that she attributed to separation anxiety. The doctor was able to intellectually identify the cause of her distress and could treat the physical manifestations, but continued to be wrought by guilt over the separation. This sense of guilt was magnified by her family's and friends' expressed disapproval over the situation. Societal values were strongly communicated to the doctor that mothers should stay home to nurture their babies and not voluntarily place themselves in situations that could cause such a separation. The doctor resolved this conflict for herself by forming a self-help support group in her unit for all parents, mothers and fathers, who were experiencing distress because of separation from their children. This prompted the military unit to recognize the need to provide some type of counseling and support for military personnel in this situation.

Most of the reservists deployed in Desert Storm came from the demographic category known as the "sandwich generation," the generation caring for children and aging parents. Hastily arranging coverage to care for elderly relatives was stressful and disruptive. Activated reserve personnel had to arrange supports for activities of daily living for adult relatives such as home health care, transportation, physical assistance with grooming and toileting, meal preparation or delivery, shopping, and even nursing home placement. This required dealing with government agencies that provide community-based services, most of which had policies and procedures (and waiting lists) that were not amenable to the immediate need for planning and service provision. Reservists noted the stress caused by bureaucratic forms and processing that added time pressure, since often they had only days or even hours to make arrangements. In some cases, the type of services being provided by the reservists to aging relatives was not available from local agencies, public or private. Old family conflicts were sometimes exacerbated as relatives squabbled over family obligations and lack of past and present support in assisting aged and infirm family members. Hard choices, such as nursing home placement, that had been avoided previously now had to be made under considerable stress to the solider, the aged relative, and other family members.

Coast Guard reservists reported expecting a 6-month tour, which seemed to cause less stress because more permanent interim arrangements could be made. In contrast, some reservists had made temporary arrangements based on the projected 90-day absence that could not be extended. Often, new accommodation had to be made at long distance. The military initially projected a short deployment, in part, hoping to preclude reservists' having to make permanent changes. They hoped to avoid the type of situation fostered by the Berlin crisis of 1961, during which some reservists—expecting to be on active duty for 1 year—closed businesses, liquidated assets, quit jobs, and moved their families, only to be deactivated in 30 days (National Secretary for Defense Reserve Affairs 1991).

The Stress of Anticipation of War

Many issues in the Persian Gulf War contributed to worry, fear, and concern. Among the most compelling were the threat of nuclear engagement, chemical warfare, long-range missile attack, and terrorist activity. Of particular significance for reservists is the finding that worry was positively associated with pre-war burnout among Gulf War soldiers (Kushnir and Melamed 1992). The stress of preparing to mobilize for war may have diminished the coping resources available to the members of the deployed forces.

The most prominent stressor related to call-up was fear of injury or death. This fear was neither uncommon nor unwarranted among reserve forces. Although many served as support personnel rather than as combatants, modern warfare rendered them vulnerable to death and injury. On February 25, 1990, an Iraqi SCUD missile landed on military living quarters, killing 22 soldiers, half of whom who were members of a National Guard unit from Pennsylvania (Vaux 1992).

Reservists were concerned about the possible use of nuclear weapons. Anxiety about nuclear exposures as a source of stress has long been documented by research (Mack 1986; Newcomb 1988). Interestingly, although Americans of all ages and both sexes report worry, women report significantly more fear and anxiety associated with the possibility of nuclear war or accident (Newcomb 1988).

Environmental health concerns in the Persian Gulf region resulted in special equipment and uniforms that were issued to reservists as they deployed from their mobilization sites (Young et al. 1992). This new and unfamiliar equipment, and the training that accompanied it, added to the stress. Prevention of heat and solar injury was emphasized to reservists. Information and training were provided about unfamiliar insect, vermin, snake bite, and parasitic possibilities (Young et al. 1992). Immunizations were provided for exotic-sounding diseases. Reservists were also briefed on the threat of enemy action utilizing nuclear, biological, chemical, and laser weapons. All of these new threats further exacerbated the stress of war, as is discussed by Fullerton and colleagues in Chapter 5 of this volume.

In research on simulated chemical warfare, Carter and Cammermeyer (1989) found a higher attrition rate, increased psychophysiological responses, and a higher rate of psychological casualty in U.S. Army Reserve personnel than had been reported in studies of active-duty, combat-experienced personnel. Unfamiliarity with the protective equipment and lack of knowledge about chemical weaponry were particular sources of stress in reservists.

The Stress Associated With Change From Reserve to Active Service

Many reservists and guard members viewed their enlistment as a great way in which to earn a little extra money, establish or increase a pension or educational benefits, procure a part-time job that fit school or work schedules, and/or get paid to socialize with friends in a setting that broke the monotony of everyday life. Few had carefully considered the commitment they were making in joining the reserve military force, never expecting that the skills they were honing in weekend and summer training sessions would be required in war. Even if thoughts of "what if" were entertained, most "part-time" servicemembers thought they would never be activated, because such action had rarely occurred since World War II.

Some reserve and guard members had very limited active-duty military experience, many being directly commissioned or enlisted into reserve service. Some members, accustomed to the part-time nature of military experience, were not prepared for belonging to the service 7 days a week, 24 hours a day. The typical long hours and intense periods of activity proved stressful, as did the loss of freedom and the need to conform to rigid schedules. The loss of autonomy and freedom of choice was particularly stressful. Unhappiness was magnified by the perception that there were inequities in service call-up and assignment policies, as well as by the inadequate state of some installations to which reservists were assigned.

The Stress of Mobilization

When one considers the losses associated with war, physical injury, disability, and death are usually the main concerns. The Gulf War was different in that the media, military leaders, and national policymakers tended to focus more narrowly on the risks associated with chemical warfare and psychological wounds. In the media, headlines such as "The Military Expects More Psychological Wounds Than Physical" appeared, and there was speculation as to the consequences of various types of chemical weapons.

Moreover, the effects of Vietnam War service had been widely publicized. Representations in the television and movie industry—in television programs such as *China Beach* and movies such as *Platoon* and *Coming Home*—depicted the wide range of war's consequences. These programs and movies showed war's impact on a veteran's ability to sustain interpersonal relationships, on parenting style, and on general mental health.

The high-tech nature of the war that was forecast, in which the servicemember was removed from the fray by operating from afar (hence, the "joystick war" moniker), belay the real threat experienced by all servicemembers, and perhaps particularly reservists. Because reservists and guard members generally served as support staff rather than as combatants, many overlooked the risks they faced.

War-related stress for reservists was predicted to result from issues surrounding call-up and mobilization rather than battle. Public debate centered on the issue of women in combat or on the impact of separating mothers from infants, with the focus on duty to care for one's child rather than on the horrors of combat. Loss became defined as the loss of family for however short a duration, the loss of nurturing of a parent, or the loss of financial security or civilian career, rather than the loss of life.

One exception, however, was in the area of the potential for chemical exposure; this threat was treated with the same anxiety as the possible consequences of nuclear attack. The unknowns of the use of chemical weapons resulted in the same worry, fear, and stress that are occasioned by toxic and nuclear accidents. In addition to concern about chemical weapons, there were also worries about environmental exposures to chemicals. In the 15 years before the Gulf War there was much public debate and medical research on the consequences of chemical contamination in war. Research on Agent Orange and the use of other defoliants had sensitized the American public to the potential dangers of chemical exposure—not only to the soldier but to the soldier's family as well. Families suffer with the soldier, experiencing the pain of infertility and fearing genetic abnormalities in offspring. Families of deploying personnel, in particular, feared a repetition of the legacies of chemical contamination experienced by those serving in Vietnam.

> Upon being issued protective gear for chemical warfare, a 24-year-old National Guard member sought counseling for her distress over her call-up for Desert Shield. She reported having nightmares of giving birth to deformed children. The guard member was knowledgeable about the controversy surrounding Agent Orange, because her father had served in Vietnam and her mother had followed the reports of the herbicide's putative effects on soldiers and their progeny. Receiving the protective gear and attending training sessions on response to chemical warfare had precipitated a fear that her own health and fertility might be compromised and that her future children might be affected. Far from being concerned about the possibility of her own death, the soldier became overwhelmed with the conviction that deployment to the Gulf would result in the termination of her ability to conceive and bear healthy children. The soldier was provided additional information about the possible chemical agents that might be used in

the Gulf. She also received additional training in the use of
the protective gear to familiarize her with it and to increase
her faith in its effectiveness. Desensitization to the gear was
accompanied by stress management training to help her
manage stress responses to her anxiety. Her sergeant will-
ingly assisted in these efforts, which strengthened the soldier's faith in her commanders.

The reluctance of President Bush to mobilize the reserves
attested to the sensitivity of exposing reservists to the threats
enumerated above. The expectation of a "joystick war" lulled
the American public into an expectation that soldiers would return safe and sound. Thus, attention was not focused on grief
and bereavement but rather on the stress caused by disruption
and hardship (Hobfoll et al. 1991).

On a more practical level, a frequently cited stressor for reservists was the substantial cut in salary experienced upon activation. A survey of reservists conducted by the U.S. General
Accounting Office (National Secretary for Defense Reserve Affairs 1991) found that one-half of those interviewed had a drop
in income, with the remainder either earning more or earning
about the same after they were mobilized. Because this study
included only 40 reservists, these statistics cannot be taken to
be representative of the total deployed reservist force (National
Secretary for Defense Reserve Affairs 1991).

An initial problem with processing pay records caused a delay in pay and travel reimbursement during the first few weeks
of mobilization, which exacerbated the stress and worry about
meeting financial obligations. Bills could not be paid on time.
Fear of losing a home or car, losing investments in business or
education, and being unable to provide for one's family were
constant worries for some reservists. Those in independent professional fields or who were self-employed tended to be affected
most sharply. One painful remedy was to request a financial hardship discharge; however, such requests were generally denied.
On the other hand, some reservists and guard members had financial hardship alleviated (or, on occasion, benefited) by employ-

ers that, as a matter of policy, continued to pay benefits or offered to pay the difference between civilian and military salaries.

Another source of monetary relief came from the many financial institutions, particularly banking and mortgage institutions, that had policies in place or created new policies to suspend or reduce required payment obligations for the duration of the deployment. These policies were vital for many servicemembers; indeed, the most frequently cited fear among reservists and guard members and their families was the potential loss of their home through nonpayment of the mortgage. Mortgage institutions that voluntarily initiated a payment freeze for reservists and guard members were heralded in the press. Other such ad hoc policies were promulgated by other institutions as well, including tuition reimbursements by colleges and universities and credit extensions for affected military families. However, it must be noted that not all activated military personnel benefited from these policies, and as a result, many of those that did not experienced severe financial distress.

Congress, too, was sensitive to the financial hardships experienced by reserve and guard personnel. It addressed the issue of retroactive benefits and protection (which resulted in, e.g., the Persian Gulf Benefits Act, Fiscal Year 1991 National Defense Authorization Act, Uniformed Services Employment Act, and Soldiers' and Sailors' Civil Relief Act Amendment of 1991) subsequent to Desert Storm to alleviate the stress caused by financial and employment problems experienced by reservists.[1]

---

[1]The Persian Gulf Benefits Act of 1991 and the Uniformed Services Employment Rights Act of 1991 were noted in the National Secretary for Defense Reserve Affairs report of 1991. The author of the report was Paul L. Jones, Director, Defense Force Management Issues, with major contributions by William E. Beusse, Roderic W. Worth, and Bobby L. Cooper. Legislation and amendments concerning reemployment/seniority rights have existed since World War II and have been reconsidered by Congress with each war/peacekeeping action. In this most recent legislation Congress spent more time on issues of activated medical personnel and private business owners' losses. They also increased the eviction protection for renters paying $1,200 or less a month (Soldiers' and Sailors' Civil Relief Act Amendment of 1991).

Because of legislation ensuring reservists' rights to return to the jobs they left, employment security, per se, was not a major concern among most reservists and guard members. However, those activated continued to be stressed by employer's reactions to their military obligation and by whether the "same or similar" job would be available to them upon deactivation. Time spent on active duty was seen as "out of sight, out of mind" in terms of promotion or job assignment. Those away from the job during the traditional period for raises or performance evaluation were concerned about the possibility of being "passed over" or "downgraded" as their loyalty to the employer might be seen as compromised by military obligations.[2]

> A 49-year-old reservist expressed job-related concerns. His company was "down-sizing" in his absence. He feared that his age, military obligation, and absence might result in a decision to terminate his employment or eliminate his position. He worried that his absence might not be felt sufficiently and that the company would conclude it could do without his services. He felt that his age might make him more expendable, especially because the gossip was that he was feathering his military pension with this duty. Even if he were retained, he was concerned that promotional opportunities would be foreclosed because of a perception that he "jumped ship" during a time of company crisis.
>
> The soldier was encouraged to continue communication with his company while on active duty. This was accomplished by arranging to receive newsletters, important memos, and updates prepared by volunteers. This intervention alleviated his anxiety, allowing him to correspond with co-workers about work-related issues and thereby maintain a work connection.

---

[2]Reservists told the author that they believed they were passed over for promotion or plum assignments while they were gone and that they lost ground in terms of reward opportunities as employers based such decisions on "What have you done for me lately? Since you were off this winter enjoying the warmth of a 'foreign vacation,' why should I consider you now over others who worked hard in your absence, especially people who did your job while you were gone?"

Once mobilized and deployed, some reservists found that their anxiety over being exposed to combat in the Persian Gulf gave way to the embarrassment of finding themselves assigned to nondangerous locations. For example, stories were told of the "stress" of sleeping six to a condo in Kansas or of skiing in Germany while replacing active-duty personnel assigned overseas. Other reservists were called up to staff mobilization/staging stations or served increased guard duty at military reserve and National Guard facilities in response to fears of terrorism. In some cases, reservists and guard members did not even have to leave home. Reservists who worked extended hours to ensure base security stateside were not afforded the same status as that afforded to those who were deployed to the Gulf. Yet, their families and their role in relation to civilian life were also affected by separation, financial hardship, and worry over future military demands. Many reservists and guard members reported suffering from guilt over not serving overseas or not having been inconvenienced by active-duty call-up. Some felt that there was a difference in level of support and services for those who served in the Gulf and those who served at home. Additionally, some reservists reported instances of feelings of internal organizational prejudice against reservists, especially those serving stateside.

> One reservist reported aggravation as his parents proudly extolled the military service of his brother deployed in the Gulf but dismissed his own deployment in Missouri as inconsequential and without sacrifice or hardship. In the eyes of his family, the lack of danger associated with serving as a replacement for an active-duty member negated his contribution to the war. The reservist was encouraged to educate his parents about his Desert Storm efforts. This included talking about the steps he had taken to respond to the hardships imposed by his service. He was instructed to ask his parents for support in his endeavors rather than complain about their behavior. This intervention worked: once informed, his parents responded supportively by letter and telephone.

Mobilization also resulted in problems ranging from jet lag to the threat of terrorism. Reservists and guard members were confronted with the fact that they were "not in Kansas anymore," a dramatic departure from the relative security and stability of their previous living arrangement. Getting used to military routine, the loss of privacy and freedom, and the confines of communal living further exacerbated problems faced by reservists.

The Stress of Reunion and Reintegration

Upon deactivation, the same reservists interviewed for this chapter reported that the camaraderie that had fostered cohesion now represented a source of sadness. For up to 8 months the troops had worked, eaten, bathed, and lived together. Staying in facilities where people lived 18 inches from one other resulted in the sharing of mail, reading materials, thoughts, fears, and feelings. The extraordinary bonds that developed now had to be loosened or separated. The course of readjustment depended on the extent to which the reservist experienced combat and trauma in war, the extent to which he or she was placed under emotional strain because of active service, and the extent to which the decisions made in response to deployment added to stress. Social support from families, friends, co-workers, and the American public reduced the stress associated with financial loss and occupational setbacks.

Conclusions

By its very nature, war is stressful. It is not possible to avoid much of what caused stress for reservists. The decisions and actions in preparation for war cannot be completely anticipated, nor can laws and policies be constructed to address all issues that accompany call-up and mobilization. Policy must recognize that reservists and National Guard members will experience stress associated with settling personal affairs and anticipating combat. Stress inoculation training and support programs should be developed to reduce distress and bolster positive coping mechanisms. Families of reservists and guards must also be provided with support in problem resolution and in stress reduction. Our society assumes that if programs and benefits are available, people will avail themselves of these services, yet this is often not the case. Following a disaster or any catastrophic event, individuals often do not avail themselves of support. In times of mobilization, just as in times following disasters, an active outreach program must be implemented.

The private sector made important contributions through provision of resources to address stress and related issues precipitated by military call-up. Future efforts should be devoted to planning the types of services that should be offered to military personnel and their families. Outreach programs should be designed to provide better information on where individuals can go to receive help for problems that surface.

The military must recognize that as painful as it is for an individual to make the transition from civilian to soldier, it is also painful for the family. Often, these families do not feel a sense of belonging to the military community. Similarly, it is easy for the active military community to overlook these new family members. It is vital that the military expand its ability to identify and support the families of reserve and guard personnel.

The transition back to civilian status and integration back into the workplace are also difficult. It should be recognized that some of the concerns of civilian life cannot be turned off or deferred during wartime, nor can civilian life be easily reentered. The stressors affecting the soldier and the soldier's family have an impact on the ability of reservists to perform their duties. To increase readiness, the offices of soldier and family support need to be strengthened and increased in importance. The military must recognize the trend in private business that Employee Assistance Programs reaps great benefit to any occupational effort, increasing performance and productivity, improving morale, and retaining well-trained and qualified personnel.

Issues such as the inability to meet the mortgage or to pay back the government for a student loan for tuition as a result of military service should be placed on the public agenda—by Congress or by the armed forces—but not be debated in the press. The media should be educated on how they could better support families and children affected by military service. Similarly, the adverse effects of media coverage on servicemembers and their families need further attention. Preoccupation with "Ain't it awful" and "How could they" journalism showing tearful uniformed mothers saying goodbye to children exacerbates the anguish and does not promote constructive dialogue.

Interestingly, some of the worst offenders in exacerbating parental guilt came from the very professionals whose advice they sought: child psychiatrists, pediatricians, and school personnel. It is more productive to debate public policy concerning financial protection, maternal separation, and obligation under peacetime conditions than to allow such debate to fuel and increase the stress associated with war. Public debate during the war does little to improve the situation. Programs of education, support, and counsel need to be available to all military members, whether they are deployed in combat zones or in support positions.

The decision to rely in large part on a "civilian" military force through the use of reserve and guard soldiers in Desert Storm showed rather effectively that the military as an organization no longer stands separate and apart from the mainstream of society. Rather than being an isolated entity that can easily pick up and move into action with little consequence to the people and community left behind, the military and its personnel have become integrated into the fabric of everyday life. As such, the absence of full-time and reserve armed forces personnel not only is missed but also creates problems that are unique. The continued down-sizing of our active armed forces and the increased reliance on reserve and National Guard units to field a fighting force present new challenges. Schools, financial agencies, human service organizations, and religious institutions should develop and provide services that respond to the needs of military personnel and their families.

Rather than relying on the military to "take care of their own," civilian agencies and professionals must acquaint themselves with the problems of deployment and reintegration of "civilian" soldiers. Programs for support and treatment must be developed *during peacetime* rather than being left to develop in an ad hoc, informal manner only when war appears imminent. The military family and the public need to be educated about what can be done to prevent stress and to resolve those stressors that are amenable to resolution.

With increased reliance on reserve and guard forces, military service is now very much integrated into community life across the nation. We can no longer assume that the military will take care of its own, because the "own" are ours, too. Though each war will be unique in some respect, general plans can be developed ahead of time that can be modified to handle these differences. Schools should develop separation and reunion support programs to institute in the event of mobilization. Mental health personnel need to acquaint themselves with military and combat stress issues and their treatment. Society must be educated to consider what it does to create and exacerbate the stress felt by those serving in combat to protect them and what it can do to alleviate some of these burdens.

Going to war is inevitably stressful, and so is coming home. Society, the government, and the military should address the sources of stress and implement programs to reduce its deleterious consequences. Reunion and reintegration back into civilian life bring their own stresses. It must be recognized that the effects of war do not end when the bullets stop flying; continued counsel and support should be given to soldiers who are experiencing difficulties in transition.

References

Carter B, Cammermeyer M: Human responses in simulated chemical warfare training in U.S. Army Reserve personnel. Mil Med 154:281–288, 1989

Engelage JR: Operation Desert Shield: The Deployment of Reserve Component Units to the Persian Gulf, 1990–1991. Fort Sheridan, IL, Fourth U.S. Army, 1991

Hiro D: Desert Shield to Desert Storm: The Second Gulf War. New York, Routledge, 1992

Hobfoll S, Spielberger C, Breznitz S, et al: War-related stress: addressing the stress of war and other traumatic events. Am Psychol 46:848–855, 1991

Kater V, Braverman N, Chowera P: Would provision of child care for nurses with young children ensure responses to call-up during a wartime disaster? Journal of Emergency Nursing 18:132–134, 1992

Kushnir T, Melamed S: The Gulf War and its impact on burnout and well-being of working civilians. Psychol Med 22:987–995, 1992

Mack J: The conditions of collective suicide and the threat of nuclear war. Bull Menninger Clin 50:464–479, 1986

Mowlana H, Gerbner G, Schiller H: Triumph of the Image: The Media's War in the Persian Gulf. Boulder, CO, Westview Press, 1992

National Defense Research Institute: Assessing the Structure and Mix of Future Active and Reserve Forces. Final Report to the Secretary of Defense. Santa Monica, CA, Rand Corporation, 1992

National Secretary for Defense Reserve Affairs: Operation Desert Shield: Problems Encountered in Activated Reservists. Washington, DC, General Accounting Office, 1991

Newcomb M: Background, personality, and behavioral correlates of nuclear anxiety. Personality and Individual Differences 9:379–389, 1988

Summers HG: A Critical Analysis of the Gulf War. New York, Dell, 1992

Ursano RJ, Holloway HC, Jones D, et al: Psychiatric care in the military community: family and military stressors. Hosp Community Psychiatry 40:1284–1289, 1989

Vaux K: Ethics and the Gulf War: Religion, Rhetoric, and Righteousness. Boulder, CO, Westview Press, 1992

Wadsworth R: A Persian Gulf War support group: process, viability, and flexibility. Int J Group Psychother 43:63–76, 1993

Wexler H, McGrath E: Family member stress reactions to military involvement separation. Psychotherapy 28:515–519, 1991

Young R, Rachal R, Huguley J: Environmental health concerns of the Persian Gulf War. J Natl Med Assoc 84:417–424, 1992

Deployment From Europe: The Family Perspective

James A. Martin, Ph.D, B.C.D.
Mark A. Vaitkus, Ph.D.
Malcolm D. Johnson, M.S.
Louis M. Mikolajek, M.S.
Donna L. Ray, M.S.W.

Military families living in Europe at the outbreak of the Persian Gulf War faced challenges in addition to those experienced by military families back home in the States. For many, their closest support systems lay thousands of miles away and were quickly accessible only through expensive long-distance calls. Families left behind in Europe also experienced the threat of terrorism to a much greater degree than did stateside families. Moreover, the Gulf War occurred at an especially stressful time for military families in Europe. The end of the Cold War and efforts to reduce expenditures resulted in the rapid drawdown of American forces in Germany and the downsizing of the American military, in general, creating an atmosphere of apprehension and anxiety.

It was against this backdrop of rapid change and uncertainty that American forces in Europe deployed to Southwest Asia. To

The views of the authors do not necessarily reflect the position of the Department of the Army or the Department of Defense (para 4-3, AR 360-5). This chapter is an expansion of an article that originally appeared in *Military Review* in April 1993.

carry out the United Nations plan to liberate Kuwait, the United States Army was required to deploy the VII Corps from Europe to Southwest Asia. Between November 1990 and January 1991, more than 79,000 soldiers departed Europe for the Southwest Asia combat zone. Approximately 54% of the soldiers in the VII Corps were married. Most had their families living with them in Europe. In total, more than 89,000 family members were left behind in Europe.

Sending servicemembers from Europe to Southwest Asia required planning and executing support for the families they left behind. Recognizing the unique stressors involved, military commanders in Europe placed high priority on providing support programs to these especially vulnerable families. In this chapter we discuss U.S. Army Europe (USAREUR) family support programs during the Persian Gulf deployment and the responses of the family members to this assistance.

Background

Since the 1960s American military families have been living in large numbers on military bases in Europe, primarily in Germany. During the 1970s and 1980s, with the adoption of the all-volunteer military force and the corresponding increase in the number of young married servicemembers, U.S. military communities in Germany took on the look and character of uniquely American communities. Complete with their own housing, schools, shopping centers, hospitals, social service agencies, and recreational facilities, these "little Americas" were thought to provide young American military families with the support and services required to cope with the many stressors associated with military life in a foreign culture. In addition to long duty hours, soldiers were often away from home days and weeks at a time for training exercises, leaving their spouses and children on their own in a strange and foreign setting. For some spouses, the Atlantic Ocean also seemed like a colossal barrier, and the perceived separation from extended family and familiar friendships posed a threat to well-being. Military communities provided an island of safety and security for these families.

As the 1990s began, with the fall of the Berlin Wall, the demise of the Soviet Union, and the evolution of democracy in portions of Eastern Europe, life was beginning to change dramatically for military families in Germany. The demands of military life and the stressors associated with overseas life were being overshadowed by the consequences of the so-called peace dividend, the drawdown of U.S. forces in Europe and the downsizing of the U.S. Armed Forces. Military members and their families saw ongoing unit inactivation announcements and lists of installation closures. The possiblity of being unemployed was real. In addition, the word from the States was that the economy was suffering and there was increasing unemployment. Everyone, across all ranks, felt uncertain about the future. It was in the context of these everyday stressors of military life in USAREUR that military leaders and families alike came face-to-face with the totally unexpected: the deployment of American forces to Saudi Arabia and the need to support and sustain a large population of unaccompanied family members for a prolonged period in an overseas setting. No one had ever planed for this contingency.

The U.S. Army Europe Deployment to Southwest Asia

Following the November 1990 announcement of USAREUR deployments to Southwest Asia, the decision was made to keep affected Army families in Europe. From a practical standpoint, it was physically and financially impossible to manage a mass exodus of families to the United States, especially while there was an all-out push to deploy a corps to Southwest Asia. In most cases, trying to return families to the U.S. would also have placed the spouses and children under enormous additional stress. Many did not have extended families who were willing and/or capable of taking them into their homes. Housing was not available at military installations in the States. Leaving Europe would also have involved additional personal and family disruption for spouses and children (e.g., loss of spouse employment, children changing schools). In addition, family members would have lost the support of their military member's unit, their established community and neighborhood, and the critical unit-based communication links. Each Army family in Europe has a written plan for evacuating itself (noncombatants) back to the U.S. in case of war. However, because Operation Desert Shield/Storm did not occur within Europe, the support provided by local Army communities could be sustained. With all this in mind, unit and community leaders placed a priority on providing local family support.

The families of nondeploying soldiers (more than half of the USAREUR force did not deploy) also faced increased and new stressors. For example, there were increased work hours in support of the deploying forces, and the ever-present threat of terrorism. The support strategy was fashioned around building "layers of support" to ensure that everyone (deployed and nondeployed) would be taken care of during the crisis. The plan called for erring on the side of duplication and overlapping of services to ensure that a "family safety net" was in place for all (Table 9–1).

In November 1990, the Family Support Task Force was established. This task force was chaired by the Chief of the Human Resources Division of the Office of the Deputy Chief of Staff for Personnel. This is the equivalent of the human resources office in a state governor's office. The task force met biweekly until the end of the Desert Storm period. After this time the task force continued to meet monthly until August 1991, to ensure support for the families of soldiers who remained in Saudi Arabia and Kuwait, and the soldiers deployed to Operation Provide Comfort, a follow-on United Nations effort to provide protection and aid for the Kurdish people threatened by the Iraqi military after Operation Desert Shield/Storm.

Members of the Family Support Task Force included key USAREUR staff and subordinate commands, as well as family

Table 9–1.   U.S. Army Europe family support services

Unit-based support	Community-based support
Rear detachment	Army Community Service
Family support group	Community chaplain
	Neighborhood Mayor Program
	Red Cross
	Hospital/clinic personnel
	Mental health services
	Legal Affairs Office
	Community Commander's Office
	Family housing

Note.   Many military communities established a "one stop" family assistance center that centralized all of these programs in one location to help ease and improve access.

member representatives from major military communities and units throughout USAREUR. Over the course of the deployment, this task force initiated more than 100 policy and/or program actions to address a broad range of family issues. More than anything else, the task force was a place to brainstorm good ideas. Regardless of existing military rules or regulations, the ideas received serious consideration. Creative solutions to common problems were freely shared across major subordinate command boundaries. Many of the "good ideas" were shared with military family support officials in the U.S. for possible adoption in units and communities at home, including the Army Reserves and the National Guard. The task force had the ear of the USAREUR commander in chief, and it operated with a "can do" attitude. Critical members of the task force (from public affairs to legal personnel) were able to quickly implement worthwhile suggestions.

Among its many accomplishments, the task force created a USAREUR-wide "Helpful 1" hot line. This call-in resource, staffed by volunteers in each community 24 hours a day, 7 days a week, allowed family members (and nondeployed soldiers) to ask questions or raise concerns anytime of day or night. The hot line reinforced the fact that there would always be someone to listen. The task force also established guidelines for the use of government vehicles (primarily passenger vans) for family support functions, instituted limited base support privileges for extended family members acting *in loco parentis* (primarily access to installation shopping and limited medical care), publicized how to obtain reimbursement for volunteer expenses associated with family support activities, and obtained permission for family members to use military dining facilities. Each of these efforts promoted group contact and informal social support among families.

Multiple Assessment of Family Support Issues

Community Assessment Team Visits

To better understand the contribution of community support, a series of assessments were intitiated. The USAREUR Inspector General Community Support Assessment Team visits included individual and group interviews with unit leaders, community leaders, and family members. The visits were carried out by a team of staff members using a purposively selected sample of communities that had been affected by the deployment. The team found that, by and large, the family support groups were in place and that rear detachment and community agencies were working hard to support their families. In most cases, the family support group leader was not a "volunteer"; rather, the group leader was usually the spouse of a senior unit leader. Often, the group leader assumed this role based on her husband's position rather than on her own desire or ability. Sometimes this dual status as the commander's wife and the group leader caused conflict with the unit's rear detachment commander (e.g., "Who is really in charge here?"). In addition, some junior enlisted wives felt "left out" by this leadership structure.

Typically, a small core group of family members seemed to be doing all the work. Some of the leaders and the members appeared overburdened. Roles were not always clearly defined among the group leaders, the rear detachment commanders, the chaplains, and the array of other community helpers involved in the family support activities. Some family support group leaders complained that they had received little training in community support services for family members. Finally, a few family support group leaders experienced frustration in trying to meet the needs of a small number of demanding and dependent family members.

Nearly all communities pooled their helping resources into a "one stop" family assistance center (FAC). These FACs were resourced and tailored to meet the informational and practical assistance needs of the deployed soldiers' families. Some Family Support Task Force members were concerned that existing community agencies (e.g., Army Community Service, Red Cross, Chaplains' Programs) lost their unique identification and that nondeployed families sometimes felt their needs were unimportant because of the constant focus on "deployed spouses." The Family Support Task Force noted that a few communities set up large, 24-hour–a–day centers when there was no need for this level of effort. It also noted burnout among some individuals when they tried to operate the FAC single-handedly.

Information flow to and from Southwest Asia was the major concern of the family members of the deployed soldiers. Delayed mail was a major problem. Family members often felt confused by the various (and frequently changing) official and unofficial guidance on mail restrictions. They had little confidence in alternative means of communication (fax and e-mail). Once direct AT&T lines were established from Southwest Asia to Germany, commercial telephone calls (from their deployed spouse) became the most reliable (if not always accessible or affordable) means of communication.

The commercial calls could provide rapid information, but they were also expensive for the family and presented possible security problems. There was serious concern among military leaders that a soldier in the theater of operations might inadvertently divulge important intelligence information in a call home—information that might be overheard by enemy intelligence operatives. There was also concern that unrestricted telephone access might increase rumors and, importantly, undermine reliance on the official casualty notification system. Many were concerned that a family member in Germany might hear of his or her spouse's death or injury inadvertently or that the family member might receive inaccurate information concerning his or her spouse's status. Phone costs did become a significant problem for some families. Fortunately, serious security problems did not occur. Also, the number of casualties was not large, and the casualty notification system was able to operate as intended.

Overall, family members were satisfied with unit and community support. Partly because of the availability of such support, very few family members elected to return to the U.S. either just before or during the deployment (approximately 7% to 8% returned). The Family Support Task Force noted the financial problems that were arising for some families because of the increase in telephone credit card bills resulting from calls to family and friends in the U.S. and calls from spouses in Southwest Asia. The task force also found that family members of deployed soldiers who had been attached to another unit were at special risk of not being adequately supported. There were also a few cases in which the soldier's unit had been inactivated (gone out of existence as part of military downsizing) after the soldier had been attached to another unit and deployed with this new unit. As a new member in a unit, or no longer officially attached to a unit, the family often had no local unit support.

Family Support Group Leaders Survey

In March 1991, a study of family support group leaders was conducted by the U.S. Army Medical Research Unit—Europe. The study was based on an anonymous mail survey of the family support group leaders (see preceding subsection). The survey was designed to elicit the group leaders' experiences in maintaining group activities and communication with family members, as well as perceptions of support from the unit's rear detachment (elements left behind) and the community agencies. A total of 442 sets of the survey were distributed to randomly selected family support group leaders. The response rate was 48%, representing responses from 83 company and 48 battalion family support group leaders, for both combat and support units.

Closed and open-ended survey questions were used to explore a variety of issues, including the leaders' demographic characteristics, the structure and operation of their family support groups, and relationships with unit and community leaders and service agencies. Family support group leaders were asked about the positive and negative aspects of their role as a group leader and the impact on their own well-being. Finally, they were asked to comment on the adaptation of family members to the stress of the Operation Desert Shield/Storm deployment. The information presented here focuses on the women operating at the two key levels of the unit support program, company and battalion family support groups. (A company would usually have 50 to 75 families, and a battalion, 200 to 400 families, depending on the size and type of unit.)

Based on this survey, 10% of the company and 4% of the battalion family support group leaders had been "elected" to their position. On the other hand, 51% of the company and 42% of the battalion leaders said that they were appointed because of their spouse's role (as commander or other senior leader). All of the group leaders who responded to the survey were women. The majority of respondents indicated that their unit had a family support group before the deployment to Southwest Asia and that many of the present leaders had been in the role of family support group leader for more than a few months. For example, 49% of the company leaders and 54% of the battalion leaders had held their family support group positions for more than 6 months.

The survey found that not all of the respondents were as busy with family support group activities as was expected. Only 25% of the company leaders and 40% of the battalion leaders indicated that they were working more than 15 hours per week on family support group activities. The median number of hours per week was 8 for the company leaders and 13 for the battalion leaders. Many of the leaders (46% of the company leaders and 75% of the battalion leaders) felt that their family support group activities interfered "a fair amount or a lot" with their personal life. Their open-ended comments suggested that they viewed the "unpredictability" of demands as the most difficult aspect of their role. They felt that they never knew and could not control when someone was going to call for assistance or how long a particular call might take. Personal life plans and needs often had to be put aside while they helped someone. Despite this complaint, the overwhelming majority (88% of the company leaders and 78% of the battalion leaders) indicated that they enjoyed their role as the unit family support group leader.

Most family support group leaders (95% of the company and 91% of the battalion leaders) indicated that they were able to share their burdens with other group members. The few family support group leaders who were unable to share the burden were the most likely to report feeling "burnt-out" related to the continuous demands of what appeared to be relatively few needy and/or demanding unit family members. There was also evidence that younger, less-experienced leaders in newly formed groups, who were often uncertain about what resources were available, had the most difficulty handling the leadership-related stress.

When asked about their unit's rear detachment commander, most family support group leaders surveyed were very positive. Many (52% of the company and 51% of the battalion leaders) felt that their rear detachment commander was well qualified for the task of supporting families. Only 11% of the company and 9% of the battalion rear detachment commanders were described as "not at all qualified." Seventy-eight percent of the company and 85% of the battalion family support group leaders indicated that their working relationship with the unit rear detachment commander was "excellent to good." Only 12% of the company and 11% of the battalion leaders described a "poor to horrible" relationship with the rear detachment commander. In addition, the majority of family support group leaders rated their community headquarters and agencies (e.g., Army Community Service) as helpful.

When asked in what ways their family support group efforts were successful, 77% of the company leaders and 73% of the battalion leaders indicated that the group was meeting members' emotional needs (typically defined in terms of emotionally based forms of social support). On the other hand, only 38% of the company leaders and 64% of the battalion leaders felt that the group was meeting family member information needs (typically defined as being able to provide up-to-date information on what was happening with their spouse's unit in Saudi Arabia). This distinction is important because more than 75% of both the company and battalion leaders felt that spouses attend family support meetings for information, compared with 21% and 26%, respectively, who indicated that emotional support was the primary reason why spouses attend these meetings.

Finally, when asked to comment on how unit families were dealing with the Operation Desert Shield/Storm deployment (2 to 3 months after their spouses had deployed), about 90% of family support group leaders said that they had seen very few or no serious adjustment problems among their unit's spouses. The modal response to the question "How long will family members be able to handle the separation?" was 6 months; 52% of the company and 67% of the battalion leaders gave this response. Most family support group leaders believed that if the deployment lasted longer than 6 months, the number of family problems would increase significantly.

When asked about unit spouses who returned to the U.S. to "wait out" the deployment, only 3% of the company leaders and 5% of the battalion leaders cited negative reasons for the departures. Seventy-seven percent of the company and 61% of the battalion leaders said spouses who left had returned to the U.S.

for a positive reason, typically to be with their extended family for the expected birth of a child. This was especially true when it was the first child.

Family Member Survey

A family member personal opinion survey provided another means of assessing the impact of Desert Shield/Storm on the families of deployed and nondeployed USAREUR soldiers. In February and March of 1991, more than 4,000 family members responded to a survey mailed to a random sample of families throughout USAREUR. The respondents reflected the known demographic composition of the total USAREUR family population. The responses reported here were statistically significant at the .05 level.

Many spouses of deployed soldiers were critical of the way unit leaders handled family needs during the predeployment period. Thirty-five percent felt that they were not given adequate information. More often than not, the most desired yet most difficult information to obtain was the unit's planned departure date. Many soldiers and families experienced multiple goodbyes because departures were frequently delayed and/or rescheduled. Sixty-five percent of the spouses indicated that there was insufficient time for family needs, and 41% felt that leaders were not supportive of families during this difficult period. In fact, information suggests that most leaders were very concerned about family support issues during predeployment, but they often had overwhelming operational requirements they had to meet to prepare their units for possible combat. The lack of a family support group appeared to be most common in units that do not routinely deploy during peacetime training.

When asked directly about sources of stress since their sponsors' Operation Desert Shield/Storm deployment, the spouses of deployed soldiers identified a number of issues. Those issues that were reported to cause a "moderate to a large amount" of stress are listed in Table 9–2.

Table 9–2.   Major sources of family stress during and after deployment to Southwest Asia for the Gulf War

Spouse's safety in the combat zone (86%)
Uncertainty about the length of the deployment (80%)
Concerns about living conditions for soldiers (61%)
Problems communicating with spouse in Southwest Asia (58%)

Note.   Percentages in parentheses specify the proportion of spouses responding to a U.S. Army Europe family member personal opinion survey who indicated that the item caused a moderate to large amount of stress. *Source.*   U.S. Army Europe 1991.

All respondents were asked how often they experienced a variety of symptoms typically related to depression (e.g., sadness, loneliness, trouble sleeping). These were measured by a modified version of the depression scale developed by the Center for Epidemiologic Studies. Spouses of deployed soldiers experienced significantly more psychological distress than the spouses of soldiers who did not deploy (Figure 9–1). From 10% to 20% of spouses of the nondeployed soldiers reported at least one symptom 4 or more days of the week, and 17% to 51% of the spouses of deployed soldiers experienced increased symptoms. Importantly, however, the effect of deployment status was not uniform across symptoms and was much more evident in the case of loneliness, for example, than in the case of feeling no energy or an inability to shake the blues.

Determining how to use such survey data is important. These data, rather than being used as a diagnostic indicator, are more reliably interpreted descriptively. From this perspective it is clear that these are common symptoms in this population. Spouses experiencing these distress symptoms can learn that they are not unique and that the distress they are experiencing is common to many, if not most, spouses under these circumstances. In other words, it is a "normal" aspect of their situation.

The sponsor's rank is a very good indicator of a host of sociodemographic variables (e.g., age, income, education, social class). The data depicted in Figure 9–2 suggest that, regardless of the sponsor's rank, the spouses of deployed soldiers experienced

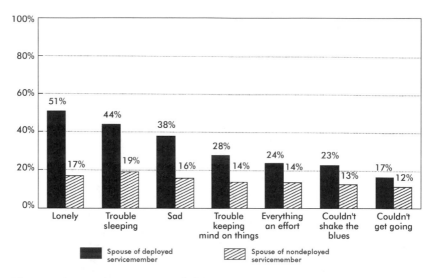

Figure 9–1. Symptoms of distress among spouses of U.S. Army Europe (USAREUR) deployed and nondeployed servicemembers, as reported on a USAREUR family member personal opinion survey during and after deployment to Southwest Asia for the Gulf War. Symptoms must have been experienced 4 or more days per week. *Source.* USAREUR Personal Opinion Survey—Family Member Survey 1991, U.S. Army Europe 1991.

higher levels of distress than did the spouses of nondeployed soldiers. As one might expect, however, older, better educated, more financially secure spouses were better able to cope with deployment stress and reported fewer symptoms. These findings provide important information for community leaders trying to target their limited resources to those most in need.

When asked about formal sources of emotional and tangible support, the majority of the spouses of deployed soldiers described a number of individuals and organizations as reliable sources of support. These included the rear detachment, the family support group, other unit spouses, the Army Community Service, the FAC, chaplains, other people in their housing area, church groups, and, for those working, their supervisors. The vast majority of spouses of deployed soldiers also indicated that others were available to assist or to just be with them. The per-

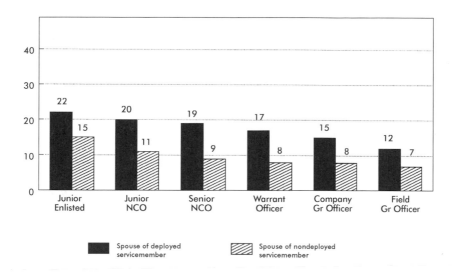

Figure 9–2. Levels of distress among spouses of U.S. Army Europe (USAREUR) deployed and nondeployed servicemembers grouped by sponsor's rank, as reported on a USAREUR family member personal opinion survey during and after deployment to Southwest Asia for the Gulf War. Symptom scores are average scores across all symptoms measured. Possible symptom scores ranged from 49 (indicating high stress) to 0 (indicating no stress). NCO = noncommissioned officer; Gr = Grade.   *Source.* U.S. Army Europe 1991.

centage of spouses of deployed soldiers confirming that there was "definite" support was substantially higher than that in the nondeployed sample: 64% of deployed spouses compared with 44% of the nondeployed group had someone to listen to them; 61% compared with 44% had someone to provide emotional support; and 52% compared with 38% could count on someone for emergency transportation.

When asked to evaluate how well they thought they were coping in a variety of life domains (i.e., family, social, and work responsibilities), most spouses said that on a day-to-day basis they were coping "very or moderately successfully." In this self-assessment, almost no differences were found between the spouses of the deployed and the nondeployed soldiers (coping with work, 85% vs. 86%; coping with family, 87% vs. 88%; and coping with social responsibilities, 68% vs. 67%, respectively). When asked about overall family adjustment to army life, again, almost no differences were found between the two groups (Figure 9–3). It appears that despite the stress associated with their sponsor's deployment and possibly because of the support they felt from their unit and community, the spouses of deployed soldiers remained very positive about their family's overall adjustment to the demands of army life.

Discussion

The family support experience in U.S. Army Europe during Operation Desert Shield/Storm suggests a number of important issues related to family support in times of war (Table 9–3). A successful family support program starts at the top of the command structure and must be reinforced at every level be-

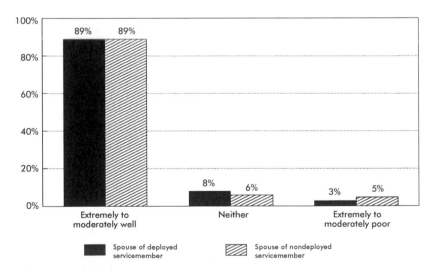

Figure 9–3. Overall family adjustment to army life among spouses of U.S. Army Europe (USAREUR) deployed and nondeployed servicemembers, as reported on a USAREUR family member personal opinion survey during and after deployment to Southwest Asia for the Gulf War. *Source.* U.S. Army Europe 1991.

Table 9–3.   Building family support during deployments

Demonstrate the interest and commitment of senior leaders, using public media to get the message out.

Bring "decision makers" together in a forum where red tape and other bureaucratic roles can be bypassed to ensure immediate action on critical issues.

Select caring and competent individuals to run things at the local level, and ensure that they have the authority to get things done.

Give family members the opportunity to participate in the decision-making process at every level. Focus on self-help.

Recognize that deployment is a stressful time for everyone and that it is normal and expectable for individuals to experience symptoms of distress.

Recognize that stress symptoms will pass and that despite these symptoms most individuals can and will continue to meet their everyday responsibilities.

low. Senior Army leaders in Europe set the tone for family support efforts of local commanders and community leaders. Senior USAREUR leaders made frequent public appearances (including on Armed Forces Network Television and Radio and in the USAREUR newspaper, *Stars and Stripes*), reassuring deploying soldiers and their families that the welfare of the soldier's family was an important priority. The data indicate that subordinate senior community leaders echoed this promise and that across Europe, unit and community staffs worked hard to fulfill this commitment. The USAREUR mission became "Take care of families!"

The many accomplishments of the USAREUR Family Support Task Force demonstrate the importance and benefits to bringing senior community representatives and command staff officers together. In an open, creative, can-do atmosphere and with access to authorities capable of cutting through red tape and normal bureaucratic procedures, the task force was able to rapidly initiate support actions to help people.

Leaving competent and caring rear detachment commanders to work with family support group leaders and community representatives also made a difference. It validated for families the senior leader's promise, "We will take care of you," and was the cornerstone for successful family support group operations. Likewise, inadequate or less well trained rear detachment commanders often found themselves overwhelmed by family support issues and frequently in conflict with family support group leaders. These commanders also had duties supporting non-deployed soldiers and their families, as well as responding to requests of the deployed unit commander—a significant challenge even for a highly competent and seasoned leader.

Many family support group leaders assumed their role in conjunction with their spouse's unit leadership positions. Most were positive about their experiences and accomplishments. Even though family support group leaders were generally not working long hours, the nature of the problems they faced (e.g., births, child care needs, extended family deaths, serious illnesses, accidents, financial problems) and the unpredictability of these problems were experienced as significant stressors. Fortunately, most family support group leaders reported that they had someone (either the rear detachment commander or another spouse) from whom they could receive support. The family support leaders indicated the need for better preparation for their role, especially more information about programs and benefits available to assist family members, including those related to the death or wounding of the servicemember.

The Southwest Asia deployment was undeniably stressful for spouses of deployed USAREUR soldiers. Many experienced distress symptoms, but most appear to have coped well. It is reasonable to believe that part of their successful coping was a result of the "blanket of support" provided by individual units and communities. Most family members had come to believe that there really was someone nearby to turn to in time of need, either another unit family member, a military neighbor, or someone from the rear detachment or the community support network.

These USAREUR family support efforts might not have been as successful had the Southwest Asia deployment lasted for a longer period and/or had large numbers of casualties resulted during the actual ground combat phase of Operation Desert Storm. Many community service support services consisted of only a few persons, and these individuals were also family members and potential victims of loss themselves. This situation made for a very fragile community family support system. Fortunately, USAREUR did not have to face either of these challenges.

The Southwest Asia deployment reconfirmed for most units and communities the fact that relatively few families often consume disproportionate amounts of resources. It also demonstrated that in times of crisis, most people "rise to the occasion" and that it is always better to encourage coping rather than to treat anyone as a helpless victim.

Very early in the deployment, USAREUR leaders recognized that soldiers who did not deploy (and their families) also faced some unique stressors. Many soldiers felt left out. They also felt unappreciated despite increased duty demands and ignored because of all the attention paid to Desert Shield/Storm soldiers and their families. USAREUR leaders attempted to directly address these issues. Although not relieving all the pain and resentment, they encouraged open discussion of these issues. They also attempted to recognize everyone's contribution, whether individuals served in Southwest Asia or remained in Europe. Leaders made rewards such as soldier (and family) vacations at an army recreation center in the Alps available to everyone. Leaders also went out of their way to promise soldiers that service in USAREUR during the war would not become a negative discriminator for promotion and other selection boards.

Conclusions

In this chapter we have looked at family support during Operation Desert Shield/Storm. We examined information from three related family support assessments carried out during the USAREUR Southwest Asia deployment. Information from these studies suggests that unit and community support efforts were keys to success and that family members of deployed soldiers both were more stressed than those whose spouses were not deployed and coped well despite the added stress associated with their spouses' deployment to the war zone.

Because of the massive turnover of personnel and units immediately following Operation Desert Shield/Storm (based on the Army's European drawdown of forces and its continued personnel downsizing), it was not possible to examine any long-term effects of this deployment on these families. We expect that this experience had both negative and positive effects on those involved. Although it may not be possible to study these former USAREUR family members, it is important that future Army and other Department of Defense surveys of Army families include both questions that will identify individuals who were in Europe during this period and questions that will provide the opportunity for self-assessment of the long-term positive and negative aspects of this experience.

For the time being, it is important to make resources available to all levels by empowering and resourcing unit rear detachment commanders and family support group leaders. In most cases, these individuals are the key to successful family support. Rear detachment commanders must know how to help and must care enough to help. Family support group leaders and rear detachment commanders must share the burden, and the community service agencies must be ready and willing to back them up. Finally, it is clear that no family support system can meet every need or expectation.

Selected Readings

Bowen GL: Families in blue: insights from Air Force families. Social Casework 8:459–466, 1985

Bowen GL, Neenan PA: Sex-role orientations among married men in the military: the generational factor. Psychol Rep 62: 523–526, 1988

Carlson EC, Carlson R: Navy Marriages and Deployment. Lanham, MD, University Press of America, 1984

Coates CH, Pellegrin RJ: Military Sociology: A Study of American Military Institutions and Military Life. University Park, MD, Social Science Press, 1965

Decker KB: Coping with sea duty: problems encountered and resources utilized during periods of family separation, in Military Families: Adaptation to Change. Edited by Hunter EJ, Nice DS. New York, Praeger, 1978, pp 113–129

Fletcher L, Giesler K: Relating Attitudes Toward Navy Life to Reenlistment Decisions. Alexandria, VA, Center for Naval Analysis, 1981

Hill R: Families Under Stress: Adjustment to the Crisis of War Separation and Reunion. New York, Harper, 1949

Hunter EJ: Families Under the Flag: A Review of Military Family Literature. New York, Praeger, 1982

Johnson A: Supporting family members during deployment. Soldier Support Journal 11(4):14–16, 1984

Jolly R: Military Man, Family Man. London, Brassey's Defence Publishers, 1987

Lewis C: Dealing with uncertainty: American military families in Europe, in Forum International, Vol 5. Edited by Kuhlmann J (Sessions of Research Committee 01: Armed Forces and Conflict Resolution, XI World Congress of Sociology, International Sociological Association, New Delhi, India, August 1986). Munich, SOWI (Sozialwissenschaftliches Institut der Bundeswehr), 1987, pp 3–45

Martin JA: The wives of career enlisted service members: application of a life stress model. Unpublished doctoral dissertation, University of Pittsburgh, 1983 [University Microfilm International 1416, 1984]

Martin JA: The wives of COHORT soldiers: initial information from a longitudinal study of the Army's New Manning System. Medical Bulletin of the U.S. Army 42:14–18, 1985

Martin JA, Ickovics JR: Challenges of military life: the importance of a partnership between the Army and its families. Military Family 6(6):3–5, 1986

Martin JA, Ickovics JR: The effects of stress on the psychological well-being of Army wives: initial findings from a longitudinal study. Journal of Human Stress 13(3):108–115, 1987

McCubbin HI, Dahl BB: Prolonged family separation in the military: a longitudinal study, in Families in the Military System. Edited by McCubbin HI, Dahl BB, Hunter EJ. Beverly Hills, CA, Sage, 1976, pp 112–144

McCubbin HI, Lavee Y: Minority families' adaptation in stressful environments: critical strengths and supports. Paper presented at the National Conference on Social Stress Research, Durham, NH, June 1986

Moskos CC: The all-volunteer military: calling, profession or occupation? Parameters 7:2–9, 1977

Nice DS: The Course of Depressive Affect in Navy Wives During Family Separation. San Diego, CA, Naval Health Research Center, 1979

Orthner DK: Families in Blue: Implications of a Study of Married and Single Parent Families in the U.S. Air Force (USAF Contract No F33600-79-0423). Washington, DC, Office of the Department of the Air Force, 1980

Orthner DK, Pittman J: Family contributions to work commitment. Journal of Marriage and the Family 48:573–581, 1986

Schneider R, Gilley M: Family Adjustment in USAREUR: Final Report. Heidelberg, West Germany, U.S. Army Medical Research Unit—Europe, 1984

Segal MW: Enlisted family life in the U.S. Army: a portrait of a community, in Life in the Rank and File: Enlisted Men and Women in the Armed Forces of the United States, Australia, Canada, and the United Kingdom. Edited by Segal DR, Sinaiko HW. Washington, DC, Pergamon–Brassey's, 1986, pp 184–211

Segal MW: The military and the family as greedy institutions. Armed Forces & Society 13:9–38, 1986

Segal MW, Kammeyer KCW, Vuozzo JS: The impact of separation on military family roles and self-perceptions during peacekeeping duty. Paper presented at the meeting of the Inter-University Seminar on Armed Forces and Society, Chicago, IL, October 1987

Snyder AI: Sea and Shore Rotation: The Family and Separations. A Bibliography of Relevant Material. Pearl Harbor, HI, Mental Health Clinic, Naval Regional Medical Clinic, 1977

U.S. Army Europe (USAREUR) Pamphlet 600-2: USAREUR Personnel Opinion Survey 1991: General Findings Report, Vol 1 (Family). Headquarters, U.S. Army, Europe, 1991

U.S. Army Medical Research Unit—Europe, Operation Desert Shield/Storm Family Support Group Leader Assessment. Unpublished report, 1991

VanVranken EW, Jellen LK, Knudson KHM, et al: The Impact of Deployment Separation on Army Families (Report NP-84-6). Washington, DC, Walter Reed Army Institute of Research, 1984

Vernez G, Zellman H: Families and Mission: A Review of the Effects of Family Factors on Army Attrition, Retention, and Readiness (Rand Note N-2624A). Santa Monica, CA, Rand Corporation, 1987

Wickham J: The Army Family. Washington, DC, Headquarters, Department of the Army, 1983

10   Preparation for Psychiatric Casualties in the Department of Veterans Affairs Medical System

Arthur S. Blank, Jr., M.D.
Laurent S. Lehmann, M.D.

Although the Persian Gulf War resulted in relatively few American casualties, this was not the outcome that had been anticipated. Indeed, military planners prepared to receive tens of thousands of dead and wounded. Veterans Affairs (VA) hospitals were an essential element in designing medical care for Gulf War casualties. Fortunately, casualties were light and the contingency plans did not have to be implemented.

The United States' experience in the Gulf War, however, probably represents an exception to the usual outcome of warfare rather than a new rule upon which to forecast casualties. It is important, therefore, that lessons learned in preparing to care for large-scale casualties not be lost. Moreover, since the end of the draft, there have been ever-increasing numbers of health care providers who have not been exposed to the military or to VA activities. This chapter, in which we discuss the preparation for vast numbers of psychiatric casualties by the VA medical system, can serve as a guide for those who follow.

Background

The Department of Defense–Department of Veterans Affairs Contingency Plan

The Department of Defense–Department of Veterans Affairs (DoD-VA) Contingency Plan was established by Public Law 97-174 in May 1982 to furnish VA medical backup to the military medical system in case of war or a national emergency affecting military personnel. Associated with the three other major components of VA (medical care for veterans, veterans' benefits, and the national cemetery system), this fourth mission of VA was enhanced by major reductions in military hospital beds in the continental United States, from approximately 500,000 during World War II to 175,000 during the Vietnam War, to approximately 16,000 at the onset of the Persian Gulf War. Coordinated by the VA Emergency Medical Preparedness Office (EMPO) (EMPO 1990a, 1990b), VA operations of the contingency plan for the Gulf War specified that up to 25,000 VA beds would be available for casualties at 77 primary and 82 secondary receiving hospitals identified under the plan, proximate to air bases in the continental U.S. designated to receive casualties.

Additional features of the DoD-VA Contingency Plan include mobilization of all VA hospitals as needed, monitoring of numbers of current patients available for transfer or discharge in order to free beds for an emergency, and consideration of impact of call-up of VA physicians, nurses, and other personnel who are members of the Ready Reserve. The DoD-VA Contingency Plan was activated on August 29, 1990, shortly after the Iraqi invasion of Kuwait. Early priorities included establishment of reporting and mechanisms for monitoring beds and staff at local, regional, and national levels, and formulation of plans for further mobilization of medical, surgical, and psychiatric services. Operational messages from VA headquarters in Washington, D.C., in August 1990, identified chemical agent injuries as a priority, initiated clinical preparations for treatment, and identified certain facilities as primary or supporting facilities for chemical agent injuries (EMPO 1990a). A clinical inventory of VA medical, surgical, and mental health units was carried out. Combat-related services such as orthopedic surgery, burn units, and head trauma care, as well as PTSD services, were identified as part of the network for the first time.

As movement of U.S. forces and preparations intensified in October 1990, the Mental Health and Behavioral Sciences Service, Readjustment Counseling Service, and Social Work Service, all of which are in the VA Central Office (VACO), were directed to commence all needed preparations for mobilization and training of special teams to lead the reception and treatment of psychiatric casualties from the Persian Gulf. These preparations were carried out under the direction of the authors of this chapter.

Veterans Affairs Psychiatric Services in Place as of 1990

The VA operates a large network of inpatient units, partial hospitalization programs, and outpatient clinics for treatment of the full range of psychiatric disorders, including substance use disorders. These programs comprised approximately 150 inpatient psychiatric services, 127 partial hospitalization programs (37 day hospitals and 90 day treatment centers), and 153 mental hygiene clinics as of 1990.

Veterans Affairs Traumatic Stress Treatment and Readjustment Counseling: Elements in Place as of 1990

Throughout the Vietnam War and for several years immediately following, with few exceptions, VA did not provide diagnosis and treatment of acute stress reaction, posttraumatic stress disorder (PTSD), and other conditions that led to readjustment difficulties in war veterans. This lack of preparedness, which was also characteristic of most private-sector mental health professionals and agencies, contributed to the emergence of a large number of cases of PTSD and readjustment problems affecting employment and family functioning among 3.1 million men and women who had served in the U.S. military in Southeast Asia.

In 1979, the U.S. Congress and VA responded to this major public health problem in the Vietnam veteran population by establishing community-based outreach and counseling centers (Vet Centers) to furnish counseling and psychiatric services for PTSD, along with a broad range of social care readjustment services. A few years later, Congress responded further by establishing specialized PTSD clinical teams (PCTs) at many VA medical centers, along with specialized psychiatric inpatient units (SIPUs) and substance abuse PTSD teams (SUPTs). They also established the National Center for PTSD, a multisite training and research consortium. In addition, during the 1980s, VA carried out recurrent training on postwar readjustment and treatment of PTSD for professionals throughout the medical care system.

As a result, at the outbreak of the Persian Gulf War, VA had on hand nearly 1,000 well-trained psychiatrists, psychologists, social workers, psychiatric nurses, and professional and paraprofessional counselors in its 171 hospitals and clinics and 196 Vet Centers. There was a very high level of sophistication about the nature of combat and its stressors, particularly in the specialized inpatient PTSD units, PCTs, and Vet Centers. This pool of expertise included hundreds of Vet Center staff who themselves had served in Vietnam. There were also additional Vietnam War–era veteran mental health professionals who had direct experience with psychiatric combat casualties and the military medical evacuation system. Further, during the 1980s, the Vet Centers and PCTs, as well as some staff from inpatient and partial hospitalization programs, had gained experience and expertise concerning acute stress reactions by working with disaster victims throughout the U.S. These expert clinicians were widely distributed throughout the VA system and provided a pool of psychological trauma expertise at all critical sites. Thirty-one of the 78 facilities designated to receive casualties had some form of specialized inpatient or outpatient PTSD treatment program in-house at the outset of the Gulf War, and most had a community-based Vet Center.

Notification and Inception of Preparations

In September 1990, at VACO, the Mental Health and Behavioral Sciences Service, a staff office with responsibilities for psychiatry services systemwide, and the Readjustment Counseling Service, a line office supervising VA's community-based counseling centers for war veterans (Vet Centers), were instructed to mobilize and train selected mental health and readjustment counseling staff for reception and treatment of psychiatric casualties from the Persian Gulf. This effort, as was the case for all VA medical and surgical preparations, was to be developed for a worst-case scenario of 50,000 casualties, including 5,000 psychiatric casualties. Consultations among VA's EMPO, various operations officials, and the present authors produced agreement that the leading edge of preparations for psychiatric casualties would be the rapid training of a three-person team at each of 70 medical centers selected as the first recipients of troops medically evacuated from the Gulf (either directly or via military medical facilities in Europe).

Needs Assessment

Preparation for treatment of psychiatric casualties was begun by specifying the subpopulations who, given the circumstances of events in the Persian Gulf, would most likely present for care to VA facilities. These included the following:

- Active-duty military personnel evacuated from the war zone for inpatient care and outpatient follow-up and disposition.

This group would include troops evacuated for medical disorders and surgical injuries as well as "psychiatric casualties."

• Returned personnel in need of debriefing for an acute stress reaction outside a medical context.

• Family members and significant others of combat medical/surgical casualties in need of counseling.

• Returned ex-prisoners of war and their family members or significant others.

• Discharged Persian Gulf veterans needing debriefing and early treatment for an acute stress reaction or PTSD.

• Released civilian hostages requiring debriefing, counseling, or other care.

• VA or Department of Defense medical staff in need of assistance for occupational stress, especially in the event of mass casualties.

Identification of Key Issues

First priority was placed on rapid data gathering to establish understanding and management strategies for the following key issues:

• Lines of coordination within VA professional services (Psychiatry, Psychology, Social Work, and Readjustment Counseling) and between these VA services and related services in Army, Navy, and Air Force.

• Roles and readiness progress of VA clinical elements (Medicine, Surgery, Infectious Disease, Nursing, etc.), logistical elements (EMPO, Administration, etc.), and the air evacuation system.

• Basic outlines of military medical systems within the war zone, Europe, and the continental U.S.

• Army, Navy, and Air Force combat stress capacity in the war zone and along the evacuation chain, and current doctrine for interventions.

- Background on unitary deployment, weapons, equipment, strategy and tactics, and characteristics of the opposing forces.
- Nongeneric, theater-specific psychological stressors, both direct and background (e.g., chemical and biological weapons, rapidity of deployment, climate, cultural differences between Kuwait/Saudi Arabia and U.S).
- Psychological stressor implications of various possible political military scenarios.
- Emergency medical-surgical training and treatment preparations under way.
- The range of mental health and counseling services available at designated reception sites.
- The identification of networking to support clinical services for casualties.

Planning of Training

The Advisory Group

Because members of the acute stress teams were geographically spread over 70 locations, a planning and consulting group was established that included representatives of the VA Social Work, Mental Health, and Readjustment Counseling Services, VA Office of Academic Affairs (responsible for educational programs), EMPO, and the Chief Combat Stress Branch, U.S. Army; professionals from the behavioral sciences at Ft. Sam Houston and VA's National Center for PTSD; the director of a VA medical facility specialized inpatient unit for PTSD; a former career Navy psychiatrist; and psychiatry faculty from the Uniformed Services University of Health Sciences (USUHS) in Bethesda, Maryland. This group met by conference call over a 3-month period and provided analysis and counsel regarding important clinical, training, and administrative issues.

Further Analysis

The Last War

We noted that 5 of the 15 members of our advisory group had served in Vietnam and had had experience with casualties and/or military mental health services during that era. Additionally, the Vet Center member of each VA medical center acute stress team as well as some members from the other mental health services had also served in Vietnam. Thus, a considerable amount of previous war experience could be drawn upon at all levels of VA preparation.

To avoid preparing for the last war instead of this one, however, a continuously updated list of key features of the Vietnam and Persian Gulf Wars was prepared and maintained. Attention was paid to both general and specific similarities and differences, with particular emphasis on features relevant to psychological stress (Tables 10–1 to 10–6). This reference document was distributed throughout the VA system. In this document it was noted that the Persian Gulf conflict differed from the Vietnam conflict in many ways, including the following: prominent role of reservists and National Guard; threat of heavy combat with standing forces en masse; threat of chemical and biological warfare; desert locale; older average age of combatants; large numbers of women personnel in the theater; and the suddenness and speed of the war, mobilization, and deployment. The last-war comparison document proved to be valuable in activating prior experience for new application while avoiding overgeneralizing from the past.

The Role of Psychiatrists

Throughout the VA medical care system, treatment of PTSD in war veterans and assistance for acute stress reactions are highly interdisciplinary in character. Most assessment and treatment are provided by care providers other than psychiatrists: social workers, psychologists, nurses, masters-level counselors, and paraprofessional counselors. This reflects the relative numbers

Table 10–1. Contrasts between the Persian Gulf and Vietnam Wars: strategies, tactics, and conditions

	Persian Gulf War	**Vietnam War**
Location	Southwest Asia	Southeast Asia
Duration	Several months	11 years
Climate	Desert	Tropical
Topography	Little cover	Much cover
Enemy	Distinct military forces	Enemy partly mixed with general population
Number of troops deployed in theater	545,000	3.1 million
Tour of duty	No limitation	Limited
Deployment	By unit; rapid	Individually; gradual
Strategies and tactics	Fewer rear-area terrorist attacks	Frequent rear-area terrorist attacks
	Threat of chemical warfare	No threat of chemical warfare
	Rear-area air attacks (SCUDs)	No rear-area air attacks
	More armor	Less armor
	No guerrilla war	Guerrilla war
	Terrorist attacks outside war zone	No terrorist attacks outside war zone
	More high-tech weaponry	Less high-tech weaponry

of these clinicians in the VA. Each PCT is required to have at least one psychiatrist.

However, as the needs of impending psychiatric casualties and (in terms of psychiatric services) of medical-surgical casualties were contemplated, all staff were reminded of the crucial role of psychiatrists in the diagnosis and differential diagnosis of acute conditions of casualties of war. Psychiatrists' importance was related to the need to rapidly diagnose both medical

Table 10–2.   Contrasts between the Persian Gulf and Vietnam Wars: political

	Persian Gulf War	Vietnam War
Public support for war	More	Less; opposition greater
Draft avoidance	Not an issue	Widespread
UN involvement	Coalition	No coalition
Outcome	Victory	Not victory; withdrawal
Public attitudes toward troops	Mostly positive	Extensively negative

conditions that mimic acute psychiatric conditions and stress reactions that can easily be confused with other psychiatric disorders. The assessment and treatment of acute conditions in casualties differ markedly from the treatment of chronic PTSD, a clinical situation in which evaluation can be conducted more leisurely and discursively. Therefore, a decision was made early in the process to require that one member of each acute stress team be a psychiatrist.

Realities of the War Zone

A review of Vietnam War–era experiences and the state of VA medical system readiness at the onset of Operation Desert Storm also indicated a pressing need to educate staff on the realities of the combat zone. This process included discussions of generic stressors and the unique stressors of the Gulf conflict. A training emphasis was placed on orientation to military equipment, tactical scenarios, and weapons. Mobilized predeployment reservists and returned personnel were included in the training exercises as much as possible. Along the same line, the planning groups had briefings from officials at USUHS and the Acting Consultant for Psychiatry to the Army Surgeon General, among others, on operations and possible scenarios in the Gulf.

Table 10–3. Contrasts between the Persian Gulf and Vietnam Wars: social and economic

	Persian Gulf War	**Vietnam War**
Economic impact	More economic pressures; reservists and National Guard left higher-paying jobs	Income reduction less frequent
Derivation of troops	Professional military, reserves, National Guard, no draftees	Significant proportion of draftees
Average age of troops	Possibly higher	Average age = 19.5 years
Marital status	More troops married	Fewer troops married
Deployment of married couples	Yes	No
Deployment of female troops in war zone	Many more female troops in war zone (34,000 within 7 months)	Only approximately 7,500 female troops in war zone over 11 years
Media coverage	More immediate, via satellite transmission	Less immediate, with no satellite transmission
Deployment of parents	Possibly more parents deployed	Possibly fewer parents deployed
Availability of sperm banks	Yes	No

Training Drives Operations

The logistical arrangements required to select and bring together staff from throughout the U.S. for training on very short notice resulted in the authors and the advisory group becoming quickly involved in the operational side of preparations throughout the VA system. This involvement occurred, in part, because a commitment to readiness was stronger centrally in the organization (VACO in Washington, D.C.) than in the field

Table 10–4. Contrasts between the Persian Gulf and Vietnam Wars: psychiatric

	Persian Gulf War	**Vietnam War**
Number of military psychiatric personnel deployed	More military psychiatric personnel deployed	Fewer military psychiatric personnel deployed
Inclusion of PTSD diagnosis in DSM	Yes (for 11 years)	No
Public awareness of traumatic stress effects and postwar readjustment processes	Wide public awareness	Little public awareness
Availability of VA readjustment and PTSD services	Available for 11 years before the war	No service available before the war, and none available for 7 years after war (up to 15 years for some persons)
Availability and use of alcohol and drugs	Little alcohol or drugs in theater	More alcohol and drugs
Employee assistance programs (EAPs)	Available in some locations for family members	No EAPs available
Emergence of self-help groups	Quick	Delayed

Note. PTSD = posttraumatic stress disorder; DSM = *Diagnostic and Statistical Manual of Mental Disorders* (American Psychiatric Association).
Source. Arthur S. Blank, Jr., M.D., and Gustavo Martinez, D.S.W.

during the early phase of preparations. The VACO was also more active because the selected three-person acute stress teams did not uniformly gain attention and status in their facilities until after the training conferences and postconference activities that are discussed in the next section. In the autumn of

Table 10–5. Contrasts between the Persian Gulf and Vietnam Wars: Department of Defense–Veterans Affairs (DoD-VA) medical

	Persian Gulf War	**Vietnam War**
Number of military medical beds in continental U.S.	14,000	175,000 (1964–1975)
Availability of DoD-VA Contingency Plan	DoD-VA Contingency Plan for possible receipt of casualties	Plan not developed

Table 10–6. Similarities between the Persian Gulf and Vietnam Wars

Enemy had advance reputation for ferocity
Opposing forces led by a dictatorial government
U.S. had technological superiority
Advance threat of terrorism within the theater
High number of casualties on opposing side
Some unplanned collateral damage to civilians in air war
Local culture significantly different from that in U.S.

Source. Arthur S. Blank, Jr., M.D., and Gustavo Martinez, D.S.W.

1990, denial of the reality that war might be impending was fairly common (though by no means universal) among leadership at hospitals; by December 1990, the denial had melted away. The training effort, in fact, functioned as an initiating force for operational preparations throughout the system.

Faculty

For training of the acute stress teams, faculty roles included 1) didactic instruction, 2) teaching clinical methods via lecture, discussion, and case discussion, and 3) planning and emotional support provided in small groups convened to process learning, pending tasks, and reactions. Faculty were chosen with all three functions in view.

Traumatic Stress Training Conferences

In December 1990, in Indianapolis, Indiana, VA provided 36 hours of training over a 3-day period to approximately 70 participants from 23 medical centers. This training was repeated for 140 participants from the remaining 47 facilities at Northport, New York, in February 1991. The latter conference ended just as the ground war began in the Persian Gulf (Fenev and Anetrella 1990, 1991).

All participants in the training were expert in the diagnosis and treatment of chronic PTSD in war veterans and therefore began the sessions with a good knowledge base on providing services to war casualties. Additionally, many had experience in responding to acute stress reactions in civilian disasters, and one-third of the participants had served in Vietnam, providing additional experiences on which to build.

The curriculum for the initial training conference is outlined in Table 10–7.

Briefing From Department of Defense Operations

A briefing from a high-level officer from the theater operations section in the Pentagon introduced the VA health care staff to the reality of the war and was a major foundation for all subsequent training and preparations at home stations. This briefing included information not yet available in the media and, as was the case for all presentations, was videotaped for further use.

Venue

The first conference was held at a major Army post, which added verisimilitude for VA personnel, allowed participants to try out protective clothing (mission oriented protective posture gear), and enabled attendance by members of a mobilized reserve evacuation hospital soon to depart for the Gulf.

Table 10–7. Curriculum for the initial Veterans Affairs (VA) traumatic stress training conference just before the Persian Gulf War

- VA–Department of Defense emergency medical system
- Military operations in the Persian Gulf: briefing by Department of Defense operations
- Military medical system and echelons of care
- Infectious disease in the Middle East
- Wounds (including battlefield, battalion aid station, and medical clearing company films from the Vietnam War)
- Chemical injuries and protective gear and procedures
- Stressors on the battlefield: Vietnam and Persian Gulf
- Chemical protective gear and decontamination procedures: demonstration
- Mission oriented protective posture gear: trying out
- Combat stress and battle fatigue principles and practices
- Current military medical equipment and hospital design: a review
- Psychiatric, medical, and surgical casualties: clinical overviews
- Diagnosis and assessment of acute stress reactions
- Psychological responses to wounds
- Pharmacological treatment of acute stress reactions and other acute psychiatric disorders
- Acute psychotherapeutic management
- Sodium Amytal interview
- Inpatient debriefing groups
- Family treatment and assessment
- Special populations: ethnic minorities, women
- Stress and burnout in medical-surgical staff: provision of help to this population
- Case studies
- Design and implementation of postconference training of the staff at hospitals
- Planning for contingencies: overflow, support, consultation

Returned Aviator

The first training conference included a helicopter pilot who had just returned from the Gulf after having been in the theater for several months. He provided formal and informal in-depth orientation to participants throughout the conference. By chance, this individual was also a Vietnam War combat veteran and helped the participants recalibrate the Vietnam experience for the war at hand.

Pickup on Systemwide Preparations

Mobilization of the VA medical system had been under way for 2 months by the time of the first training conference and for 4 months by the time of the second conference (see below). Thus, the VA participants brought with them reports of accomplishments and obstacles in the mobilization process at their home stations. Numerous meetings at the training conferences made it possible for these experiences to be pooled and for solutions to be designed with the assistance of faculty and peers. This process also gave input to VACO officials, who then implemented midcourse corrections systemwide. The solutions that emerged from small group sessions included several psychosocial support tactics. For example, a plan was proposed for meeting family members of casualties upon their arrival at hospitals. Another plan called for enlisting National Guard and reserve members from the communities around VA hospitals to assist with reception of casualties. The servicemembers were requested to dress in their units, thus facilitating a more gradual transition from a military to a civilian environment.

Participants recognized the importance of providing support for hospital staff in the form of stress management and morale-building activities. Other groups targeted for assistance included Vietnam War veteran physicians and nurses from the private sector, who were contacting VA hospitals to volunteer their services for Gulf veterans.

Core Training Issues

In addressing the mental health needs of Gulf War troops, special areas of concern were noted; the harsh, unfamiliar desert environment with its heat and sand, and the anticipated isolation of U.S. troops from the local population, whose customs were significantly different from our own, were examples. There were concerns about the effects of new types of warfare: the physical and psychological effects of chemical and bacteriological warfare, and the psychological impacts of massive burns and amputations that were the anticipated outcomes of large-scale tank battles. There were also concerns about the impact of the war on servicemembers who had experienced PTSD in previous conflicts that might be reactivated in this new deployment. Another focus of attention was the effect of the war on those patients already in treatment: veterans of previous wars suffering from PTSD.

Training was not limited to issues related to PTSD, because it was recognized that there would be a range of stress reactions among psychiatric casualties, including brief reactive psychoses, adjustment disorders, and unusual presentation of other major and minor psychiatric illnesses. It was hoped that there would be fewer drug- and alcohol-related problems because of the isolation of U.S. troops and the restrictions of the Saudi and other Allied nations against these substances.

The anticipated mixture of disorders that would be seen formed the basis for the principles of evaluation and treatment of psychiatric casualties: Do not diagnose precipitously; do not medicate precipitously. The Department of Defense concept of "battle fatigue" as a normal reaction to the extreme stress of combat was consistent with the VA perception of PTSD as the pathological expression of what were once adaptive coping mechanisms.

A "debriefing" approach was suggested similar to that used with disaster victims and with survivors of the bombing of the Beirut Marine barracks. This technique allows recognition of emotions associated with the stressors and development of a cognitive grasp of the stress event in the context of support from peers with similar experiences. This supportive psychoeducational approach may also prevent premature labeling of the survivor as a "psychiatric patient." There was also an emphasis on awareness of the needs of families, including the families of deployed troops who were currently experiencing psychological, social, or economic distress. It was emphasized that families of the wounded would have to be educated by caregivers about their loved one's injuries in a sensitive manner and be involved, as much as possible, in a helping role during the recovery process. Finally, attention was paid to the needs of caregivers, including the clinicians themselves as they dealt with acutely psychiatrically disturbed Gulf War returnees, and those with disfiguring and disabling wounds. There was a perceptible sense of distress among these experienced clinicians who constituted our trainees, and particularly among the Vietnam War–era and –theater veterans, who once again would face the horrors of acute combat trauma.

Focus on Wounds

It was believed that we might face large numbers of combat casualties, especially burns and amputations, as a result of armored warfare. The special needs of female soldiers who might suffer such disfiguring injuries in their Persian Gulf combat support roles were explored. The training exercises furnished the participants with an extensive exposure to wounds via battlefield medical films and presentations by surgical personnel. Some participants who had been field or hospital medics in Vietnam shared their personal experiences with this exposure. For nonmedical mental health staff participants who had not previously had much experience with physical trauma, this exposure was a valuable—if sometimes painful—preparation.

Case Conference

Cases were formulated to convey clinical situations that the acute stress teams and their colleagues might confront. These cases were discussed in small groups. Insofar as possible, group leaders with prior war-zone or medical evacuation experience were used. Many of the cases that were used in the conference were composite real cases from prior wars, revised to fit the present conflict. These scenarios were based upon anticipated combat situations. The clinical and administrative topics that were covered by the cases are shown in Table 10–8.

The following are two examples of cases used, accompanied by explanatory material furnished to the group leaders in advance of group discussion. Each case was accompanied by a list of questions directed toward the clinicians who would be caring for casualties.

Case 1

You are asked to see a patient on the surgical ward in consultation. The consultation request appears as follows: "20-yr.-old Marine lance corporal evacuated following loss of lower right leg in combat. Recently amputation revised to AK [above the knee]. Heavy combat exposure. Past 2 days insomnia, combat nightmares, etc. Suspect combat stress reaction/PTSD. Please evaluate."

Table 10–8. Clinical issues for case discussion at the Veterans Affairs (VA) traumatic stress training conferences before and during the Persian Gulf War

- Causes of delirium; differentiation from acute stress reaction, acute psychotic state, etc.
- Medical and surgical causes of acute psychiatric symptoms
- Management of acute schizophreniform disorder
- Assessment and treatment of acute posttraumatic stress disorder, with and without significant dissociative symptoms
- Detection and management of recurrent depression
- Evaluation of suicidality
- Diagnosis of hidden substance abuse, withdrawal states, and medical complications
- Differentiation of psychiatric disorder from nonpsychiatric withdrawal from effective performance
- Management of acute Axis I psychiatric disorder in presence of Axis II disorder with significant impairment of functioning

On your review of the patient's current hospital chart, it becomes clear that for the past 2 days he has awakened at night, and reports nightmares of combat that he describes vividly; he has been awake much of the night and falls asleep periodically during the daytime. He mentioned to the staff that when sitting in the dayroom sometimes people passing in the hall look like Saudi Arabians for a minute. He has been trying to read the newspaper this morning but couldn't concentrate.

You check the military record, which reveals that the patient was involved in very intense ground combat. A number of his comrades were killed, including two from a grenade explosion, which had shattered his lower leg and damaged his knee. Prior to this event, his unit had been overrun or nearly overrun, and the patient had had to lay still in a trench for an extended period, lying under the bodies of two dead buddies, fearing discovery by the enemy.

A conversation with the nurse reveals that although an attempt had been made at the theater hospital to get by with a BK [below-the-knee] amputation, complications had required a further operation 6 days ago, resulting in an AK amputation. The nurse indicates that the patient's sleep difficulties began shortly after that operation, and she comments that his barbiturate has been increased in response to the continuing sleep problem. She also mentions that this morning in particular, the patient has been restless and complaining, especially about some loud laughter and talking from some other patients. Until today, however, except for occasional forays to the dayroom, all he wanted to do was to lie in bed doing nothing.

The following is the additional information furnished group leaders for Case 1:

The classic features of early, prodromal delirium are restlessness (especially at night), daytime somnolence, insomnia with vivid dreams or nightmares, hypersensitivity to light or sound, fleeting illusions or hallucinations, and distractibility, all of which are evident in this patient. All of these except perhaps the daytime somnolence are common in acute stress reaction or acute PTSD. The patient might have delirium, acute stress disorder, or both. Various post-op factors (embolism, drugs, an electrolyte problem) or barbiturate can cause delirium. The maneuver of asking the patient to draw a clock with the hands placed at a certain time can be a sensitive test for early delirium, showing subtle distortion before there are gross changes in mental functioning.

The questions pertaining to Case 1 and directed toward the clinicians who would be caring for casualties were as follows:

1. As you prepare to interview the patient, what initial differential diagnosis do you have in mind?
2. What are some possible causes of various diagnostic possibilities?
3. What one test of the mental status exam might help clarify the diagnosis?
4. What particular behavior of this patient might be an unconscious reenactment of an aspect of a traumatically stressful situation?
5. Might an electroencephalogram contribute to diagnosis? How?

Case 2

Captain Brown is a 45-year-old helicopter pilot sent back from the theater following a leg fracture (tibia and fibula) sustained in an accident (fell in a trench while horsing around at night). The fracture was extensive but was set successfully without complications in the theater; the patient was sent back for extended convalescence. The record indicates that he had been a helicopter crew chief in Vietnam. In the Middle East his unit was set up near a hospital, and his brother is a physician who was assigned to that hospital.

The medical record also indicates that the patient was a high-performing and conscientious pilot, although during the last few weeks before his accident he had almost continuous involvement in combat and a couple of narrow escapes. It is noted incidentally that he had survived a crash caused by enemy fire in Vietnam. While in the hospital in the Middle East, the patient commented to a nurse, "I have to admit, I've been tense most of the time since I've been here."

The orthopedic resident tells you that when the patient was admitted 2 weeks ago, he was entirely normal psychiatrically and seemed quite comfortable, intelligent, and affable. However, 3 days ago he began to become irritable and belligerent, complained of feeling anxious, and had some difficulty sleeping. The immediate precipitant for the consultation request is that this morning the patient complained of attacks of depersonalization, about which he was very upset. As the resident is telling you that he thinks the patient may be having a combat stress reaction (patient has been talking about some harrowing episodes), the nurse yells down the hall, "Dr. Hones, we've got a problem with Captain Brown here."

The following is the additional information furnished group leaders for Case 2:

Patient has been taking diazepam (Valium) since his arrival in the Middle East (obtaining the drug from his brother) in connection with chronic anxiety. He had worked up to a significant daily dose. The anxiety may have been connected with residual traumatic stress effects from his Vietnam experiences. Shortly after arriving back in the U.S., his Valium supply ran out. He decided to go without and was too embarrassed to mention the habit to anyone. His symptoms the past few days are standard benzodiazepine withdrawal symptoms, and what has just happened is that he has had a seizure.

He needs to be restarted on a benzodiazepine and tapered slowly. He also needs a thorough psychological evaluation (generalized anxiety disorder vs. PTSD). Whether he should return to the Middle East will depend on the outcome of the psychological assessment. He needs some information about the features of the benzodiazepines.

The questions pertaining to Case 2 and directed toward the clinicians who would be caring for casualties were as follows:

1. What do you think may have just happened?
2. What pharmacological intervention may he need over the next week or two?
3. What should be the overall psychological approach to his situation and difficulties?
4. If the war is still on after the patient's Fx is healed, what would your opinion be about his going back to the Middle East?

Liaison With Military

Liaison between VA hospitals and military units was essential to coordination of return to duty or discharge from service, including medical discharges. In the Persian Gulf War, VA preparations included efforts by all VA facilities to establish liaisons with nearby Army, Navy, and Air Force stations. Administrative procedures for establishing these links were clarified in the context of readiness training. The inclusion of uniformed services officials from USUHS, Ft. Sam Houston, the Pentagon, and other facilities stimulated systemwide VA–Department of Defense coordination.

Media Interest

The VA mental health mobilization for the Persian Gulf War attracted media attention, including a request from national network television for coverage of training conferences. Television coverage would have interfered with training objectives and detracted from the privacy required for staff to deal with sensitive topics, and therefore was not permitted. Reporters were welcomed at a field exercise in which press coverage would not be a disruption.

Recommendations to Management

Assembling small teams from multiple locations during the course of a mobilization creates a window for observation of how the mobilization is proceeding systemwide. Because the first acute stress team training conference occurred several weeks into the mobilization, faculty and operations officials in attendance were able to formulate recommendations that were routed back through the Director of VA Emergency Medical Preparedness and then the Chief Medical Director (VA's top medical official), to the Secretary of Veterans Affairs. The recommendations included

1. Establishment of expert-level mobile training and consultation teams to visit any medical center that is in need of assistance after casualties begin to be received.
2. Conversion of the Persian Gulf War acute stress teams into standing, permanent multidisciplinary teams that are ready for future mobilization.
3. Attention to the needs of female casualties in a previously largely male medical environment.
4. Requests to the veterans service organizations for assistance to military patients and their family members.
5. Creation of consultation-liaison teams for psychiatric consultation on medical and surgical casualties.

Completion of the Formal Training Program

During the several-week interval between the two training conferences, the military situation in the Gulf developed quickly. Large numbers of troops were deployed to the theater as the United Nations forces prepared for a ground war. VA's preparations for psychiatric casualties continued at a rapid pace. A training program was developed incorporating videos of the first training conference. More documents addressing clinical issues were prepared by various elements, including a guide to pharmacological treatment of acute stress reaction and other acute disorders prepared by the National Center for PTSD (Friedman et al. 1991). Multiple systemwide conference calls were held, in which the acute stress teams participated. At the second training conference in February 1991, a live television satellite broadcast was conducted by training faculty from the conference site to all VA medical facilities. This occurred within 72 hours of the initiation of the ground war.

Subsequently, the 70 acute stress teams organized the mental health, social work, and readjustment counseling services at their facilities to provide excellent care for the expected evacuees. By means of recurrent briefings at their home stations, the teams established awareness of the psychosocial aspects of medical-surgical care throughout the total clinical and administrative spectrum. Finally, distribution of training conference videos throughout the VA medical system completed the preparation.

Lessons Learned

During the lead-up to the Persian Gulf War, for the first time in its history, the VA's medical care system was called upon, under the DoD-VA Contingency Plan adopted in 1982, to mobilize for large-scale care of medical, surgical, and psychiatric evacuees from a war zone. In addition to multiple medical, surgical, and administrative responses undertaken by VA between August 1990 and February 1991 (Table 10–9), VA Psychiatry, Psychology, Social Work, and Readjustment Counseling Services implemented mobilization and training of 70 three-person acute stress teams to lead the treatment of psychiatric casualties at 70 VA hospitals and to provide for comprehensive psychosocial and consultation-liaison services for patients and their families.

In the end, because of the early termination of the Gulf War, VA facilities were not utilized, and all care could be provided by the military medical system. Coming 17 years after the end of war in Vietnam, and 8 years after the institution of official VA

Table 10–9. Chronology of key events in Veterans Affairs (VA) and Department of Defense (DoD) health services preparedness for the Persian Gulf War

August 1990	Iraq invades Kuwait.
	Activation of DoD-VA Contingency Plan, with identification of VA facilities for receipt of casualties.
September 1990	Inception of planning in VA Central Office (VACO) for psychiatric casualties and readjustment assistance for returnees from the war in the Persian Gulf.
October 1990	Identification of chemical agent receiving sites. Selection of key medical, surgical, psychiatric and readjustment personnel; decision to provide rapid training for personnel at these sites.
November 1990	First medicine, surgery, and infectious disease training activities.
December 1990	Second round of medicine, surgery, and infectious disease training activities.
	First traumatic stress training conference.
	Activation of working groups on clinical services emergency preparedness, psychiatric casualties, family support, and readjustment.
January 1991	Systemwide preparedness activities.
February 1991	Second traumatic stress training conference.
	Systemwide satellite broadcast.

medical system responsibility to provide acute care for war casualties, the Persian Gulf mobilization revealed that the responsible services could become ready to provide care for a large number of psychiatric evacuees on a directed timetable and could achieve such readiness with considerable commitment and enthusiasm. A decade of program development for PTSD in Vietnam War veterans, occurring at the initiative of Congress, had produced within VA a large cadre of expert clinicians who understand the nature of war and its psychosocial stressors.

Several lessons were learned from experiences of the Persian Gulf conflict:

1. VA medical facilities and their attached community-based Vet Centers should have standing, permanent, acute stress teams. These teams should be multidisciplinary (including Psychiatry, Psychology, Social Work, Readjustment Counseling, Nursing, and Chaplain Service professionals at a minimum) and should lead responses to civilian disasters and maintain readiness to lead mobilization of the facility in case of war.

2. Mobilization to provide acute psychiatric care for active-duty personnel enhances VA's service to veterans and should be done in further conflicts. The attention and energies of VA Mental Health, Readjustment Counseling, and related services became riveted on the task of preparing for psychiatric casualties. For this reason, and because of a widespread commitment to avoid a repetition of the professional neglect of Vietnam War veterans in the 1970s, during the Persian Gulf postwar period, VA has mobilized an extensive outreach effort to veterans of the Persian Gulf War. VA Vet Centers (now 202 in number) had seen more than 35,000 returnees from the Persian Gulf for readjustment counseling and psychotherapy for PTSD by mid-1993, and VA's PTSD clinical teams and specialized inpatient PTSD programs are similarly meeting the needs of Persian Gulf veterans (see Chapters 18 and 19, this volume, for further, more detailed discussion of these programs). So VA's new role of providing acute care during wartime (brought to a fine point, but fortunately not needed, during the Persian Gulf events) has served the purpose of accelerating and simulating the traditional role of furnishing care to veterans for war-related psychological problems.

3. The acute stress teams should maintain close liaison with proximate military installations, so that setting up liaison for return to duty or discharge of active-duty patients hospitalized at VA facilities is easy and rapid.

4. All ongoing PTSD-related training activities throughout VA should include a module or component on acute traumatic stress, including war stress.

5. Standing organizational elements such as the acute stress teams, and any preparations for reception of casualties in case of war or disaster, should recognize a central role for psychiatrists in the evaluation and diagnosis of persons with acute psychiatric conditions.

6. Patient-centered psychosocial tactics, including but not limited to the following, should be key elements in VA medical care for wartime casualties: a) providing immediate attention to families of recently injured personnel, b) drawing on veterans organization members, and c) involving uniformed National Guard members and reservists from the hospital's community.

7. Particularly in the case of sudden war with rapid mobilization, unrealistic denial of impending emergency can occur, even in a health care system officially tasked with providing care for casualties. Denial probably becomes more widespread the longer the interval since the last war or disaster. Denial is usually present in those who have not previously experienced an emergency and can be overcome, especially with input from those who have served in a war zone or who have directly assisted with care of the injured along an evacuation chain.

8. Intensive and rapid training at the onset of an emergency produces acceleration of readiness in a highly constructive manner.

9. Telecommunications, including phone conferencing and television satellite broadcasts, can also accelerate systemwide preparations. VA preparations for the Persian Gulf War tapped only slightly the potential of telecommunications in achieving an effective mechanization of a medical system. The use of short-notice telephone conferencing is critical to coordinating preparation. Systemwide activation would have been furthered by daily satellite TV broadcasts from the training conferences for specialized teams back to their

home stations. Satellite broadcasts can easily include telephone call-in for questions and comments from the receiving audience to the presenters, which would result in an effective mechanization of a medical system. Availability of short-notice telephone conference. For a rapid, large-system mobilization, two-way satellite video/audio would be the optimum method for accelerating both training and operational preparation.

In closing, it is useful to review what was learned about the essential elements of a training program on the management of acute psychiatric casualties of combat. First, it is important to remember that the responses of psychiatric casualties of combat can be similar to those found in survivors of civilian disasters. For this reason, the approaches developed for helping Gulf War returnees have been useful for VA medical center and Vet Center clinicians in assisting victims of recent natural disasters, such as hurricanes and earthquakes. Be sure that your facility or organization includes mental health services in its disaster plans and drills. Many current texts on emergency care pay little attention to the mental health needs of survivors, but this is changing. The VA Emergency Medical Preparedness Office is working closely with the VA National Center for PTSD and with the Department of Health and Human Services to ensure that there is awareness of and training for the mental health needs of disaster victims.

Second, educate your staff about the existing emergency preparedness plans and the role of your facility in these plans. Include information about the numbers of staff of different disciplines who may be called up to active duty in the reserve or National Guard and who therefore may not be available for service at the facility. Describe the logistics of medical evacuation, with particular attention to established airheads for reception of casualties, ambulance services, and your facility's plans for transfer of current patients to other VA or non-VA facilities to make room for incoming casualties. Describe support and co-ordination plans with other health care providers in the community.

Third, describe the principles of evaluation, diagnosis, and treatment of incoming casualties, including those with identified psychiatric problems as well as those with physical injuries. Emphasize the importance of taking the time to make accurate diagnoses rather than rushing to diagnose and treat prematurely. Note the differential diagnosis of the acute psychiatric reaction and disorders that may be encountered. Describe, as best you can, any features of the combat environment that might impact on the types of casualties or stressors experienced by the casualties your facility receives. Teach a debriefing approach that is supportive and can help the survivor to gain better control over stress-related symptoms and, hopefully, prevent the development of further pathology. Note the value of group treatments and the importance of the family in recovery. Use whatever educational resources are available, including consultation and media from VA National Center for PTSD and local staff members from VA medical centers or Vet Centers who are experienced in care of acute psychiatric casualties, as well as experts from neighboring military hospitals and bases.

Fourth, train your staff to be sensitive to reactions of family members and to prepare them as they first are reunited with their injured survivor. Have staff continue to be available to assist them. The needs and concerns of families require special attention. In many instances the family may become a valuable helper in the recovery process. In community disaster situations, extended family or community support activities may be very helpful in containing or reducing psychiatric sequelae with assistance from clinicians.

Finally, remain aware of the psychological needs of the clinicians who will be caring for psychiatric and physically injured casualties. Teach your staff to recognize the stress and potential emotional reactions they may experience in dealing with significant numbers of severely and acutely ill casualties, many of whom may present in ways that are different from those of the patients they are used to seeing. Describe what support systems and approaches have been established to help them adapt to addressing these patients' needs.

Disasters—and, for the foreseeable future, wars—will always be with us. We may find some solace in knowing that we have a greater understanding today of the nature and management of the acute psychiatric disorders that may develop from these stressors than ever before.

References

Emergency Medical Preparedness Office (EMPO): Circular 10-90-107 and Supplement No 1. Washington, DC, Department of Veterans Affairs, August 1990a

Emergency Medical Preparedness Office (EMPO): Fact Sheet. Washington, DC, Department of Veterans Affairs, November 1990b

Fenev A, Anetrella L: Intervention in Traumatic Stress: VA/DoD Contingency. Project Code 91VJ. Northport, NY, Regional Medical Education Center, Department of Veterans Affairs, December 1990

Fenev A, Anetrella L: Interventions in Traumatic Stress: VA/DoD Contingency. Project Code 91WC. Northport, NY, Regional Medical Education Center, Department of Veterans Affairs, February 1991

Friedman MJ, Charney DS, Southwick SM: Psychopharmacotherapy for Recently Evacuated Military Casualties. White River Junction, VT, National Center for PTSD, Department of Veterans Affairs, 1991

11 Deployment Stress and Operation Desert Shield: Preparation for the War

Kathleen M. Wright, Ph.D.
David H. Marlowe, Ph.D.
Robert K. Gifford, Ph.D.

In this chapter we describe the stresses experienced by soldiers as they prepared for war during Operation Desert Shield, the buildup period to the Persian Gulf War. Information gleaned from interviews conducted during this tense period of uncertainty has provided important data on soldiers' adaptation, morale, cohesion, family relationships, and concerns, as well as on potential problems they encountered.

As Desert Shield progressed, units settled in to the desert, awaiting augmentation by Seventh Corps American forces from Germany. Other support elements, primarily reserve units, were also arriving to help build the theater infrastructure. The equipment and supplies necessary to sustain these forces were also brought into the theater.

The infrastructure of the theater matured rapidly. It became useful for mental health personnel to consider this as an evolving community, characterized by a series of developing relationships that occurred at the level of small, unit-based work groups. In turn, these small groups of infantry squads and armor crews were part of larger platoons and companies linked together at increasingly complex and diverse levels of organizational structure within the theater. From this perspective, indicators of community mental health were assessed at the level of the small work group, whose members lived and worked together.

The examination of issues and reactions of groups within the context of evolving community structures encourages attention to the nature of developing relationships within the group. It also facilitates observation of the influences directly affecting these relationships that come from outside the group's immediate boundaries. The use of community functions as indicators also offers a perspective from which to design and implement preventive interventions, recommend changes in existing policies, and address the need for alternative strategies.

In this chapter we offer the reader an opportunity to observe the effects of anticipatory stress and its ramifications for groups and individuals. The experiences and perceptions of combat and support units stationed in the Persian Gulf during the early months of the deployment are compared based on interview data collected during Operation Desert Shield. The organizing focus for these interview data was provided by community-based indicators, which permitted an ongoing assessment of the overall mental health status of the units then in the theater. Several parameters—including group adaptation to the transition of the deployment, the overall morale and confidence of group members, and their perceptions of the bonding, cohesiveness, and instrumental and affective support that had developed within the group—were examined as a basis for assessment of functioning. Influences that were external to the group but that directly affected the functioning of its members included the status of their family relationships and the quality of the relationships developed between the group and its leaders. Based on the analysis of these observations and interview data, we present clinical, research, and community-based recommendations that can inform the actions of civic and military leaders, clinicians, and family members during future military contingencies.

Background on Deployment Research

The emerging emphasis on international peacekeeping missions sponsored by the United Nations has expanded the potential role of the U.S. military in constabulary and low-intensity conflict operations (Etzold 1990; Janowitz 1960; Moskos 1976; Segal 1989; van Doorn and Mans 1966). As mobilization and deployment of units for relatively diverse and potentially long-term missions have assumed increasing significance, so have related research efforts focusing on unit morale and the bonding of unit members as critical indicators of adaptation. For example, in 1982 the Walter Reed Army Institute of Research began to study U.S. Army units deployed for 6-month periods to the Sinai Desert as part of the United Nations–sponsored Multi-National Force and Observers Peace-Keeping Mission. Using a psychosocial perspective, investigators in these studies assessed unit cohesion (i.e., the developing relationships and bonding of unit members with each other and with their leaders), unit morale, and the adaptation of combat-trained soldiers to a constabulary role. Results indicated that despite initial concerns about action-oriented combat troops adjusting to this new role, the direct experiences of living and working together in the new assignment resulted in these troops' increasing effectiveness as peacekeepers (Segal and Gravino 1985). In addition, soldiers began to perceive their participation in this mission as important for their career goals, and they revised their views of "soldiering" to include peacekeeping (Segal and Meeker 1985). These positive changes in soldiers' attitudes toward their new mission and adjustment to their redefined role were also reflected in more sophisticated political discriminations and judgments about the peacekeeping role as an alternative to combat (Meeker and Segal 1987; Segal and Meeker 1985; Segal et al. 1984, 1987).

Researchers also examined the effects of boredom and isolation on soldier adaptation and morale, attempting to discern the implications of such experiences for deployed units. Recommendations emphasized the importance of preparation of troops for such missions. It was urged that the length of such deployments be weighed against the potential for decreased effectiveness, and the value of using recreational and travel facilities in the area as an antidote was stressed (Harris and Segal 1985; Segal et al. 1984). As different types of U.S. Army units assumed the Sinai peacekeeping mission, research expanded to include unit-related comparisons and longitudinal follow-up of their adaptation from predeployment training to redeployment home. This research was designed to assess the long-term consequences of the soldiers' experiences (Segal et al. 1990). These studies found that soldiers coped with their predeployment concerns by seeking as much information as possible about the area. Correspondingly, recommendations from postdeployment follow-up emphasized the importance of predeployment training and the inclusion of more information as part of this preparation.

The researchers also noticed changes in soldiers' perceptions and attitudes following the deployment. These changes included a greater sensitivity to the effects of deployment on their families and increased self-confidence in their own professionalism. Related studies assessed the impact of telephone communication with family members back home on soldier morale. Telephone contact during deployment was a mixed blessing for soldiers. Given the phone's widening availability and importance for forward-deployed soldiers (Applewhite and Segal 1990; Ender 1992), further work needs to be done in this area.

The increasing numbers of young, married servicemembers resulted in significant research efforts devoted to assessing the psychological and psychosocial effects of deployment separation on military personnel and their families. One example of this research was the 2-year, extensive, large-scale study of the Atlantic Fleet sponsored by the Office of Naval Research (Archer and Cauthorne 1985, 1986). In this work investigators assessed stress and coping in approximately 4,000 deployed U.S. Navy personnel and their waiting spouses, as well as evaluated morale and job performance changes over the course of deployment. Major findings emphasized the critical work-family overlap for servicemembers and their spouses, and the strong influence of each on the other's attitudes, perceptions, and eventual adaptation to the deployment was noted. Results from this study led to the development of an assessment checklist for servicemembers and their spouses to help them identify potential problem areas before deployment in order to prevent more serious difficulties during the separation. This study also recommended community interventions and referral resources for waiting families.

Recognition of the significant effects of deployment on military personnel and their families continued with research efforts focused on family functioning while the servicemember was absent. Although separation proved stressful for military families, the majority had developed healthy adaptation patterns to deployment (Eastman et al. 1990). A subgroup of families, however, were identified as "at risk." Families who were considered to be at risk scored higher on life stresses and indicators of poorer functioning, such as increased conflict and control, and lower on indicators of family cohesiveness and organization. Based on correlational data, the authors could not conclude which came first—the life stresses or the poorer functioning and less effective coping. However, it was noted that higher-risk families were younger and had been married fewer years.

The effects of role disruption on family functioning during deployments and subsequent readjustment upon return of the absent soldier-spouse have been a consistent theme in the military family literature since World War II. Hill's (1949) classic study assessed the stresses of separation and reunion for returning veterans and their families. McCubbin et al. (1974) continued this focus in their work with families of Vietnam War veteran prisoners of war, examining the stresses of role transitions in families after prolonged separations. This research emphasis has persisted in recent studies of family separation of soldiers deployed to the Sinai Desert (Jones and Butler 1980; Vuozzo 1990). Correspondingly, research evaluating the effects of parental absence on child development has enjoyed a prominent place in the deployment literature. Studies have assessed such outcomes as changes in cognitive functioning (Hillenbrand 1976) and the emergence of behavior problems in children during the parent's absence (Gabower 1960) or upon return home (Gonzalez 1970), and have recommended family interventions to prevent long-term adjustment problems (Amen et al. 1988; Shaw 1987).

More recently, community-based studies have emerged in the deployment literature. Research comparing family adaptation in different types of communities has shown that the community context can mediate the negative effects of deployment separation on family functioning through support of the spouse left behind. Correspondingly, knowledge of and confidence in this support can relieve some of the concerns of those deployed (McGee 1991). There has been a growing emphasis on service delivery and the role of the community in supporting the families of deployed military personnel. Anticipation of family support needs and of the potential problems that may arise during deployment, such as information flow, financial concerns, and mail and telephone contact, has been described (Moore-Bick 1991). On a larger scale, Chetkow-Yanoov and colleagues (1984) have discussed the design and assessment of various family services and programs. Finally, research on soldier and family responses to deployment strongly supports the importance of predeployment preparation (Buttz 1991; Hegge and Tyner 1982; Smith and Hazen 1991). This preparation should include information programs for families and realistic exercises and training for soldiers (Lenorovitz 1990; Moore-Bick 1991). Practical guidance for unit leaders and care providers related to the different phases of deployment is also useful. The development of a supportive community structure of services and programs to sustain families left behind facilitates adjustment to separation and adaptation to a new environment, as well as helps prevent negative psychological outcomes. (For a more comprehensive review of military family research, see the selected bibliographies prepared by the Military Family Resource

Center, Ballston Center Tower Three, Suite 903, 4015 Wilson Boulevard, Arlington, VA 22203-5190.)

During Operations Desert Shield/Desert Storm, the selection of topics addressed in interviews with soldiers was informed by critical categories gleaned from the literature. The issues of soldier adaptation, morale, cohesion, and the effects of family separation were discussed with soldiers. Given the sudden escalation of events requiring the immediate preparation of units and their equipment for the Operation Desert Shield deployment, there was not sufficient time for extensive preparation of soldiers and their families. As the following discussion will show, most of the significant concerns raised by soldiers interviewed during Operation Desert Shield related to family issues. The soldiers perceived by unit leaders and service providers to be most at risk were those who were younger and newly married, those in troubled marriages or relationships, and those with extensive worries about their families back home. Soldier concerns about their spouses and children, and about their parents and younger siblings, remained a predominant theme throughout the deployment. Although many positive changes occurred in soldier adaptation as the theater matured, worries about family safety and security and the pain of separation remained.

The WRAIR Research Program

In 1989, the Department of Military Psychiatry of the Walter Reed Army Institute of Research (WRAIR) established a program of research on traumatic stress to determine the psychological sequelae of combat and combat losses for soldiers. The deployment of U.S. Army units to the Persian Gulf in August 1990 provided the opportunity to extend the research program by following units from the time of their initial notification to deploy through the final outcome of the operation. The intent was to capture the phases of Operations Desert Shield/Desert Storm as they unfolded, providing a longitudinal assessment of soldiers and their families. The main focus of the research was on the psychological consequences of the experiences of deployment and combat.

In September 1990, the initial phase of the Desert Shield/Desert Storm research program began. A team from the Department of Military Psychiatry visited the Persian Gulf theater of operations and identified salient issues to inform the design of instruments for continued monitoring of soldier and unit adaptation to the deployment (Gifford et al. 1991, 1992). A semistructured interview guide and survey questionnaire resulted from this initial assessment. In November 1990, a second team visited the four Army divisions then in theater, conducting semistructured individual and group interviews. Approximately 1,300 survey questionnaires were collected from soldiers in each of the divisions and their support units.

The semistructured interview format followed a chronological description of soldiers' experiences and reactions from the time they were first notified of the deployment, through their preparation and leave-taking, to their arrival in Saudi Arabia. The objective was to elicit soldiers' perspectives on certain issues: adaptation to the deployment, unit morale, the development of cohesion, family and personal relationships, and concerns and potential problems. As discussed in the previous section, these areas were conceptualized as providing information about the general mental health status and functioning of deployed units and would serve as indicators of the unit members' adjustment.

The results summarized below focus on the interviews conducted in November and December 1990 and on those reactions and perceptions most widely and consistently expressed by soldiers. Whenever possible, vignettes provided by soldiers illustrate critical themes, unique stressors, and emerging contextual factors contributing to adjustment. Because of the different structure, tasks, and experiences of combat versus support units, the results are organized in two sections: 1) soldier issues in the four Combat Arms Divisions and 2) issues from the corps-level support organizations.

Operation Desert Shield: The Maturing Theater

Combat Units

Adaptation

The primary concern raised by soldiers during the first research team site visit in September was their uncertainty about the duration of the deployment. In the November–December visit, the transition from an open-ended deployment to one with a terminal point became the critical factor positively affecting soldier adaptation and morale. Also during this time, a number of additional influences on soldier adjustment converged. These included the rapid maturation of theater, corps, and division infrastructures required to meet the demands of an expanding force; the increase, as part of this maturation, of life support and stress-mediating structures (e.g., unit designed camps, fundamental amenities, days off, creature comforts, telephones); and the effects on soldiers and units of extended, uninterrupted training and living together under conditions of hardship.

These developments occurred within a context of external events; decisions made at higher levels outside the theater had significant impact on soldier adaptation. For example, critical decisions in the November–December time frame included Secretary Cheney's announcement of the Desert Shield deployment "for the duration," the imminent arrival of Seventh Corps units from Germany in theater, and the United Nations resolution sanctioning the use of force against Iraq. For soldiers, the rapid development of the theater coupled with the political developments resulted in a focused anticipation of combat. The soldiers perceived combat as the event that marked the end point of their deployment and their imminent return home.

Morale

Morale is used here to refer to the soldiers' overall perception of and commitment to mission and unit, sense of well-being, and general acceptance of the conditions of the deployment and of a potential combat scenario. It does not refer to fluctuating feelings, moods, or responses to momentary problems. In most units, morale had improved since the research team's initial assessment in September 1990. In September, morale was generally high; in November, it was higher still. Soldiers in almost all companies interviewed typically rated their morale at about 7 to 8 on a 0- to 10-point scale. They pointed out that it was as high or higher than it had been at their home stations. Generally, soldiers attributed their high morale to their belief that there was now an end to the mission and that when they got the job done they would go home. Although initially a blow, the statement that they would be in Saudi Arabia "for the duration" ended extensive and sometimes damaging rumors about rotation dates home. This decision reinforced a sense of purpose and made the deployment appear closed rather than open-ended. As many of the initial differences between units and organizations in theater regarding the quality of life support, and morale, welfare, and recreation amenities decreased, so did feelings of resentment and deprivation.

Soldiers reported that the major contributors to their personal morale were mail; showers; tents; rest areas; hot food; cold drinks; being able to live as squads, crews, or platoons in self-improved areas; entertainment; and some free time. Visits to the resort area at Half Moon Bay, home visits to civilian families who worked in Saudi Arabia, and the special celebration at Thanksgiving were all great morale boosts. Wherever telephones were widely available, soldiers and leaders reported them to be a major contributor to morale. The opportunity to call home often resulted in rapid solutions of family problems and maintained critical emotional linkages and feelings of well-being. For most soldiers, the initial burst of telephone calls was followed by self-regulation in the rate of calling.

Soldiers viewed contributions to morale as symbols of caring and respect for their needs on the part of their leaders. Even small changes and improvements assumed great symbolic value. During this time, almost all standard indirect measures of morale, such as disciplinary actions, sick call visits, accidents, and intragroup conflicts, were extremely low. The assessment by a group of platoon sergeants, leaders at the small unit level, reflected the conclusions of many soldiers interviewed:

> Overall morale is pretty high. Good morale and cohesion are due to the proximity factor and the high interdependency in squads and platoon. Sharing hardships is important. There are new soldiers in the unit, but you would never know it. Living together in hardship also builds cohesion.

Cohesion

Soldiers did an extraordinary job taking care of each other at the unit level. Both the research team, based on their observations, and the soldiers interviewed concluded that both the cohesion of unit members and their bonding to squad leaders and tank commanders were very high. Above the small work group, at the squad and crew levels, cohesion was relatively high and improving. Cohesion increased as a result of living, working, training, and solving problems together in a challenging and isolated environment. Soldiers came to know and trust each other both as professionals with respected technical and combat skills and as friends and sources of support. Interviews with four-man tank crews revealed the importance to these individuals of "integrity," or keeping the members of a crew together.

> Bonding: Knowing what he'll say or do before he does it. We become "interchangeable parts." This helps the new soldiers fit in more quickly. They help each other in terms of family problems. We keep an eye on each other. Being together 24 hours a day is high cohesion building.

Soldiers reported across-the-board improvements in cohesion, communication, morale, and combat confidence since their arrival in Saudi Arabia. But they also talked about the need for privacy and a chance to get away at times. In interviews,

soldiers described a series of informal cultural rules and strategies for ensuring a minimum of interpersonal conflict under
crowded and stressful living conditions. Almost all confronta-
tions were turned into jokes and dealt with humorously rather
than antagonistically. They also reported a greater tolerance of
differences in themselves and in their groups. Aggression was
channeled into athletics or into wrestling matches. As one soldier said, "You do not want to fight with the man who will cover
your back!" Cohesion appeared highest in those groups that had
been together for the longest periods. One of the members of an
armor platoon, composed of four tank crews, in which almost
all of the soldiers had served for at least 1 year, put it this way:

> Our platoon is the backbone of the company. We're confi-
> dent in our leaders and in ourselves. We're friends and be-
> lieve in and trust each other. We take care of each other and
> take it seriously. We're completely cross-section-trained,
> any of us can do any job in the platoon. We treat each other
> as family: we're like brothers, we share problems, we joke.
> And like a brother, when I get angry at him[,] we wrestle in
> the sand pit.

In most cases, bonding had developed between soldiers and
their leaders. Soldiers reported bonding most strongly to those
who participated and led by doing, who shared available news
and intelligence with them regularly, and who treated them with
the moderate informality, intimacy, and care that are considered
appropriate in a potentially dangerous precombat situation.
Soldiers did not bond to leaders when they had doubts about
their leaders' competence, an evaluation based on their leaders'
performance or perceived lack of common sense. Problems in
bonding were most marked in units that received large numbers
of midlevel noncommissioned officers (NCOs) as fillers and attachments immediately before deployment or as replacements
in theater. In units that experienced such turnover and turbulence, soldiers invariably said that they wanted a tough, all-out
training exercise to test new and untried unit leaders.

By November, most soldiers no longer perceived the deployment as a field training exercise. Life in Saudi Arabia became normal routine, "the regular daily way we live." Soldiers referred to bases and camps as "home." They often used the word "here" to cover both Saudi Arabia and their home post in the United States. With the anticipation of imminent combat, field exercises away from the large fixed camp areas became more valued. The unit field sites were viewed as embodying more freedom and as a place in which positive relationships between soldiers and leaders were encouraged. Related to this issue was the observation that while at their field sites these individuals had ingeniously solved a number of living problems, as well as a number of equipment and field maintenance problems. Many expressed the hope that these solutions were being recorded and transferred to others in theater and to incoming units.

Family and Personal Relationships

During the November–December time frame, most problems surfacing in the deployed force seemed to be family related. Chaplains and soldiers perceived the group most at risk to be young, recently married soldiers with pregnant wives and soldiers in relationships that were troubled before deployment. Rumors of widespread marital breakup and perceptions of increased incidence of "Dear John" letters had negative effects on morale. Concerns persisted even when the rumors proved to be untrue. Apprehension about the safety and security of their homes and families was raised by rumors reportedly spread by replacements coming in theater, who described increasing crime in their former communities. In a number of cases, soldiers worried about their children's or younger siblings' reactions to the threat of war and loss. Long-term child care arrangements for deployed single parents or dual-career couples and custody issues for divorced parents were relatively infrequent, but distressing, problems. A tightly bonded four-man tank crew discussed the potential implications of such concerns and how to cope with them:

> People [e.g., the crew] depend on you. We may have prob-
> lems, but when it's time to do our job . . . I may have some
> tears in my eyes before I go to sleep, but that's alright. I
> have the right to do that. Leave home problems at home,
> prepare yourself for what is coming. One man in a crew can
> get a whole crew killed, that's a "no go." If we go to war, leave
> family problems behind you. Talk to other crew members
> about it. If you are the type to dwell on problems, you're
> a risk to the people over here. We have a couple of loners
> in the platoon. Sitting by themselves in the dark. Other
> crew members keep an eye out and try to interact. . . .
> We're not complainers. We're not suffering here. We're just
> anxious to do what we have to do. We live better than any
> other Army in the field.

Family support groups, established back at the home posts, received conflicting reviews from soldiers across units. Some soldiers seemed to know little about the groups or their spouses' participation in them, whereas some perceived the family support group as working well and could explain their spouses' role and responsibilities. On the other hand, a number of unit leaders described their spouses as severely stressed by the demands, responsibilities, and continuous work in family support. Some soldiers were concerned about leaving families at a new post just before deployment, with little knowledge of the area or community. Soldiers most comfortable with arrangements at home either had spouses with an established support system or had spouses who returned home to their family of origin.

On the whole, contact with spouses by mail or telephone remained a primary source of support and was critical for morale for the overwhelming majority of married soldiers. Letters provided tangible contact with home. The telephone provided an opportunity for more intimate contact and reassurance, as well as immediate participation in problem solving. Lack of communication, either because of slow mail delivery or because of lack of access to telephones, was very frustrating for soldiers and hurt morale.

Concerns and Potential Problems

In November, units with the highest confidence appeared to be those with the most extensive knowledge about Iraqi combat capabilities and the best ways to overcome them. When soldiers had an exaggerated image of Iraqi strength, they were more anxious, and, alternatively, when soldiers were casually dismissive of Iraqi military potential, they tended to be overly complacent. In November, soldiers appeared to be pacing themselves. They reported that they did not want to "peak too soon," and some expressed fears about growing stale with overtraining or about losing their edge as a result of constant "over-alertness." As one soldier put it, "My edge requires time to be laid back before I go all out." A few leaders seemed counterproductive in their attempts to prepare their soldiers psychologically for combat. For example, some soldiers were deeply shaken by leaders who talked to them about the large numbers who would be killed in combat, rather than emphasizing that although there would be casualties, they would try to bring everyone home alive.

Many soldiers interviewed in November were negatively affected by casualty estimates in the media. They did not understand the nature of such projections and believed that the casualty figures of 20,000 to 50,000 used in the press referred to soldiers killed in action rather than to battle injuries of any sort.

One commander's method for preparing his soldiers is worth mentioning because it was perceived by them as extremely helpful during this phase of combat anticipation. Circulating around the areas where they lived and worked, he was constantly visible.

> We have a great plan and excellent chain of command. . . .
> I emphasized we were so far ahead of the Iraqis in terms of
> equipment and training. . . . They trusted me. I was trying
> to encourage healthy self-confidence. Healthy respect. Re-
> lationships are based on mutual respect. . . . I would tell
> them: You are American heroes. You're the point of the
> spear. Each of us is counting on one another. Interdepen-

dence. You'll write history, as warriors. Don't do anything
to diminish what you have already accomplished. I knew
they were ready. . . . I kept card files on each soldier and
their families for details about their lives. It is astonishingly
important to them. Showing them they would not be put at
undue risk. It shows: This leader really cares about me.

Soldiers often spoke about the general political situation in
Saudi Arabia. Some questioned why they were there, what the
national interest and objectives were, and the reasons they were
going to war. Typically, soldiers said, "I don't want to fight for
cheap gasoline, but I will fight for democracy because I'm an
American, and for human rights in Kuwait, or to keep that bas-
tard from getting nukes."

Many soldiers were deeply concerned that the deployment
would hurt their reenlistment options and futures in the Army
since they could not complete training or education requirements that were necessary to be competitive for promotion.
Many leaders were worried and angry about the possibility of
downsizing and a mandatory reduction in force. A number of
soldiers spontaneously brought up the fear that they would go
to war, survive, and then "get a pink slip as I come off the plane
at home." This issue had great potential to hurt morale.

In November, relative deprivation had improved, but the
perception that there were "double" standards continued to
erode soldier mood at a different level. Letters and news articles
from home implying that the entire theater shared the living
conditions, food, and amenities of rear echelons or other services rankled. Forward-deployed soldiers knew and appreciated
the fact that they lived differently for operational reasons. However, they wanted people at home to know what they had
achieved while "living tough." Their perception of "double"
standards was also reflected in anger over reports of officers being sent home for school or to change command.

One indicator of possible overconfidence, or perhaps just
haste to get the job done and go home, was inferred from discussions about the imminent arrival of the Seventh Corps from

Germany. Although many soldiers looked forward to the arrival of the Seventh Corps, a number dismissed it as unimportant, asserting, "Just let us go and get the job done." The most enthusiasm occurred in units in which the rationale for Seventh Corps' deployment to the theater had been explained to soldiers in terms of casualty minimization. One final issue that surfaced in the interviews concerned reports across units that midlevel sergeants were showing the greatest strain and were the most likely to get into arguments. It was unclear why these NCOs were the most distressed.

Although the possibility of combat became increasingly certain during this time, soldiers still wanted to know how long they would be deployed if there were no war. There was general agreement that if there had not been a war or an announcement about rotation plans within 6 months after initial deployment, there would have been a massive morale problem. A summary of issues raised in the interview assessments of community functioning for soldiers in combat units is presented in Table 11–1.

Support Units

The topics discussed in this subsection are drawn from individual and group interviews conducted with corps-level personnel from seven support organizations representing four different functional areas (ordinance, postal, medical, and graves registration).

Adaptation

Some support units interviewed were accustomed to deployment and were well established shortly after arrival in theater. They had comfortable living conditions, primarily because of their experiences from prior deployments that guided decisions about what to bring with them (e.g., extra tentage, showers, VCRs, tapes, and washing machines). Other support units were not as well equipped or self-reliant and as a consequence were more dependent on other organizations for support. For

Table 11–1. Issues raised in the interview assessments of community functioning for soldiers in combat units

Adaptation	Ambiguity about deployment ended Sense of purpose emerging Infrastructure of theater developing and amenities improving
Morale	Feelings of relative deprivation decreased Communications with home improved Symbols of leader caring evident
Cohesion	Unit member bonding very high Rules and strategies to moderate conflict emerging Bases and camps becoming home
Family relationships	Mail and phone contacts important Worries about family safety evident Family transitions before deployment a concern
Concerns and potential problems	Iraqi military potential viewed unrealistically Concerns about "losing their edge" over time evident Confusion about casualty rates evident Rationale for the deployment and combat Concerns about future careers in the Army evident

some, living conditions worsened when they moved away from the concentrated headquarter areas to their field sites.

None of the support soldiers interviewed liked the crowded quarters that were transiently occupied upon arrival in Saudi Arabia. The transient quarters were large open warehouses or areas set up with thousands of tents. The support soldiers described the stresses of living with strangers, the lack of privacy and crowding, not having control of their own areas, and, in particular, not having their own showers and latrines that they could maintain in good condition. Latrines and showers at field sites, maintained by the unit itself, were spotless in comparison with facilities in the warehouses or tent cities.

Most of those interviewed in the support units felt confident in their skills and well trained to perform their jobs. However, once in theater, the workload for these units was heavy and generally increased over the course of the deployment. Routinely, the majority of soldiers assigned to these units worked 14- to 18-hour days. Shiftwork was organized with semipermanent day and night shifts, rotated every 2 to 3 weeks. This arrangement worked reasonably well. However, for units quartered in open warehouses, individuals on the night shift had trouble getting to sleep during the day because of the noise and commotion of transient soldiers co-quartered with them while waiting to be sent to various receiving units in the theater. Some support soldiers worried that their leaders were not attending enough to safety issues. Their concerns focused on increased probability of accidents given the intensified rate of work, greater workloads with attendant fatigue, and inability to recuperate during time off.

The support units interviewed contained both men and women. In general, women claimed that sexual harassment was not a problem. Some of them would have preferred to live with their units in mixed groups rather than living in an all-female area with strangers. Others preferred the alternative for the additional privacy. The general consensus was to give the women both options: establish a separate area for those who want it, and permit those who do not to stay with their units in a mixed area. Mixed-gender units typically exhibited siblinglike relationships reminiscent of those found in a college dormitory or an Israeli kibbutz. As one female soldier noted, "I know their wives, they know my husband. We are friends and there can't be any playing around."

Morale

Pride in their tangible accomplishments in building the theater's infrastructure from the ground up sustained morale in the support units surveyed. In addition, being able to live comfortably through one's own efforts, in an austere environment and often despite perceived lack of support from higher levels, raised morale. For example, morale was particularly high in one reserve unit in which the majority of the soldiers had been with the company for a long time. Unit members brought skills from civilian life (e.g., carpentry, electrical work, plumbing) that made adaptation to the theater easier. The newer members of the unit called up for the deployment were young, highly motivated, and, typically, in college or graduate school. In addition, two of the unit leaders were former Vietnam War veterans who knew the system of the "big" Army well, were expert and creative "scroungers," and were able to obtain anything unit members might need.

As found in the combat units, the duration of deployment emerged as a critical issue affecting morale among support units. Reserve and National Guard soldiers in the support units perceived 180 days as their maximum tour length and viewed extensions beyond that as, at best, an extreme hardship for themselves and their families. They believed their morale and productivity would drop dramatically if they were extended beyond 180 days without some defined end in sight. They also were concerned about keeping their military orders current in order to hold open civilian jobs and maintain interest rates with creditors until their return home. At the time, they had orders in hand for only 90 days. They reported that some employers and creditors were threatening not to extend job protection and credit benefits beyond 90 days unless they were shown updated documents. Reserve personnel anticipated the same problems again if their deployment in Saudi Arabia was extended past 180 days.

Cohesion

Cohesion varied much more across the different support units interviewed than it did across the combat units. In reserve units, cohesion seemed to be diminished by attachment of large numbers of active-duty personnel or other augmentees, a necessary requirement given the workload. For several of the support units in which cohesion was high for unit members, cohesion with leaders was problematic because of new, inexperienced, and frequently changing leadership at the company level and above. Cohesion in several units also suffered because of mergers, frequent moves, and changes in command. Some units had lost all sense of relationship and connection to their higher organizations, which further contributed to their sense of isolation.

Family and Personal Relationships

Reservists, as noted, focused on 180 days in theater as their "duration," and so did their families. These soldiers were deeply concerned about how their families would cope emotionally and financially if their deployment extended beyond this time. Most would not even acknowledge the possibility of being deployed longer than 6 months and quickly changed the subject when the issue was brought up. Personnel who were self-employed at home were particularly worried, as were soldiers who were single parents and concerned about potentially or actually unstable child care arrangements.

Concerns and Potential Problems

Many support soldiers perceived their units as overextended. They worried that they would be used up physically and psychologically and that they would fail at critical points in the future, if or when combat occurred. Soldiers in both active-duty and reserve support units that were attached to other organizations for the deployment described themselves as "orphan units." They asserted that they had never "trained the actual mission" they were required to perform in the deployment with their new organizations. Some did not have the necessary equipment to work optimally. Members of one unit stated that they had never had exposure to or practice for the potential stressors unique to their combat mission (e.g., rate and volume of work, long hours, shifts, living conditions).

As noted for soldiers in combat units, active-duty personnel in support units were worried about the future downsizing of the military. Some had passed the date upon which they were to leave the service, being retained in place for the deployment. They had missed an important period of transition for new jobs and living arrangements. Soldiers past their transition dates, as well as those facing reduction, wanted the option of remaining on active duty for a period of time (e.g., up to 90 days after return home) to get their lives in order and make plans for the future. Soldiers who planned to reenlist wanted assurance that places would be available for them in the special schools or programs they needed in order to be competitive, to begin after "the duration." A summary of issues raised in the interview assessments of community functioning for soldiers in support units is presented in Table 11–2.

Conclusions

Findings from the Operation Desert Shield phase of research of the WRAIR Research Program conducted in November–December 1990 included a theater context that had matured considerably since the initial deployment in September. The results from this phase of research, summarized in Table 11–3, encompass the stressors identified by the research team in September and the critical changes discovered during the second assessment in November and December.

Theater infrastructures continued to develop in November, but much had been accomplished in a very short period of time. With the upcoming arrival of the Seventh Corps, combat and support units already established were eager to share what they had learned. Despite the cultural constraints and austerity of their physical environment, soldiers communicated a sense of pride in the creative solutions they had discovered. As the theater developed and amenities improved, even small changes assumed symbolic significance. Improvements made by soldiers at the unit level transformed field sites in the desert into "home,"

Table 11–2. Issues raised in the interview assessments of community functioning for soldiers in support units

Adaptation	Importance of prior experience in field or deployment training exercises evident
	Workable male/female living arrangements evolved
	Concerns about fatigue and accidents because of heavy workloads and long hours evident
	Crowded living conditions for many units apparent
Morale	Pride in building theater infrastructure emerging
	Tangible accomplishments from work experienced
	Many units living comfortably through their own ingenuity and efforts
	Uncertainty about tour length evident
	Concerns about jobs and creditors at home evident
Cohesion	Cohesion more variable than in combat units because of greater turbulence in leader and unit member changes
	Sense of isolation and feeling unconnected from chain of command evident in some units
Family	Worries about family's ability to function expressed
Concerns and potential problems	Concerns about failure at critical points should combat occur expressed
	"Orphan units" feeling untrained for their support requirements

and externally directed improvements demonstrated leader and chain-of-command caring and concern.

Most critical for soldiers during this period was that the stress of uncertainty about the duration of the deployment and

Table 11–3. Operation Desert Shield deployment stresses and changes

Key stresses: early phase	Uncertain tour length
	Ambiguous demands: precombat preparation vs. garrison environment
	Lack of communication with families at home
	Information deprivation and rumors
	Austere living and harsh desert conditions
	Lack of respite away from other unit members
	Cultural isolation and ambivalent perceptions
Changes: maturing theater	Improving amenities: important as symbols and in their own right
	Decrease in perception of deprivation relative to other units
	Focusing events: "for the duration" announcement and January 15 UN deadline to Iraq
	Units' referring to field sites as "home"
	Enhancement of unit confidence and cohesion by training and close living

the ambiguity surrounding their eventual mission were resolved. Focusing events and times provided closure. Secretary Cheney's announcement of "for the duration," and the January 15 deadline given to Iraq by the United Nations, clarified soldiers' uncertainty about their role and purpose. When the soldiers became convinced that "the road home led through Kuwait," their energy became more and more focused on their units and on their training. As unit members lived and worked together under conditions of hardship, their cohesion, confidence, and morale improved, providing the backdrop for their adaptation.

Most soldiers were deployed to the Persian Gulf as members of relatively intact units, leaving their families within a structure of community support represented by unit-level family support groups and the rear detachment command, a cadre of unit members, who would be the interface between the deployed soldiers and their families at home. Although some spouses returned to their families of origin, many remained at the military installations, embedded in a well-defined structure of community social support that would sustain them in the months to come as the deployment moved into the combat phase of Operation Desert Storm.

Correspondingly, the soldiers, supported within the context of their units, developed deepening relationships while building new communities in the desert of Saudi Arabia as they waited for events to unfold. Both the evolving soldier communities in the desert and the communities of families waiting at home may be compared with other communities responding to disaster or crisis. Each illustrates adaptation through various transformations arising from common experiences of separation and loss that affect all the members of the community. The shared experiences of soldiers and their families in both contexts reinforced the bonds between group members, providing a basis of mutual support. In both contexts, an assessment of group cohesion, morale, and adaptation over time served as indicators of community adjustment to a crisis situation and of the capacity of the community to sustain itself should the crisis continue or worsen. Both the community of families and the community of deployed soldiers changed during the course of Operation Desert Shield as decisions made by world leaders led toward war. This evolving set of circumstances focused each community on sustaining its members throughout the prolonged deployment and the eventual crisis of combat.

Recommendations

The following are recommendations based on findings from the Operation Desert Shield phase of research of the WRAIR Research Program conducted in November–December 1990.

Community

Communities should be aware that soldiers activated to serve in reserve units and their families may be at higher risk during and following the deployment than active-duty servicemembers.

Some reasons for this increased risk may include the more disruptive circumstances of the deployment for reservists and their families: the deployment was unexpected, relatively sudden, and marked throughout by significant financial and job-related concerns. In addition, as described earlier in this chapter, because reserve units were predominantly support units, reservists had different experiences than did soldiers in combat units during Operation Desert Shield. They experienced differences in workload, living arrangements, and role and mission clarity. Adaptation to the deployment for some of these units may have been more difficult and prolonged given that, at least initially, less of a supportive, cohesive structure existed for members of these units than for members of combat units. Soldiers in many reserve units also experienced a longer separation period from their families than did those in combat units, remaining in Saudi Arabia to support the redeployment home and close the theater.

Given this matrix of stresses, there are several interventions that communities might consider: predeployment preparation efforts, with community reassurance of soldiers and families of ongoing support for the duration of the deployment; community outreach efforts to families of reservists who may have special needs or require special assistance; and, following redeployment home, special recognition by the community of contributions and sacrifices made by reservists and their families.

Using a community perspective and considering the military unit as a community of small interlocking work groups suggest that the unit can serve as a transitional context, providing a recovery environment as soldiers support one another after sharing a common set of experiences in Operations Desert Shield/ Desert Storm. Keeping units intact following the cessation of hostilities provides stability for unit members so that they can prepare together for redeployment home. Information addressing family reunion issues and readjustment to their former work environment at the installation can be provided and discussed during this time, as well as can debriefings about combat experiences and other significant deployment-related events.

Clinical

Unit-level care providers should be aware of the deep sense of attachment that developed in the desert among soldiers in cohesive units during Operations Desert Shield/Desert Storm, and anticipate their sense of loss when various ones among them leave the unit. Related to this are the implications for new soldiers who come to replace these veterans and the potential difficulty of their integration. Consultations to unit leaders, in which awareness of these issues is raised and interventions suggested, might be useful in preventing future problems.

Clinicians working with Desert Storm veterans should consider the possibility that adjustment to the predeployment and deployment phases of Operation Desert Shield may have been more stressful for soldiers than the eventual combat phase of the operation. For example, this broader context included the stresses of readying units and equipment for a rapid deployment; leaving families suddenly and unexpectedly, sometimes with little personal time to prepare and say good-bye; experiencing a prolonged period of adapting to a new environment initially characterized by uncertain tour length, ambiguous demands, lack of communication with home, and isolated and austere living conditions; and anticipating combat. In addition to these significant stresses were soldiers' career concerns about their future in the Army given the plans for downsizing, which for many soldiers became a reality after they returned home. Under these circumstances, it may be difficult for veterans to perceive any recognition or appreciation for their sacrifices. Adjustment following these events may be marked by anger and bitterness that have little to do with exposure to combat.

An important finding from pre– and post–Desert Storm interviews that may provide a more balanced perspective for soldiers experiencing adjustment difficulties was the positive outcomes and changes that soldiers experienced during their time in Saudi Arabia. They described greater confidence in their abilities to cope, an enhanced sense of self-worth, and a developing awareness of priorities about what is important in their lives. Along with these indicators of growing maturity was their belief that they were contributing to a significant international event. Overall, soldiers managed their work and relationships remarkably well in circumstances characterized by uncertainty, austerity, and anxiety. Recalling these strengths and what they learned during this time may help them evaluate the costs and benefits of their Desert Storm experiences.

Research

Research studying the outcomes of soldier experiences in Operations Desert Shield/Desert Storm should include an assessment of the positive changes noted above. Increased self-confidence and tolerance of others, greater maturity, decisions about values and priorities, and changing perspectives on family and career issues were frequently mentioned by soldiers in interviews. Even when enumerating the stresses, fears, and difficulties of the deployment, they did not regret the opportunity to be a part of it. Such research should, if possible, include longitudinal follow-up, because awareness of many changes may become increasingly significant over time.

Future Directions

The research on the deployment phase of Operation Desert Shield discussed in this chapter is one component of an extensive research program being conducted by the Walter Reed Army Institute of Research in which the consequences of the Gulf War for servicemembers and their families are being assessed. The program continued through the combat phase of Operation Desert Storm and then followed units and soldiers previously interviewed and surveyed after their return home in Summer–Fall 1991, and again 1 year later in 1992. Currently, data collection is completed for the combat units and analyses are ongoing. Future plans include final follow-up of Army Reserve and National Guard support units, and expansion of the research to selected samples of active-duty, reserve, and National Guard personnel representing the other military services. With these efforts, the database for Operations Desert Shield/Desert Storm will include approximately 40,000 service-members representing hundreds of different units and organizations.

In addition to data collected for servicemembers, the research extends to military families with interviews and survey questionnaires designed to examine stresses, life events, and coping during the deployment, and readjustment problems after soldiers returned home. A study of children of deployed parents and an evaluation of community and installation-based family support services and programs represent other projects within the program.

Major efforts in the post–Desert Storm data collection and analyses are focusing on the epidemiology of psychological sequelae of deployment to combat and will include consideration of factors contributing to self-development and maturity, as well as influences affecting risk for postcombat stress disorders and symptoms. Providing an etiological taxonomy of the broad range of reactions to such traumatic events may facilitate the design of treatment models for mental health and community care providers in the active force, the Veterans Administration, and civilian society who may work with these soldiers/veterans or their families in the future.

References

Amen DG, Merves E, Jellen L, et al: Minimizing the impact of deployment separation on military children: stages, current preventive efforts, and system recommendations. Mil Med 153:441–446, 1988

Applewhite LW, Segal DR: Telephone use by peacekeeping troops in the Sinai. Armed Forces and Society 17:117–126, 1990

Archer RP, Cauthorne CV: An investigation of the effects of deployment-related factors on performance and psychosocial adjustment (Technical Report No ONR 00014-84-C-0666). Arlington, VA, Office of Naval Research, Navy Manpower Research and Development Program, 1985

Archer RP, Cauthorne CV: A final report on an investigation of deployment related factors on performance and psychosocial adjustment (Technical Report No 86-1). Arlington, VA, Office of Naval Research, Navy Manpower Research and Development Program, 1986

Buttz CL: Preparation for overseas movement: lessons learned. Mil Med 156:639–641, 1991

Chetkow-Yanoov EG, Reisner N, Rubin A: Emergency centers in Israel: a small community organizes to cope with war related crises. Disasters 8:297–301, 1984

Eastman E, Archer RP, Ball JD: Psychosocial and life stress characteristics of Navy families: Family Environment Scale and Life Experiences Scale findings. Military Psychology 2:113–127, 1990

Ender MG: GI phone home: the use of telecommunications by the soldiers of Operation Just Cause. Paper presented at the 87th annual meeting of the American Sociological Association, Pittsburgh, PA, August 1992

Etzold TH: National strategy and mobilization: emerging issues for the 1990s. Naval War College Review 43(1):19–30, 1990

Gabower G: Behavior problems of children in Navy officers' families. Social Casework 41:177–184, 1960

Gifford RK, Martin JA, Marlowe DH: Operation Desert Shield: adaptation of soldiers during the early phases of the deployment to Saudi Arabia. Paper presented at the biennial meeting of the Inter-University Seminar on Armed Forces & Society, Baltimore, MD, October 1991

Gifford RK, Marlowe DH, Wright KM, et al: Unit cohesion in Operation Desert Shield/Storm. Journal of the U.S. Army Medical Department, November/December 1992, pp 11–13

Gonzalez VR: Psychiatry and the Army Brat. Springfield, IL, Charles C Thomas, 1970

Harris JJ, Segal DR: Observations from the Sinai: the boredom factor. Armed Forces and Society 11:235–248, 1985

Hegge FW, Tyner CF: Deployment threats to rapid deployment forces (Report No 82-2). Washington, DC, Walter Reed Army Institute of Research, Division of Neuropsychiatry, 1982

Hill R: Families Under Stress: Adjustment to the Crisis of War Separation and Reunion. New York, Harper & Brothers, 1949

Hillenbrand ED: Father absence in military families. The Family Coordinator, October 1976, pp 451–458

Janowitz M: The Professional Soldier: A Social and Political Portrait. New York, Free Press, 1960

Jones AP, Butler MC: A role transition approach to the stresses of organizationally induced family role disruption. Journal of Marriage and the Family 42:367–376, 1980

Lenorovitz JM: Desert Shield deployment shows need for realistic training in harsh conditions. Aviation Week and Space Technology 133(13):50–51, 1990

McCubbin HI, Dahl BB, Metres P, et al: Family separation and reunion: families of prisoners of war and servicemen missing in action (Cat No D-206. 21:74–50). Washington, DC, U.S. Government Printing Office, 1974

McGee CP: Impact of Operation Desert Shield/Storm on reserve component families. Paper presented at the biennial meeting of the Inter-University Seminar on Armed Forces & Society, Baltimore, MD, October 1991

Meeker BF, Segal DR: Soldiers' perceptions of conflict likelihood: the effects of doctrine and experience. Journal of Political and Military Sociology 15:108–115, 1987

Moore-Bick JD: Operation Granby: preparation and deployment for war. The Royal Engineers Journal 105:260–267, 1991

Moskos CC: Peace Soldiers: The Sociology of a United Nations Military Force. Chicago, IL, University of Chicago Press, 1976

Segal DR: Recruiting for Uncle Sam: Citizenship and Military Manpower Policy. Lawrence, University of Kansas Press, 1989

Segal DR, Gravino KS: Peacekeeping as a military mission, in The Hundred Percent Challenge. Edited by Smith CD. Washington, DC, Seven Locks Press, 1985, pp 38–68

Segal DR, Meeker BF: Peacekeeping, warfighting and professionalism: attitude organization and change among combat soldiers on constabulary duty. Journal of Political and Military Sociology 13:167–181, 1985

Segal DR, Harris JJ, Rothberg JM, et al: Paratroopers as peacekeepers. Armed Forces and Society 10:487–506, 1984

Segal DR, Harris JJ, Rothberg JM, et al: Deterrence, peacekeeping, and combat orientation in the U.S. Army, in Challenge and Deterrence in the 1990s. Edited by Simbala S. New York, Praeger, 1987, pp 41–53

Segal DR, Furukawa TP, Lindh JC: Light infantry as peacekeepers in the Sinai. Armed Forces and Society 16:385–403, 1990

Shaw JA: Children in the military. Psychiatric Annals 17:539–544, 1987

Smith AM, Hazen SJ: What makes war surgery different? Mil Med 156:33–35, 1991

van Doorn J, Mans JH: United Nations Forces on legitimacy and effectiveness of international military operations. Paper presented at the Section on "The Professional Military Man and Militarism" at the Sixth World Congress of Sociology, Evian, France, 1966

Vuozzo JS: The relationship between consistency in focus of coping and symptoms among wives experiencing geographic marital separation and reunion. Unpublished master's thesis, University of Maryland, College Park, 1990

12 Family Notification and Survivor Assistance: Thinking the Unthinkable

Paul T. Bartone, Ph.D.

In this chapter I focus on military personnel who provide various kinds of support and assistance to the families of killed and wounded soldiers. The U.S. Army has developed extensive programs and policies for the processing of war casualties and for providing help to the survivors (Bartone and Ender 1994). Recent research has shown that individuals who perform these casualty support duties often find them highly stressful and can experience a variety of deleterious psychological sequelae.

Following traumatic events, the focus of attention for treatment providers and researchers alike is usually the immediate victims, those directly exposed. This is generally true whether the stressors are related to war (e.g., Kulka et al. 1990; Lifton 1967; Ursano et al. 1981) or to civil disasters (e.g., Lindemann 1944; Titchener and Kapp 1976). With respect to civil disasters, there is a growing concern with traumatic effects on helpers and

The views of the author do not necessarily reflect those of the Department of the Army or the Department of Defense (para. 4-3, AR 360-5). The author gratefully acknowledges the many helpful comments on the manuscript provided by Jocelyn V. Bartone, Evelyn H. Golembe, Mark A. Vaitkus, and the volume editors.

rescue workers (e.g., McFarlane and Raphael 1984; Taylor and Frazer 1982) and on those who provide other kinds of assistance to the immediate victims. A number of studies have shown that those giving practical and psychological support to victims can themselves suffer severe ill effects (Berah et al. 1984; Keating et al. 1987; Raphael 1986).

The experience of war can be traumatic not only for soldiers but also for family members worried about their loved ones' safety. Sadly, every war brings to some families the dreadful news that a loved one was killed or seriously injured. Although U.S. casualties in the Persian Gulf War were relatively low, given the scope of the operation and the large number of troops involved, there were still 467 U.S. soldiers wounded in action and 293 killed. Seven hundred sixty American families got official bad news of some kind, and 293 were notified that their loved one was dead.

The Persian Gulf War presented an opportunity to study stress, coping, and adaptation in U.S. Army casualty workers who assisted many of these unfortunate families. In what follows I provide an overview and summary of studies conducted during and shortly after the war that examined responses to stressors associated with U.S. Army casualty processing and family notification and assistance duties. I first focus on the individuals who work in the casualty operations center. They process casualty data, locate next of kin, and notify families by telephone of the status of wounded soldiers. Next I consider Army officers who notify next of kin of the death of their loved one. Despite evidence from other occupational groups (e.g., police officers [Eth et al. 1987]) that informing families of a loved one's death is an extremely stressful duty, Army death notifiers have not been previously studied. Finally, I examine Army casualty assistance officers. These are individuals appointed to provide long-term personalized support to families of deceased soldiers. I present case material as well as statistical results and, in a general discussion, describe common themes that cut across casualty support activities. This leads to some practical recommendations for those involved in working with casualties and assisting families, as well as for leaders and treatment providers.

U.S. Army Casualty Operations Center Workers

A little-known, peculiarly challenging military job is performed by those responsible for administrative processing of casualties and information related to casualties. The largest concentration of Army casualty workers is found at the Army's central Casualty & Memorial Affairs Operations Center. The Persian Gulf War raised concerns in this unit about the possible psychological effects of wartime casualty operations on personnel performing these duties. Before the beginning of the offensive ground operation (Operation Desert Storm), unit leaders invited psychologists from the Walter Reed Army Institute of Research to conduct research on casualty operations that might yield valuable lessons for the future.

Army casualty operations center workers collect, organize, verify, relay, and record detailed information regarding soldiers who are sick, wounded, or killed. Their primary goal is a human service one: to ensure that families are notified in a timely and sensitive manner of the condition of their loved ones, and to help these families receive benefits and assistance. Under ordinary circumstances, the casualty operations center office is staffed by about 20 full-time workers who maintain a 24-hour, 7-days-a-week operation. As the Persian Gulf crisis developed in the autumn of 1990, this small permanent staff was augmented by about 80 additional personnel drawn primarily from the Army Individual Ready Reserves. Among their other duties, casualty personnel notify by telephone families of soldiers who are wounded in action or very seriously ill. The duties of the casualty operations center workers are summarized in Table 12–1.

Using self-report surveys, observations, and interviews, investigators examined the casualty operations workers both before and after the major ground offensive (Bartone and Fullerton 1992). The primary stressors reported early in the research differed somewhat from those reported later. The main sources of stress during both time periods are listed in Table 12–2. During

Table 12–1.   Duties of U.S. Army Casualty & Memorial Affairs Operations Center and regional casualty office workers

Receive official reports of serious injuries, illnesses, and death to Army active-duty personnel.

Verify accuracy of reports.

Check personal data records to identify next of kin.

Notify next-of-kin by telephone in the case of serious injury or illness

In the case of death, relay information to regional casualty office for personal notification of next of kin.

Provide follow-up and updated information on casualty to family.

Prepare and issue certificate of death and related official documents.

Ensure that family receives certain benefits.

---

the Gulf War, intense media coverage on the subject of casualties created additional pressure to process casualty notifications rapidly. Rapid notification is a desirable aim that sometimes conflicts with the need to verify the accuracy of information before proceeding with notifications.

To operate more efficiently and to be able to handle the large numbers of projected casualties, the casualty operations center was reorganized for the wartime situation. Special areas were designated so that workers could focus on specific tasks, such as notification of the families of soldiers who had been wounded in action, communicating with the home bases of major projected casualty regions (e.g., Fort Hood, Texas), or processing death records. The wounded-in-action (WIA) area was widely regarded as the place where the most stressful work took place. A description from an interview with one worker in the WIA section illustrates several of the key sources of stress for this group:

> There were 23 of us in a crowded room with no windows. The air circulation system made an awful noise, but didn't do much for the heat. It was small and noisy, with lots of people talking at once. The hardest thing I had to do was call people to tell them, right out of the blue, that their son

---

Table 12–2. Major stressors of U.S. Army Casualty & Memorial Affairs Operations Center and regional casualty office workers

---

Before war

Fears of being overwhelmed by large number of casualties

Fears of soldiers being victims of chemical and/or biological weapons

Training and integrating augmentees into existing staff structure

Reorganization of operations center to handle massive casualty flow, including installation of additional phone lines

Time pressure ("Will we be ready on time?")

During and post war

Telephonic notification to family of seriously wounded soldiers

Having incomplete information; unable to answer family's questions

No feedback on eventual outcome ("Did I help at all?")

VIP requests for information (e.g., from Congress, White House)

Perception of senior leader "micromanagement"

Media attention

Crowded working conditions

---

or daughter was wounded. You never know how they're going to react. Sometimes they get angry, and start cursing at you. Sometimes they just get real quiet, and sometimes they break down crying. There's not much you can say to help. One lady wanted me to pass a message to her son who was wounded in Saudi, but there was no way for me to do that. She got real mad, and said, "You people can blow up the world seven times over, but you can't send one little message to my son?" It's not a good feeling. Sometimes I feel now like I want to call some of these people and ask them, "How is your son? Was our information accurate? How far off the mark were we?" We don't get any feedback. How did our cases turn out? We never know.

Most of these workers reported that the hardest part of the job was telephoning families to inform them of a serious injury or illness. These workers usually had a clear understanding of the steps that needed to be taken but were reluctant to be the bearer of the bad news and the immediate cause of the family members' emotional pain and grief. For some, this was intensified by a sense of "corporate guilt" for the war-related suffering of these families.

The perception that senior leaders were "micromanaging" by paying overly close attention to the details of the operation and not permitting subordinates to do their jobs was common:

> We were micro-managed down to our toe-nails. De-briefing sessions should have been ongoing. The "pucker-factor" kept going up and up and up. It peaked with the SCUD attack and then stayed up due to leader response. We got some outrageous taskers, for example, to phone families every 24 hours and give them a report on the soldier's condition, even if there's no change. Some families don't want to be called again and again. But it was a requirement, we had to do it. You feel awkward calling these people to say "Hi, we have nothing new to tell you, but we love you." They don't like it either.

The impact of this kind of stress on the workers' health and well-being was investigated more systematically with use of survey data. Having survey data on groups before and after the period of heaviest casualties permitted a kind of naturalistic field experiment, with two quasi-independent samples: a control group of "low exposed" workers ($n = 50$) whose health and well-being had been assessed during the pre-war period (in early January 1991, before the allied ground offensive) and an experimental group of "high exposed" workers ($n = 47$) whose health and well-being had been assessed after the war (in May 1991). (The samples are quasi-independent in that 17 cases were common to both groups.) The health and well-being of the low-exposed group were measured during their training period, before any exposure to wartime casualty operations; the high-exposed group all had worked in casualty operations throughout the period of the heaviest casualties during the war. In addition to identifying the sources of stress for these workers, the goal was to determine the effects of exposure to wartime casualty operations on the psychological health and well-being of the casualty operations workers and to explore the potential stress-moderating value of psychological and social resources (Bartone and Fullerton 1992).

The low-exposed and high-exposed groups did not differ in age, race, sex, education, or marital status. However, members of the high-exposed group were, on average, of lower rank than those in the low-exposed group. Compared with typical samples of Army soldiers, casualty operations workers tend to be older (median age = 37), better educated, and higher in military rank. About 44% of each of the two groups were female, and about 40% were black. Both groups were composed largely of Army reservists who had been activated to augment a normally small regular staff. Many (about 40%) had volunteered for casualty operations duty.

Results of Student's *t* test comparisons show that the high-exposed group reported significantly more psychiatric symptoms ($P < .01$), more negative affect ($P < .01$), and lower total psychological well-being ($P < .01$) (Table 12–3).

Curiously, at the same time, the high-exposed group reported higher morale ($P < .01$) and positive affect ($P < .14$; trend) than the low-exposed group. Nonparametric contrasts (Mann-Whitney U test) were applied to the "work" social support scales, because the two samples were found to have different variances on these measures. This approach revealed that the high-exposed group perceived significantly higher support from peers at work than did the low-exposed group. Data from clinical interviews support the interpretation that individuals became more friendly, close, and supportive over time as they worked long hours together on emotionally difficult and challenging tasks.

Previous research suggests that those who volunteer for casualty operations duty, compared with those who are conscripted for such duty, may be more resilient to casualty-related stressors (Bartone et al. 1989). Further examination of the high-exposed group revealed few differences between casualty op-

Table 12–3. Comparison of the health and well-being of "high exposed" and "low exposed" casualty operations workers during the Persian Gulf conflict

	High-exposed	Low-exposed	P
Morale	3.93 (1.20)	3.90 (0.79)	<.01
Negative affect	7.45 (3.86)	6.91 (2.38)	<.01
Positive affect	13.12 (3.59)	12.72 (2.87)	<.14[a]
Psychological well-being	5.66 (6.43)	5.70 (4.27)	<.01
Symptoms	10.85 (9.59)	7.81 (6.30)	<.01
Peer social support at work[b]	28.27 (8.06)	23.94 (6.79)	<.01

Note. Measures of health and well-being in the two groups compared by use of Student's *t* test (two-tailed); Values presented are means and, in parentheses, standard deviations.
[a]Trend.
[b]Unequal variances; Mann-Whitney U test used.

erations volunteers and nonvolunteers. Volunteers were more likely to be single and white and report a greater willingness to continue working in casualty operations. Nonvolunteers reported getting more social support from friends outside of work. Those in the high-exposed group who made telephonic notifications to families were less willing to continue working in casualty operations than others and relied more heavily on social support from their own families.

The next step was to test for stress resistance resources or moderators. Correlational analyses were performed within each of the two groups, the high-exposed and the low-exposed. If social or psychological resources are important as stress moderators, they should be more strongly related to mental health indicators for the high-exposed (high-stress) group than for the low-exposed (low-stress) group; theoretically, such "moderator" variables should exert greater influence on outcome variables when stress conditions are high. The psychological resource examined in this study was personality "hardiness," which presumably facilitates the formation of positive cognitive constructions of stressful life events and circumstances. Originally developed by Salvatore Maddi and Suzanne Kobasa Ouellette

(Maddi 1967, 1970; Kobasa 1979; Maddi and Kobasa 1984), the concept of personality hardiness is grounded in existential psychology and personality theory (Keen 1970; Kierkegaard 1849/1954; Kobasa and Maddi 1977). Theoretically, as a function of their own psychosocial developmental history, hardy (authentic) persons are more open to experience on a variety of levels and are more solidly grounded and confident in their sense of self and place in the social world. The critical implication for stress research is that hardy persons are not as easily threatened or psychologically disrupted by ordinarily painful aspects of the human condition. This theoretical underpinning sets hardiness apart from such superficially related constructs as "optimism" (Scheier and Carver 1985) or "hope" (Snyder et al. 1991), which generally posit a much simpler process whereby stressful or painful experiences are disregarded or ignored. Of particular relevance to the domain of combat stress and war-related casualties is Maddi's (1976) suggestion that the hardy person is not as vulnerable to the threat of imminent death. Empirical studies have confirmed that personality hardiness is a promising individual-differences variable that seems to influence the relationship between psychosocial stress and health outcomes (see, e.g., Bartone 1989b; Contrada 1989; Kobasa et al. 1982; Roth et al. 1989; Wiebe 1991).

Perhaps partly as a function of its theoretical depth and complexity, the construct of hardiness has proved difficult to measure (Funk 1992). The present work utilizes a refined 30-item hardiness scale (the Dispositional Resilience Scale) that corrects many of the problems of earlier hardiness measures (Bartone 1991; Bartone et al. 1989). The scale measures the three general characteristics of commitment, control, and challenge that Kobasa (1979) suggested hardy persons possess; each of the characteristics is measured based on 10 items. The Dispositional Resilience Scale is fully balanced for positive and negative items, with an equal number (15) of each. The correlation between the 30-item form and the 27 nonoverlapping items from the original hardiness scale (Kobasa 1979) (6 alienation from self, 2 alienation from work, 7 powerlessness, 10 security, 2 cognitive structure) is –.74 (Bartone 1991). Scores on the short form have demonstrated appropriate correlations with theoretically related (convergent) and unrelated (discriminant) variables and are generally predictive of continued mental and physical health under a variety of environmental stressors (e.g., Bartone 1989a; Bartone et al. 1990). For example, scores on this measure were found to discriminate Army disaster assistance workers who remain healthy from those reporting stress-related symptoms over time (Bartone et al. 1989). Also, in a recent study of Persian Gulf War veterans, investigators found that the combined effects (interaction) between scores on this hardiness measure and combat exposure predicted health outcome in a regression model (Bartone et al. 1992b).

Results show the correlations between hardiness and morale, positive affect, negative affect (–), and well-being are indeed substantially stronger in the high-exposed group than in the low-exposed group (Table 12–4), a finding that supports a stress-moderating interpretation. Of the social support measures, only support from family and support from friends outside of work correlated with the mental health indicators more strongly in the high-exposed group than in the low-exposed group. This does not indicate that social support at work is unimportant (the within-group variance on work support measures is somewhat restricted, and this limits the power of correlational analysis to reveal effects), but it does suggest that for casualty workers under high-stress conditions, support from family and from friends outside of work for some reason becomes more important. Perhaps support received when away from a highly stressful job such as casualty support operations helps the individual maintain a sense of normalcy and encourages attributions of positive meaning and value to the unpleasant duty.

These findings show that exposure to wartime casualty operations leads to some negative psychological effects, as indexed by psychiatric symptoms, negative affect, and total psychological well-being. Support among co-worker peers apparently develops over time and is an important social resource for those

Table 12–4. Correlations between "resource" variables and mental health variables for low-exposed (n = 50) and high-exposed (n = 47) casualty operations workers during the Persian Gulf conflict

Exposure group:	Morale Low/High	Positive affect Low/High	Negative affect Low/High	Total well-being Low/High	Symptoms Low/High
Hardiness	.39*/.59**	NS/.66*	NS/−.50	.31*/.67**	−.30*/−.37*
Support from friends outside of work	NS/.39*	NS/.38*	NS/NS	.31*/.36*	NS/NS
Support from family	NS/NS	NS/.31*	NS/−.36*	NS/.39**	NS/NS

Note. NS = not significant.
*P<.05; **P<.01

exposed, as is support from family and friends. Paradoxically, the high-exposed group actually had higher morale and greater positive affect than the low-exposed group. This finding supports Bradburn's (1969) argument that positive and negative affect are distinctive components of psychological well-being, rather than opposite ends of a single bipolar dimension, and that both can be high at the same time. Under the right conditions, exposure to the stress of casualty operations can apparently lead to a positive sense of meaning and accomplishment reflected in higher morale and positive affect, even while some psychological distress associated with witnessing the pain, suffering, death, and grief of fellow human beings is experienced. The findings regarding personality hardiness suggest a possible psychological pathway in the underlying stress-illness mechanism, wherein persons high in hardiness are more inclined to extract positive meaning from unpleasant, negative events. The degree to which social forces in organizations (e.g., support, cohesion, leadership) can influence and reinforce such positive attributions is an important issue in need of further research.

Death Notification Officers and Casualty Assistance Officers

Another investigation examined responses to the stressors associated with Army death notification and survivor assistance during Operation Desert Storm (Bartone et al. 1991; Bartone et al. 1992a). Studies conducted following the fatal crash of a chartered Army jet in Gander, Newfoundland, in 1985 (all 248 soldiers aboard were killed) showed that many officers who provided assistance to bereaved families suffered substantial psychiatric distress as a consequence of their duties (Bartone and Wright 1990; Bartone et al. 1989). These negative effects were smaller for casualty workers who reported good social support systems of their own and for those possessing the cognitive/personality style of "hardiness."

The Persian Gulf War also afforded the chance to extend these findings to war-related casualty operations. Of special interest were Army death notification officers, a group not previously studied despite evidence from other occupational groups (e.g., police officers) that informing families of a loved one's death is an extremely stressful duty (Eth et al. 1987). Although few studies are available on those who make death notifications to family members, it does appear that this is especially difficult duty for people to perform. For example, Eth and colleagues (1987) found that Los Angeles police officers were highly apprehensive about death notifications and felt unprepared for such duty and that apprehension increased rather than decreased as the number of notifications an officer had made increased. Charmaz (1976) made similar observations regarding coroners and their deputies who make death announcements, and Hall (1982) noted that law enforcement officers generally are poorly trained or educated for this aspect of their jobs, a situation that appears to add to stress levels. Physicians also have been noted to have a very difficult time informing family members of a sudden death (Robinson 1981).

In the Army the initial family notification of a death is made in person by an officer or noncommissioned officer (NCO) in full dress uniform. This individual, the death notification officer, informs the family of the soldier's death, provides whatever details are available, and offers the condolences of the Secretary of the Army. Notification by way of a personal visit, as opposed to a telegram or telephone call, is meant to convey a greater sense of appreciation and respect for the sacrifice of the deceased soldier and the family. The notification officer is given the following instructions: "As a notifier, you represent the Secretary of the Army. You are expected to be courteous, helpful, and sympathetic toward the next-of-kin in this sensitive mission. Your presence should soften the blow, if possible, and show the Army's concern for its personnel, their dependents, and their next-of-kin" (Department of the Army 1987, p. 3).

Army death notification officers have one overriding function: to personally visit the closest family member(s) of the deceased and provide a respectful, accurate notification of death. The notifying officer is required to wear a formal military dress uniform to symbolize this respect. An important goal of the Army casualty system is to provide timely notification to families, in most cases within 24 hours of the death itself. Once the correct family member has been located, the notifying officer gives a brief, factual statement on the circumstances of the death and offers a formal statement of condolence. Although most notifications are made alone, a chaplain may accompany the notifying officer if one is available. The interaction with the family is kept brief, unless there are special circumstances. Ideally, relatives or friends are available to lend support to the family member(s). Before leaving, the death notification officer informs the family that a casualty assistance officer (CAO) will call shortly to assist with arrangements and any needs of the family. Following the notification, the notifying officer immediately contacts the CAO to inform him or her the notification was made, verify address and telephone number, and provide any other information relevant to providing assistance to the family.

The CAO telephones the family and arranges a time to visit. The general function of the CAO is to provide immediate and ongoing assistance to the next of kin in settling the affairs of the deceased, in arranging financial benefits and entitlements, and in addressing other issues that relate to the servicemember's death. The duty can last as long as a year. CAOs are given this guidance: "You are charged by the Secretary of the Army to render all reasonable assistance needed to settle the personal affairs of a deceased soldier. The quality of your service must reflect your full attention to duty and to the next-of-kin. It will lessen the emotional and financial strain borne by the next-of-kin during a period of great trauma" (Department of the Army 1987, p. 5).

In the first meeting with the family, the CAO obtains the family's wishes regarding funeral arrangements and location. Once this is determined, the CAO facilitates the transport and receipt of remains and assists the family in planning the funeral and any memorial services. The CAO also assumes responsibility for ensuring that the personal effects and belongings of the deceased soldier are returned to the family. The CAO presents the family with any military awards the soldier may have earned and such items as the flag that covered the coffin if the family chose to have a traditional military funeral. A very significant aspect of the CAO role involves helping the family obtain whatever benefits or entitlements they may be due, whether from the Army or from other agencies (e.g., Veterans Administration, Social Security Administration).

Depending on the needs of the family, the duties of the CAO can continue for a year or more. In most cases, however, the duty lasts for 3 to 6 months. Because the occurrence of fatalities is not predictable, death notification and casualty assistance duties are performed by officers and NCOs on an "as needed" basis. It is an additional duty, and one for which the individual frequently receives no special preparation or training.

In March–April 1991, surveys were administered to Gulf War CAOs and death notification officers. Time 1 surveys were distributed through Army Casualty Operations channels in both the U.S. and Europe. Measures were thus obtained on psychiatric symptoms, illness, psychological well-being, and several other variables of concern for 206 respondents (about half of whom were CAOs and the other half of whom were death notification officers). Next, interviews were conducted at two locations. These interviews provided a more detailed view of the important issues and sources of stress for casualty workers and helped to define the questions for the Time 2 survey. The latter survey was mailed to all initial respondents in July–August 1991, about 6 months after the first survey was administered. Approximately 60% (122) of the initial respondents completed and returned Time 2 surveys. This response rate is considered extremely good, given the high mobility of the active-duty Army population. (For further discussion, see Bartone and Fullerton 1992; Bartone et al. 1991.)

The primary sources of stress for Army death notification officers were compiled from survey and interview results and are listed in Table 12–5.

Table 12–5.   Primary stressors of death notification officers

Uncertainty about how the family will respond (grief, crying, anger, violence, shock, heart attack?)

Notifier's uncertainty about how he or she will perform ("Can I handle this? Will I maintain my composure?")

Fragmented family situations (divorced parents, ex-spouse, etc.)

Wrong address, nobody home, family already heard from another source

Identification with the event ("It could have been me")

Guilt, delivering worst possible news

Feeling powerless to help or make things better

The following excerpts from the interview material illustrate the kinds of problems encountered by Army death notifiers:

Case 1 (Death Notifier, Senior NCO)

All the E-7's [master sergeants] in our unit got put on the list [of potential death notifiers]. It's the kind of duty you can't train for; you shouldn't force people to do it. Some people are just not cut out for this kind of thing. You have to give the family the saddest news, and do it with respect and dignity. I got called at two A.M. . . . They didn't have an address, just a Rural Delivery Number. I drove out there and started looking. It was very dark and hard to see. Finally, I stopped at a fire station and asked. Luckily, some fellows there knew where Mrs. ——— lived. As soon as she saw me, I could tell she understood why I was there.

Case 2 (Death Notifier, Senior NCO)

The training I got told me what you need to say, in a set pattern. I was worried about how to say the words, without sounding like a heartless robot. My casualty was a Staff Sergeant, a very good NCO. His wife grew up in a military family, and the father is retired military. The casualty was shot in the upper thigh area and bled to death. There were three of us that went to the house, myself, the chaplain, and another NCO. The NCO stayed in the car. We weren't sure of the exact address. It was a bad deal, going through the neighborhood knocking on doors. She [the widow] came walking around the corner and saw us; she knew, bad news was in her eyes. You ask yourself, if she falls apart, what will you do? The chaplain asked if there was anyone we could call. Her mother lived down the street. She assured us there was nothing more to do. She was nervous, but she made my job easier by being strong. The chaplain held her hand and said a prayer. Afterward I thought, did I do enough, did I do it the right way? When you do it, there's no time for small talk.

Case 3 (Death Notifier, Officer)

I got the call about 1500 hours. My casualty was the driver in a head-on collision. I went to the address, but the name on the quarters didn't match the name I was given. There was a rumor she was living with her sister. We did some checking, and called back to D.A. [Department of the Army] Casualty Branch. They called and verified the soldier's address, and that the wife was living there. So I went back to the house, with a chaplain. There was nobody home, so we began to inquire around the neighborhood as to the whereabouts of the Next-of-Kin. The regulation says to do this, but I think it's a bad idea. I scared two women to death, going around the family quarters in (dress uniform) greens with a chaplain. We found the woman, she was living with her sister. She didn't speak English, but the sister did. The woman went completely to pieces. She could not express herself in English. We were there only 10 minutes. I didn't sleep much that night, and the next day felt sad and melancholy. I kept thinking about how fleeting life is.

Occasionally the family had already heard about the death through non-Army channels by the time the notifier arrived. This was frustrating and problematic for the notification officers, because it left them suddenly unprepared for the encounter and forced to react spontaneously to a surprise situation. Some families had received inaccurate or unverified information regarding the death—for example, through media reports—that the notifying officer was unable to clarify or respond to. Sometimes the official information on the death was later contradicted by news reports, as in the following case:

Case 4 (Death Notifier, Senior NCO)

When I went out to make the notification, the wife was at church with her parents. We waited at the house. It was awkward for all of us. The daughter really fell apart. She collapsed, and just said, "No, Daddy, no" over and over again. If a person falls, you have to catch them, but Army policy says you can't have physical contact. The father went to the floor with her and just held her for awhile. The first coherent words out of her mouth were "What happened?" It wasn't appropriate then to give the canned speech, "The Secretary of the Army regrets to inform you . . . ," so I just told them what happened as I knew it. He was killed by an enemy mine. Later, a news story said it was a friendly mine, a cluster bomb someone picked up for a souvenir. The family will remember that forever.

Although notifiers were generally relieved that their contact with family members was brief, for most it was an experience not easily forgotten:

While I was in the house I saw his [the casualty's] photo. I kept asking myself, did I know him? Did he do something stupid [such as pick up an unexploded bomb]? How is the wife going to get along? I went home and just watched TV for two hours. I had a lot of trouble sleeping that night. I was wondering, could I have done something else to make it less painful for her? I just kept going over it again in my mind.

In contrast to the notification officers, whose contact with the family was of brief duration, the CAOs had extended contact with family members. The primary stressors for CAOs, which overlap somewhat with those for notification officers, are listed in Table 12–6.

Table 12–6.   Primary stressors of casualty assistance officers

Extended exposure to death-related emotions, grief, anger of
  family members
Sense of inadequate training, preparation
Slow communication of information through official Army channels
Belief that senior leaders/agencies are "micromanaging"
  (redundant phone calls)
Perception that awards and other recognition to soldier and his or
  her family are not forthcoming from Army
Slow return of remains to family, especially when body was
  severely damaged
Exposure to remains (e.g., inspection of casket contents upon receipt)
Family conflicts surrounding funeral arrangements, apportioning
  of benefits, etc.
Unwelcome attention of media and politicians
Return of personal effects to family
Personal identification with deceased and his or her family
  ("It could have been me")
Competing work demands; trying to do two jobs at once

The following case interviews show some of the issues of
concern for CAOs during and after the Persian Gulf conflict:

Case 5 (CAO, Senior NCO)

The deceased was a Specialist, and the next-of-kin was his
24 year old wife. ———— [the soldier] was playing Trivial
Pursuit with a group of soldiers in the barracks downstairs
when it [an Iraqi SCUD missile] hit. Though the wife was
the "next-of-kin," the soldier's mother and father needed
help too. What made it hard was there was a rift in the family, soldier's parents and wife didn't get along. My first visit
to the parents was very difficult. The mother says: "The
Army killed my son!" You have a helpless feeling—telling
a person the worst possible news, and there's nothing you
can do to make it better for them. The first concern was
getting the body back. . . . I helped the family plan out the
funeral for Thursday. The remains were viewable, and they
had an open casket wake for two days. The mother stood at
the head of the casket for 5 hours, both days. She said to

me, "People look at me like I should be crying. Am I supposed to cry?" She talked a lot about her anger.

The Dover folks did a good job making the remains viewable. During the funeral, the mother started stroking the soldier's face, and the face started breaking apart. The black under the make-up started to show through. This was very tough on everyone. The mother went to pieces on me. The funeral director had to clear the room and then repair the face. You have to be real careful about letting people touch the body.

The parents were angry at the Army for their son's death, and they called their congressman. I've had numerous calls from . . . [the congressman's] office. The parents were struggling financially, living in a trailer. I think they resented the wife getting all the insurance money. They were very secretive about a memorial parade for their son in their home town, didn't tell me or the wife until the very last minute.

I'm getting a lot of pressure from my own unit, my commander wants me "back to work." He says: "The burial is over, you're finished, get back to work! See you at 5:45 on Saturday morning for drill!" This makes it tough. The family still needs my help. There are financial burdens too. I've made lots of long-distance calls from my home phone, used up lots of gas. I had told the family they would get a special memorial wall display ["shadow box"], but then it was denied by the Army. So the NCOs in my unit are paying for one to give to the family.

Returning the personal effects was hard. I brought them to the wife. The wallet was still wet from cleaning, and smelled like a fire. There was a gold chain, had a drop of blood on it, and several letters that hadn't been mailed. This was hard on the wife, but she was glad to get them.

I don't know when my CAO duties are completed. What date do I use? There are lots of issues still pending, unresolved, such as awards. I'm very close to the family. They hear things in the news and call me to ask if it's true. For example, they heard an auto dealer was selling cars at cost to members of the unit. When does it stop?

Case 6 (CAO, Warrant Officer)

I got [the] call about noon that I was to be the CAO. They gave me the pertinent information. The soldier was 23 years old, single, and in the Army because she wanted to be. It was a large family, mother, father, 4 brothers, sisters, 3 grandparents. On my first visit, the whole family was there. I didn't know if I could keep my composure. The dad couldn't talk to me at all then. The mother did. Later they switched, and the mom couldn't talk to me, but the dad did. Disposition of remains was the major issue for the family. The "Disposition of Body" form is very important. "Remains" was a problem word for the mother. She said to me: "Don't call my child that!" As a CAO, you need to go over the Disposition form prior to sitting down at the kitchen table with the family.

There was some delay in getting the remains returned from Dover. . . . The body wasn't back yet, so they couldn't focus on details very well. News people were there too, which frightened the family. The deceased was finally identified through dental records. The body was too severely damaged to be viewable. The parents had a lot of trouble with this and wanted to look inside the casket. They asked for my advice, and I told them[,] "It's better to remember her as she was." The funeral director knew the family, which made my job much easier. The funeral was with full military honors, and I got a flag for each family member. The flag meant a lot to them. They didn't hold the military responsible for what happened. There was a one-day viewing (closed casket). A close friend gave the eulogy.

The family had asked that no reporters be allowed at the funeral, but the media didn't respect that. Two reporters snuck in. One in particular, a UPI man, was very insensitive to the family, pushing a microphone in their faces and the whole bit. At the church reception, a reporter took the grandmother away from me, pretending to be a friend of the deceased. She got the grandmother talking. The family found out later it was a reporter who never knew the deceased. They were very upset by that. Nearly every time

I called the house their line was busy. Reporters were calling constantly. The family asked me what to do about the media? I advised them to buy an answering machine to screen their calls, which they did.

One problem I have is with redundant phone calls. If I call the unit with some information, I'm also required to call D.A. [Department of the Army Casualty Center, Washington, D.C.], [and] ———— [the regional casualty center]. All these phone calls take time away from the duty of helping the family! Also, right now we are waiting for the death certificates to arrive. These are necessary for V.A. claims, getting taxes back from IRS, etc. D.A. says it will take 4–6 weeks for them to arrive. This puts another hardship on the family.

Case 7 (CAO, Warrant Officer)

I was called at 0600 and told about CAO duty assignment. The deceased was an officer who had been killed-in-action. His wife lives here, 30 years old and 7 months pregnant. Her mother is here too. I met with the Notifier at 0800 and debriefed him. I think an itemized checklist would help for this. The notifier said the wife had no idea why he was there, which was surprising considering the dress uniform. Her mother was staying with her. They live on a cul-de-sac on post.

When I got there, I went very slow with her. I gave her the Death Gratuity check (intended to defray funeral expenses), pointing out that this is not a "pay-off" for her husband's life. He had only left for Saudi in December, and the family had just adjusted to his absence. The wife took the death pretty hard. Fortunately, she had good neighborhood support and a strong Family Support Group, and her mother there too. After that first visit, I went back to the Casualty Assistance Center and was debriefed. My question was, what do I do next? The big task was to recover the remains. It took 10 days for a positive identification to be made. The body was flown from Saudi to Frankfurt and then to Dover. The people at Dover stonewalled, didn't tell us the body was there. The soldier's father had called me right away. He wanted the remains returned to him. He had gotten both state congressmen involved, and the pressure was intense. The funeral director . . . called me, wanted to know when he would get the body. The father wanted to set the date for the funeral. The funeral director convinced the family not to view the remains. I'm pretty sure he was there, but there probably wasn't much left. He was flying low and fast, and he crashed and burned. A sore point with the family is the death was listed as a non-combat death. The initial reports . . . said it was an accident. But those in the aircraft behind it said it was taking enemy fire. The guy killed was 28 years old.

I drove the widow to the airport here so she could fly to the funeral, but the airport was jammed with spring-break travelers. I asked an agent for priority in getting the widow a flight, but was refused. They sent her to the end of the line! But she made it. After the funeral, things improved for her exponentially. I noticed she was able to talk about her husband's death more objectively, without breaking down.

There was lots of press at the funeral. They [the family] had a two day wake. A reporter got into the wake, and wrote up a story. . . . They did the funeral with full military honors. The nature of the death was real important to the parents. . . . they wanted it to be recorded as a combat death. They are still pushing to get it changed. The Center told me that combat or non-combat classification of death affects how the family feels about the loss, awards, etc. Awards was another sore point for the wife. There were so few killed-in-action, the system was certainly not clogged. She couldn't understand why it was taking so long to get the awards he was due. The company commander of the soldier's unit never wrote a letter or provided any message of condolence to the family, and never put him in for any awards. Neither did his group commander. I'm going to write a letter myself to the father.

When the Form 1300 [death certificate] arrived I noticed several typing errors . . . they had the rank wrong; the town was misspelled. I worked to get that fixed. That's a very important document. It turned out I was able to get the deceased promoted posthumously. This didn't come down on orders, but on a special certificate. I presented it to the widow, it made her very happy.

I got no special training as a CAO, other than an outdated video. There's so much that you have to know to do it well. You also need to have the right personality for it . . . not everyone can be a good CAO. I think we should have trained, professional CAOs who specialize in assisting families. Outside of war and mass casualty situations, we should have professional CAOs.

Case 8 (CAO, Senior NCO)

The case I was given was a KIA [killed-in-action]. My first meeting with the family I was very nervous, had trouble talking. The family's first question was "When is the body coming back?" I stayed only 20 minutes. The body was in bad condition. We had to wait for the body, which was very difficult. There was little information coming from Dover. Finally, the death was confirmed by dental records and fingerprints. Dover waited until the last minute to tell me the remains were coming, I got very little notice. This made it hard to plan the funeral. The issue of viewing the remains came up. The D.A. Pamphlet doesn't tell you what to do when remains are badly damaged. The parents wanted to see the remains, but changed their minds at the last minute. The widow insisted on seeing them. The face was completely reconstructed. Dover did a good job on the body. I went for a walk with the father after the remains came back. During that walk I think he accepted the death for the first time.

. . . A lot of coordination is necessary. The arrival of remains has to be coordinated with funeral arrangements. Many phone calls have to be made. Every time we do something, such as pick up the body, we have to notify a long list of agencies. . . . A lot of this is unnecessary, micromanaging. CAOs should be issued a calling-card along with blanket TDY [temporary duty] orders [equivalent of authorization for business travel].

> The training I got was poor, the films they showed are old and out of date. For example, the part on military honors at funerals needs to be updated. I'm thankful the family I helped didn't have children. I have a 2 year old son—I don't think I could do it if there were children involved. The greatest stress is the coordination, the excessive phone calls, and the family conflicts. Also, my normal job duties are pressing on me right now. Some requirements can't be put off. My reserve center monthly reports have been late. The training calendar must get done. We're getting close to May . . . , and the workload is going up.

Several common themes emerge regarding the experience of CAOs, based on these four cases of CAOs during and after the Gulf War. In addition to the essential difficulty of coping with strong family emotions related to the death, CAOs describe feelings of being unprepared and ill-trained for the duty, frustration associated with the often slow transfer of information, and a sense that senior leaders and agencies are "micromanaging" the CAOs' activities. Most also feel that inadequate recognition is paid to families and deceased soldiers in terms of awards and letters from leaders representing the military organization. Other common difficulties involve waiting for the return of remains to the family and direct and indirect exposure to bodies in badly damaged condition. Conflicts within families regarding funeral arrangements, disposition of remains, personal effects, and benefits can cause great difficulties for CAOs. The sometimes unwelcome attention of media and politicians increases the burden on families and on the CAOs who are trying to assist the families. The actual return of personal items such as wallets, wedding rings, and photos is often wrenching for the family and the CAO alike. Many CAOs describe a sense of personal identification with the deceased and the family that intensifies the experience and makes it difficult to terminate the assistance activity. Finally, a major problem for some CAOs stems from the continuing demands of their regular job, which they must perform along with their CAO duties.

Correlational analysis of the Gulf War survey data for CAOs and death notification officers was conducted. For CAOs, longer contact with family members was related to lower psychological well-being ($r = -.33$, $P<.05$), and more reported sickness ($r = .43$, $P<.01$). For death notification officers, in contrast, longer contact with family members was associated with less sickness ($r = -.38$, $P<.05$). Also for death notifiers, having attended the funeral of the deceased was associated with less sickness ($r = -.35$, $P<.05$), fewer psychiatric symptoms ($r = -.32$, $P<.05$), and increased psychological well-being ($r = .33$, $P<.05$). These results are suggestive of a curvilinear relationship between exposure to grieving families and illness, wherein too little as well as too much exposure is associated with increased illness and symptomatology, at least for death notifiers.

To explore this issue further, investigators performed an analysis of covariance for death notifiers, looking at the effects of contact duration on sickness reports, with funeral attendance as a covariate. In this model the covariate was highly significant, but contact was not significant once the effects of the covariate were removed. A stepwise regression confirmed this result, showing funeral attendance as a significant (negative) predictor of sickness reports ($\beta = -.44$, $P < .01$, df $= 28$); duration of contact failed to enter the model. These results suggest that "exposure" in the sense of duration of contact with family members for death notifiers is less important than having an opportunity to attend a ritualized community mourning service, perhaps because such a service affords an opportunity to process and integrate grief that has been vicariously experienced.

Stepwise multiple regression was applied to examine the possible moderating effects of personality hardiness and social support on health outcomes for both CAOs and death notification officers. Negative affect scores from Time 1 were entered to control for possible confounding effects of neuroticism. For the total exposed group, only personality hardiness entered as a significant predictor, and it did so for both total symptoms ($\beta = -.40$, $P < .01$, df $= 51$) and psychological well-being

($\beta = .72$, $P < .01$, df = 51). When the data on CAOs and death notifiers were examined separately, social support was found to be a negative predictor of poor general health for CAOs ($\beta = -.33$, $P < .05$, df = 34), and hardiness, a positive predictor of psychological well-being ($\beta = .71$, $P < .01$, df = 34). Negative affect did not enter either predictive relationship. For death notifiers a similar pattern emerged: social support was found to be a negative predictor of total symptoms ($\beta = -.47$, $P < .01$, df = 26), and hardiness, a positive predictor of psychological well-being ($\beta = .70$, $P < .001$, df = 26). Negative affect also did not enter either of these models.

In accord with previous research findings, both personality hardiness and social support appear to reduce the psychological and health risks associated with death notification and casualty assistance. In examining Army death notification officers for the first time, it was discovered that attending the funeral of the deceased is associated with better health. One possible interpretation for this surprising finding is that ritualized, communal mourning activities serve a healing function for survivors, as many psychological anthropologists have argued (e.g., Rosenblatt et al. 1976).

Although extent of exposure, as indexed by duration of contact, is positively related to symptoms and ill health for CAOs, this relationship is reversed for death notification officers, with greater exposure related to better health. Further efforts to understand this surprising finding are needed, including exploring the possibility of a curvilinear association between exposure and related ill effects. Overall, exposure to grieving families is of much shorter duration for death notifiers than it is for CAOs, who can be involved in helping families for 6 to 12 months. Those death notifiers whose exposure is extremely brief perhaps have less opportunity to work through or resolve any vicariously experienced grief or guilt associated with delivering such painful news to widows and parents. Having some extended contact, especially in the context of formalized mourning activities such as funerals, can be beneficial in this regard. However, longer-term contact with family members, as many CAOs experience, can represent an overload of both practical and psychological demands for the caregiver, leading to increased distress and symptoms.

Summary and Recommendations

The results of these investigations confirm the stressful nature of casualty operations work during and after the Persian Gulf War and reveal an association between casualty assistance duties and a variety of negative health indicators. Sources of stress that cut across various casualty support roles are 1) exposure to death and the strong emotions of grief-struck family members, 2) trouble obtaining timely, accurate information, 3) perception of "micromanaging" by senior leaders and agencies, and 4) identification with the victim(s). Many casualty assistance workers also experience problems related to intense media attention, and family conflicts among the survivors. Death notifiers and family CAOs in particular often report feeling untrained and unprepared for this duty.

Based on the described findings and experiences of Army casualty support personnel during and after the Persian Gulf War, three general recommendations are offered for those who may be called upon to provide similar services and for those concerned with policy and treatment issues:

1. *Train and prepare casualty assistance workers in advance.* Death is an inherently unpleasant subject for most people, and one that is, in most situations, easy to avoid. But advance training and preparation are needed for casualty workers not only to ensure that they have the appropriate skills but also to foster in them a sense of being psychologically equipped to deal with death-related issues. Training programs should vary depending on the specific tasks and circumstances, but all should be well organized, be taught by experienced and knowledgeable teachers, and cover material that is germane to the expected duties. Training

aids such as videotaped vignettes can be useful, but these should be up-to-date and relevant. Role-playing is a technique that can help casualty workers develop a sense of readiness to face unusual situations. A question-and-answer/discussion period can help identify unanticipated concerns. How much training is enough will again depend on the organization and circumstances. Workers in organizations such as the Army or police agencies (e.g., Hendricks 1984) who may be called upon to provide casualty services at any time should receive regular training, as well as specialized training as situations require. An overview of casualty operations in the organization is useful in giving casualty workers a framework for understanding their own role, and reduces confusion and mystery. Printed materials containing policy guidelines, requirements, tips, checklists, and guidance on where and how to obtain additional information should be distributed. Perhaps the most useful item is the name and phone number of a local casualty expert who can answer questions as they arise. Whenever possible, volunteers rather than conscripts should be used for casualty activities because they are at lower risk for problems and are likely to be more committed to the duty. Also, experience is usually an advantage, although there is some evidence that this is not the case as regards death notification (Hall 1982). Persons with a recent death or terminal illness in their own family should not be required to perform casualty duties.

2. *Establish procedures for fast and accurate transfer of casualty information.* Many of the problems described by Gulf War casualty assistance providers relate to the slow communication of information across levels in the organization. Whether the issue is verifying the cause of death or the condition of a wounded soldier, identifying and contacting the next of kin, coordinating the return of remains, or obtaining death certificates, awards, and benefits, effective communication is critical. The communication challenge is greater when the organization is involved in global operations with offices and agencies located in different time

zones. For Army casualty operations today, the telephone remains the critical communication tool. Radio-teletype machines are still used for many official messages. Increasingly, computer-based electronic communications are speeding the flow of casualty information, but this is still an under-utilized technology. There is a need for information to flow down from the central and regional casualty operations centers to the individuals who are providing services directly to families, and for information to flow back up the chain so that senior managers know the status of cases and can provide appropriate support and resources. Unfortunately, in the absence of simple and effective procedures and methods for passing information quickly in both directions, the goal of assisting families is sometimes impeded. In some regions especially, there is a tendency to rely too much on the CAOs to make reports by telephone to multiple agencies in the organization. This can put an undue strain on the time and resources of the service provider. When this system fails, as it inevitably must at times, senior leaders with a legitimate and pressing need for casualty information sometimes respond with more insistent and rigid reporting requirements, leading to the perception of leaders who "micromanage." What is needed is an automated reporting system that permits the simultaneous transmission of status reports to multiple addressees. Several computer electronic mail systems are available that could easily be tailored to such an application. Central, regional, and local casualty operations centers should be linked with computer electronic communications. This linkage would permit the very rapid transmission of casualty data in both directions and would eliminate the need for repeated phone calls. Casualty assistance workers in remote locations and/or without access to telecommunications equipment could be temporarily issued the necessary items (e.g., laptop computer with modem) by their regional casualty office. Telephone calling cards could also be issued to facilitate the making of necessary voice calls.

3. *Offer "debriefings" to casualty assistance workers.* Besides the ongoing support of leaders and co-workers, probably the best tool for helping casualty workers cope constructively with their own reactions to death and grief is a debriefing session of some kind. Casualty assistance providers to some degree share in the pain and despair of the family, the more so as they identify more closely with the life circumstances of the deceased. This is the unavoidable cost of the duty. Most healthy people have their own support systems and coping strategies for managing this kind of stress. What the organization can do is to reinforce healthy individual strategies and provide additional opportunities to process disturbing experiences in a positive way. During its Gulf War experience, Fort Hood made effective use of the "debrief" for death notifiers and CAOs alike. After a notification was made, the notification officer met with the CAO personally to discuss what had occurred. CAOs also were encouraged to visit the local Casualty Assistance Center at any time to ask questions and/or to debrief. These were usually informal sessions that were part information gathering and part discussing reactions and problems. Many anecdotal reports support the therapeutic value of these informal debriefings. Also, notification teams were used rather than individuals. In most cases, a chaplain and an "assistant notifier" accompanied the notification officer to inform the family of the death. The team arrangement was implemented with the explicit intent of providing the notifier with a mobile support system and an ongoing opportunity to "debrief." Notifiers reported that this approach was very helpful, especially during the period immediately following the notification. One particularly helpful feature of this strategy was that notification team members could affirm for the notifier that the notification was made in a professional and supportive manner. Many notifiers worry afterward that they may have inadvertently said or done something to increase the pain of the family member.

Various formats are possible for debriefing sessions. The Fort Hood experience suggests that individual or small-group debriefings that focus on events and the communication of information have therapeutic value for casualty assistance workers. Shalev et al. (1989) provided a thoughtful examination of the event-focused debriefing and reviewed its use with soldiers exposed to combat and other stressful experiences.

The findings of the present study with respect to the stress-moderating effects of personality hardiness suggest another direction that therapeutic posttraumatic debriefings might take. Although best treated as an empirical question, healthy adaptation might be fostered even for individuals who are characteristically moderate or low on this dimension by encouraging "cognitive restructuring" along the lines of the hardy personality/cognitive style. For example, in the context of a debriefing, casualty assistance providers could be encouraged to view the duty, no matter how disturbing and painful, as a valuable learning experience that can help one grow as a person. They could also be encouraged to focus on the positive impact they likely had on the lives of the people they assisted.

By studying those agencies and individuals who provided casualty-related services and support to families of U.S. victims of the Persian Gulf War, a number of valuable lessons have been identified with application beyond the military. Many organizations and individuals must cope with casualties generated by natural disasters, famine, terrorist strikes, and accidents. By learning from the painful experiences of the Gulf War, we strive to improve policies for helping families of war victims, as well as the casualty workers who assist those families. In sharing these lessons with a wider audience, it is hoped the pain of all families who suffer the injury or death of a loved one, and that of those who help them, will be lessened somewhat.

References

Bartone PT: Hardiness, optimism, and health: a construct validity study. Paper presented at the 60th annual meeting of the Eastern Psychological Association, Boston, MA, April 1989a

Bartone PT: Predictors of stress-related illness in city bus drivers. Journal of Occupational Medicine 31:657–663, 1989b

Bartone PT: Development and validation of a short hardiness measure. Poster presentation at the 3rd annual convention of the American Psychological Society, Washington, DC, June 1991

Bartone PT, Ender MG: Organizational responses to death in the military. Death Studies 18:25–39, 1994

Bartone PT, Fullerton TD: Psychological effects of war stress on casualty operations personnel. Poster presentation at the 100th annual convention of the American Psychological Association, Washington, DC, August 1992

Bartone PT, Wright KM: Grief and group recovery following a military air disaster. Journal of Traumatic Stress 3:523–539, 1990

Bartone PT, Ursano RJ, Wright KM, et al: The impact of a military air disaster on the health of assistance workers: a prospective study. J Nerv Ment Dis 177:317–328, 1989

Bartone PT, McCarroll JE, Wright KM, et al: Personality hardiness and resiliency in high-stressed military populations. Poster presentation at the 98th annual convention of the American Psychological Association, Boston, MA, August 1990

Bartone PT, Gifford RK, Tyler MP: Psychosocial stress in Operation Desert Storm casualty assistance providers. Paper presented at the annual convention of the International Society for Traumatic Stress Studies, Washington, DC, October 1991

Bartone PT, Gifford RK, Tyler MP, et al: Stress and illness in wartime casualty workers. Poster presentation at a meeting of the Eastern Psychological Association, Boston, MA, April 1992a

Bartone PT, Gifford RK, Wright KM, et al: U.S. soldiers remain healthy under Gulf War stress. Poster presentation at the 4th annual convention of the American Psychological Society, San Diego, CA, June 1992b

Berah EF, Jones HJ, Valent P: The experience of a mental health team involved in the early phase of a disaster. Aust N Z J Psychiatry 18:354–358, 1984

Bradburn NM: The Structure of Psychological Well-Being. Chicago, IL, Aldine, 1969

Charmaz KC: The coroner's strategies for announcing death, in Toward a Sociology of Death and Dying. Edited by Lofland L. Beverly Hills, CA, Sage, 1976, pp 61–81

Contrada RJ: Type A behavior, personality hardiness, and cardiovascular responses to stress. J Pers Soc Psychol 57:895–903, 1989

Department of the Army: Casualty Assistance Handbook (Pamphlet No 608-33). Washington, DC, Headquarters, Department of the Army, 1987

Eth S, Baron DA, Pynoos RS: Death notification. Bull Am Acad Psychiatry Law 15:275–281, 1987

Funk SC: Hardiness: a review of theory and research. Health Psychol 11:335–345, 1992

Hall MN: Law enforcement officers and death notification: a plea for relevant education. Journal of Police Science and Administration 10:189–193, 1982

Hendricks JE: Death notification: the theory and practice of informing survivors. Journal of Police Science and Administration 12:109–116, 1984

Keating JP, Blumenfield M, Reilly M: Post-disaster stress in emergency responders. Paper presented at the annual meeting of the American Psychiatric Association, Chicago, IL, May 1987

Keen E: Three Faces of Being: Toward an Existential Clinical Psychology. New York, Appleton-Century-Crofts, 1970

Kierkegaard S: The Sickness Unto Death (1849). Translated by Lowrie W. New York, Doubleday, 1954

Kobasa SC: Stressful life events, personality, and health: an inquiry into hardiness. J Pers Soc Psychol 37:1–11, 1979

Kobasa SC, Maddi SR: Existential personality theory, in Existential Personality Theories. Edited by Corsini R. Itasca, IL, Peacock, 1977, pp 243–276

Kobasa SC, Maddi SR, Kahn S: Hardiness and health: a prospective study. J Pers Soc Psychol 42:168–177, 1982

Kulka RA, Schlenger WE, Fairbank JA, et al: Trauma and the Vietnam War Generation. New York, Brunner/Mazel, 1990

Lifton RJ: Death in Life: The Survivors of Hiroshima. New York, Random House, 1967

Lindemann E: Symptomatology and management of acute grief. Am J Psychiatry 101:141–148, 1944

Maddi SR: The existential neurosis. J Abnorm Psychol 72:311–325, 1967

Maddi SR: The search for meaning. Nebr Symp Motiv 18:137–186, 1970

Maddi SR: Personality Theories: A Comparative Analysis, 3rd Edition. Homewood, IL, Dorsey Press, 1976

Maddi SR, Kobasa SC: The Hardy Executive: Health Under Stress. Homewood, IL, Dow Jones–Irwin, 1984

McFarlane AC, Raphael B: Ash Wednesday: the effects of a fire. Aust N Z J Psychiatry 18:341–353, 1984

Raphael B: When Disaster Strikes. New York, Basic Books, 1986

Robinson MA: Informing the family of sudden death. Am Fam Physician 23:115–118, 1981

Rosenblatt PC, Walsh RP, Jackson DA: Grief and Mourning in Cross-Cultural Perspective. New Haven, CT, Human Relations Area Files, 1976

Roth DL, Wiebe DJ, Fillingim RB, et al: Life events, fitness, hardiness, and health: a simultaneous analysis of proposed stress-resistance effects. J Pers Soc Psychol 57:136–142, 1989

Scheier MF, Carver CS: Optimism, coping, and health: assessment and implications of generalized outcome expectancies. Health Psychol 4:219–247, 1985

Shalev A, Ursano RJ, Ingraham LH, et al: Event-oriented debriefing following traumatic exposure: S.L.A. Marshall's approach. Paper presented at the biennial meeting of the Inter-University Seminar on Armed Forces & Society, Baltimore, MD, October 1989

Snyder CR, Harris C, Anderson JR, et al: The will and the ways: development and validation of an individual differences measure of hope. J Pers Soc Psychol 60:570–585, 1991

Taylor AJW, Frazer AG: The stress of postdisaster body handling and victim identification work. Journal of Human Stress 8(4):4–12, 1982

Titchener JL, Kapp FT: Family and character change at Buffalo Creek. Am J Psychiatry 133:295–299, 1976

Ursano RJ, Boydstun JA, Wheatley RD: Psychiatric illness in U.S. Air Force Viet Nam prisoners of war: a five-year follow-up. Am J Psychiatry 138:310–314, 1981

Wiebe DJ: Hardiness and stress moderation: a test of proposed mechanisms. J Pers Soc Psychol 60:89–99, 1991

Part IV
Treatment and Management of the Effects of War

The Problems of Listening

Stephen M. Sonnenberg, M.D.

Speaking with psychologically wounded veterans of war challenges the skills of the psychiatrist, as well as other mental health care providers, for many reasons. In the Persian Gulf War, few of those who served in the theater of operations experienced psychic trauma related to combat, but some did. In this chapter I focus on the problems associated with listening to such veterans who come for psychiatric evaluation and treatment.

The core skill that the psychiatrist brings to any clinical interview is the capacity to empathize. When speaking with an individual who has been traumatized by combat experiences— a nurse or physician who tried to heal the wounded, a technician whose job it was to prepare the bodies of the dead for shipment home, a soldier wounded by a missile attack or who participated in the killing of the enemy, to mention a few specific examples—the clinician's empathic skills are stressed and stretched in specific ways. It is beyond the scope of this chapter to discuss in detail the nature of empathy. Yet it is the case that empathic responsiveness and introspective efforts to make use of such responses are basic human capacities. These capacities are often reinforced by certain developmental experiences, such as a warm and sheltered early childhood, but, on the other hand, are sometimes extinguished by a childhood characterized by overwhelming loss. It is also the case that an individual's endowment may play a role in determining one's capacity for empathy: to employ an extreme example, some sensitive individuals may turn early experiences of loss into a foundation for empathizing well with others who experience loss.

Although psychotherapeutic talent and skill are less a focus of psychiatric training than in even the relatively recent past, they still constitute core elements in the practitioner's therapeutic armamentarium. Psychiatric residents are usually beginning physicians with a greater-than-average capacity for, and interest in, understanding their own and their patients' feelings. More or less self-consciously, psychiatric trainees use and often improve their empathic and introspective tools during residency training. When one is examining the problems of listening to war veterans, then, a useful perspective is to consider the empathic and introspective tasks of the listener, the areas of likely empathic difficulty, and the causes of these difficulties (Table 13–1).

Areas of Empathic Difficulty

Erosion of the Barrier Between the Healthy and the Sick

Physicians are accustomed to treating the sick and seeing themselves as among the well. Of course, many circumstances, such as illness in the physician, can change that comfortable boundary. To understand the patient's world, the clinician uses empathic identification with the patient and introspection to study

Table 13–1.   Obstacles to empathic listening to persons who have experienced the trauma of war

Erosion of the barrier between the healthy and the sick
Guilt over war and survival
Child abuse
Hardness of soldiers and the realities of war
Fear of the killer identity
Fear of death
Guilt over unpatriotic feelings
Perception of fundamental biological change and incurablity

this identification (Arlow 1979). In this process, the practitioner often experiences a temporary erosion of the barrier separating the healthy and the sick. This is a result of the empathic clinician's realizing that he or she has personally known something akin to the patient's experience. But when the patient's illness has been caused by an outside force powerful enough to make a previously mentally healthy person ill, the healer is dramatically confronted with the realization that he or she is exquisitely vulnerable (Sonnenberg 1985).

A sense of vulnerability is at the core of why, in this kind of situation, the clinician may have difficulty working with such a patient.

Clinical Example 1

A combat veteran with posttraumatic stress disorder (PTSD) was in psychotherapy. He repeatedly told of bloody encounters with the enemy. He described his intense anxiety in the consulting room. When the memories took hold of him, he experienced intrusive, uncontrollably vivid flashbacks. After several sessions the therapist began to experience intrusive recollections of her own: flashbacks to near accidents involving her young children, which, with the aid of her imagination, progressed to serious, bloody accidents. She became more and more anxious over her thoughts and inappropriately tried to reassure her patient, emphasizing the fact of his survival. This misguided effort was consciously designed to extinguish his flashbacks and his anxiety, but unconsciously her effort was directed at dampening her own anxiety. Fortunately, she was aware that something was wrong with the way she was listening and responding, and she sought supervision. The supervisor noted that she was using her own life experiences and her imagination in ways that could be helpful to her patient. But, the supervisor noted, her effort to empathize had frightened her, and he asked her if she could figure out why it had. The psychiatrist responded that she feared that if her children were seriously injured in an accident, she was unsure that she could cope or would ever be the same again. She realized that, like her patient, she could develop a serious psychological disorder as a result of exposure to trauma. This realization had caused her to want to silence her patient or cure him magically with reassurance.

Guilt Over War and Survival

A second common difficulty in listening during therapy with persons who have experienced the trauma of war relates to the therapist's guilt over war (Camp 1993)—guilt that can be aroused and enhanced by the experience of empathizing with a patient. It is well known that those traumatized by war are often guilty over having fought, over their survival, or over what they did to survive. The psychiatrist, as a physician, has entered a medical culture that prizes life, sometimes irrationally so, as illustrated by the tendency of some doctors to advocate the use of extreme measures to prolong life in the terminally ill. This, of course, is a very complex ethical issue, one not to be addressed in this chapter. Yet it is important to emphasize that acculturation into the medical profession does involve the development of an identity that uniquely emphasizes the preservation of life. Thus, for many physicians, the notion that war may preserve more lives than are lost is an obscure concept, especially when that physician is joined in a close relationship with a patient suffering after participation in war, as is the case in psychotherapy with a member of the population that is the focus of this chapter. Again, an example of how this can create difficulties in listening will be offered, by returning to the psychiatrist previously discussed.

Clinical Example 1 *(continued)*

After she overcame her anxiety about her own vulnerability, the psychiatrist listened more effectively to her patient. The patient began to talk more about those he had killed in combat and about several situations in which comrades had been seriously wounded or killed while he survived without injury. He became quite depressed during this phase of the treatment and began to express guilty feelings to the psychiatrist: that he did not deserve to be alive. The psychiatrist, on her part, became quite sleepy in sessions and again returned for supervision. This time her supervisor suggested that she consider what her patient's guilt stirred up in her, and she returned to the imaginary theme of her children and their accidents. She had not been thinking of this consciously while with her patient, but now she imagined she would feel responsible if they were injured: she would feel that if she had been with them, it would not have happened, or that if she had been with them, she should have been more vigilant. Then, in dialogue with her supervisor, she realized that in empathic response to her patient's survivor guilt, she had unconsciously been imagining a parallel situation in her own life. This had led her to become sleepy, to avoid its conscious recognition. She also realized that as a physician she abhorred war in a special way and wished to speak out against it far more than she had ever done in reality. War caused people to die, or to be maimed, and she was dedicated to health and the preservation of life. The guilt over not having done more to prevent war made her even guiltier over her patient's plight; this guilt reinforced and was reinforced by her feelings about her children, as she empathized with her patient's guilt over having killed and over having survived without saving his comrades. Realizing all this allowed her to listen more effectively, because she understood that whatever conflicts she felt about working with her guilty patient, her responsibility was to help him work through his guilt associated with his activities in combat.

Child Abuse

Most combatants in war are young, chronologically still adolescents. Their youth places them at higher risk for traumatic reactions to stress. Psychiatrists, even early in their careers, are in adulthood. Mental health professionals today are acutely aware of the problem of child abuse and receive special training to equip themselves to recognize and treat its victims. Increasingly, then, adult-age psychiatrists treating traumatized war combatants view these patients as adolescent victims of child abuse. Further, they see the symptoms with which these individuals present—dissociation, flashbacks, problems with impulse control, for example—as similar to the symptoms of civilian victims of abuse.

Clinical Example 2

In a recent lecture on chronic PTSD, a psychiatrist noted that those in this clinical population had suffered from their conditions for decades and that they reminded him of the adult survivors of childhood abuse. A member of the audience, also a psychiatrist who worked at a Veterans Administration (VA) clinic, realized that she had never before thought of combat veterans as youths at the time of trauma. They always seemed to her to be battle-hardened, crusty men. She reported this realization in supervision and was encouraged to consider this new dimension as she listened to her PTSD patients. She then found a new perspective developing: the rage her patients felt toward the VA, and toward her as its representative, was more understandable as she realized the organization and she were for these patients the symbols of the government of a nation that had abused its young. She then responded differently. She was more ready and able to apologize to these victims, as the representative of their abuser. This had favorable therapeutic effects, as her patients became more trusting of her.

The Hardness of Soldiers and the Realities of War

The psychiatrist must become comfortable with the world of the combatant and the hardness that soldiers develop in response to war. Combat is all that one can imagine, and more: there are cruelty and sadism of the highest order, and murder and mayhem. And these become the daily fare of combatants, as well as some support personnel in the combat zone. Further, a psychologically normal reaction to these conditions is to accept them and talk about them matter-of-factly. This reaction can easily be confused with psychic numbing by the medical listener who is inexperienced with combat. Another possible reaction is that the listener concludes that the former combatant is evil.

Clinical Example 3

A traumatized combatant spoke of her experiences as a nurse in a field hospital. She had become very upset when a particular soldier came under her care. She spoke of his appearance, of how he was severely injured in an explosion. Even when he survived, and made great strides toward recovery, she remained very upset. She spoke of how he was not really disfigured, but she could not stop thinking of how his legs were scarred. The nurse insisted that this reaction of hers was unique, because she usually took the injuries of the men she treated in stride. The therapist was skeptical: she assumed that her patient was defending against recognition of just how upset she was about the totality of her war experience and that the patient's concern with this particular patient was the tip of the iceberg. In this case the therapist did not think that the nurse was evil, but she did challenge her patient to consider her attitude as a defense, and at that point therapy reached an impasse. Then, an experienced colleague suggested that the psychiatrist explore with her patient the details surrounding the patient's concern with the soldier in question. What emerged was striking. The nurse revealed that her patient reminded her in facial features of a younger brother, who had suffered a fall in play years earlier. Subsequently, that sibling had needed orthopedic surgery on both legs. She had always felt guilty over her brother's mishap, and she now recognized that the physical similarity between the soldier and her brother, both in facial features and in body parts injured and scarred, had had a specific traumatic effect on her. The psychiatrist, who had never experienced combat, came to see that those who had experienced combat might learn to take it in

stride, reacting at times to very specific circumstances that
were traumatic for a particular reason.

Fear of the Killer Identity

Freud (1919/1955) noted that in war, combatants experience
a change in their psychic makeup: their peaceful attitudes are
replaced by warlike ones, and they become ready to kill as
members of a unit under orders. When a psychiatrist listens to
and empathizes with a traumatized soldier, he or she may encounter such attitudes and may be put in touch with similar attitudes in himself or herself. At the core of such experiences the
psychiatrist becomes aware of his or her own capacity to aban-
don peaceful values and may even feel capable of killing. This
can be so upsetting that the psychiatrist withdraws from his or
her position of engagement with the patient (Lindy 1988). In
the past, more emphasis has been placed on the therapist's rejection of the patient as evil, but what is being stressed here is
that behind such rejection is an identification with the patient
as a killer and a recognition that underlying that identification
is a part of the self almost universally repudiated by psychiatrists and other healers.

Clinical Example 4

A former soldier described his experience in basic training
and his development, then and later, of a sense of being
part of a unit. He and his comrades were dedicated to one
another and to their commanding officer, and rose to
heights of courage in many combat situations, destroying
large numbers of the enemy. The psychiatrist found himself
more and more uncomfortable as he listened to these de-
scriptions, and began to feel drowsy as he worked with his
patient. On one such occasion, a moment of drowsiness
produced a dreamlike visual image: he and his children
were playing touch football. The psychiatrist did not know
what to make of all this, including the visual image, but
discussed it with several colleagues in a peer supervisory

group. With the help of the group the psychiatrist began to think of his own experiences on the football field, as a high school and college athlete. He recalled how, at times, he and his teammates became so passionate that they felt they wanted to kill their opponents. As a grown man, the psychiatrist had mused about such misguided passion, but he knew that he had come into contact with his own capacity to kill under the pressure of a peer group engaged in combat. He realized his talks with his patient had threatened to bring that awareness again into consciousness. His new awareness of these issues allowed him to listen more effectively to his patient. He could then hear more clearly how very guilty his patient felt about his combat experiences, which involved not only personal involvement in killing many of the enemy but also a sense that he had been transformed into a subhuman murderer.

Fear of Death

Related to fear of the killer identity is the fear of death. Freud (1915/1957) also noted that war makes men aware of their own mortality, which is usually denied. When the traumatized patient vividly describes his or her sense of mortality, and the deaths of comrades and enemies, the psychiatrist who does not usually deal with death in his or her medical practice is immersed in a world of the dead. Here, again, the clinician may withdraw, should he or she be unaware of fantasies and anxieties associated with the fear of death and dying. As in the previous clinical example, if the clinician does become aware of his or her own conflicts over listening to his or her patient's fears of death, discussion of that subject in the therapy will be facilitated.

Clinical Example 5

A technician who bagged bodies for transport home constantly spoke of the dead in his psychotherapy [see McCarroll et al. 1993; Ursano and McCarroll 1990]. The psychiatrist began to associate to her own experience as a first-year medical student dissecting a cadaver in gross anatomy, and she developed nightmares and a fear of her own death. Yet she vowed to continue the therapy and to forget about her feelings about death. But the therapy became stalemated, and the psychiatrist realized that she felt anxiety whenever the patient spoke about his fears of death. She further realized he had been speaking of such fears far more often than she had consciously recognized. She became so concerned over how much she had missed in this psychotherapy that she sought therapy herself. When her own treatment revealed to her the depth of her fear of death, and the neurotic reasons for it, her patient's therapy progressed remarkably. This, she knew, was because she had become a better listener.

Guilt Over Unpatriotic Feelings

Therapists, it has been noted, sometimes feel that they should work actively against war, as a result of working with those traumatized in combat. But sometimes there is another twist: the therapist feels guilty over what he or she considers unpatriotic feelings and flees the therapy to avoid them.

Clinical Example 1 *(continued)*

Let us now recall the psychiatrist who experienced guilt over not working hard enough to end war. It was noted that appreciation of this helped her to work with her patient. Yet, at one subsequent point, she did experience doubts about herself again, this time because of her feelings of being unpatriotic. There was again interference with her work, which resolved as she better understood the complexity of her conflicts over war, especially when she stood in opposition to official United States policy.

Perception of Fundamental Biological Change and Incurability

Some experts who have studied psychic trauma suggest that it can produce fundamental psychobiological change (Winnik

1968) that is irreversible, and for some psychiatrists who work with traumatized veterans of combat, experience indicates that this is sometimes so. In such cases the psychotherapist often gives up, and withdrawal from the patient causes the therapeutic effort to end without success. Recognition that trauma victims who cannot recover can still be helped by long-term support allows therapists to set realistic goals and to maintain therapeutic relationships with chronically ill veterans of war.

Clinical Example 6

After the Vietnam War, many mental health specialists who were inexperienced in working with combat veterans gave up on helping veterans with severe, chronic PTSD. However, peer support groups of former combatants sprang up around the country, and group members enlisted the support of other interested psychiatrists, psychologists, and social workers. These individuals made clear that severely disturbed veterans needed and could benefit from long-term, open-ended support. Today, there are both patients and therapists who bear witness that long-term support can be helpful, sometimes preventing self-destructive activity by troubled veterans, even when there is no expectation of fundamental improvement in those who suffer in this chronic and severe way from the effects of trauma.

Conclusions

In this chapter the problems of listening encountered by those who treat traumatized veterans of war have been discussed. The perspective from which listening difficulties have been described is the clinician's empathic and introspective function.

According to the view related here, the clinician uses his or her life experience during the empathic process. The process of empathizing can cause the clinician to feel more anxiety, guilt, depression, or other unwanted affects or states of mind in relation to current life circumstances. Given all this, it is no wonder that clinicians spend a great deal of time studying the problems they have listening, in general and with respect to specific groups of patients.

The literature on psychotherapy and psychoanalysis contains abundant material on countertransference and the therapist's resistances to understanding the patient (Schwaber 1983, 1986; Silverman 1985). Complicating that literature is the existence of various definitions of countertransference: some say it must be unconscious, some that it must relate to childhood conflicts, some that neither of those characteristics is necessary, and some that both must be present. Of course, this is but one of many examples of the complexity of definitional debate as regards this subject. For purposes of this chapter, the terms *countertransference* and the therapist's *resistances* have not been used. Rather, the focus here is that, like the patient, the therapist is a human being with his or her own conflicts, impulses, wishes, fears, anxieties, and symptoms, and that in dialogue with the patient all the therapist's life experiences and psychological processes can potentially be influenced or activated (Beiser 1984; Calder 1980). When this happens, as it inevitably does, it can cause problems in listening. Yet these problems in listening are potentially sources of valuable information for the psychiatrist: they can lead to the therapist's self-inquiry and to subsequent clinical inquiry that helps clarify what is on the patient's mind (Gardner 1983; Jacobs 1991; Kern 1978; McLaughlin 1975, 1981, 1988; Sonnenberg 1991, 1993a, 1993b).

Dealing with problems that relate to violence, destruction, and death, which war inevitably entails, is a particularly challenging clinical situation for psychiatric physicians, who come from a medical tradition in which death is the ultimate enemy. As has been described, the clinician may very well experience unconsciously his own unwanted conflicts surrounding aggression and mortality. That trauma causes the healer to feel particularly vulnerable has also been noted.

A point that also needs to be made is that in each of the clinical examples there was an incomplete discussion of the forces within the therapist that made listening more difficult.

Every clinician has many points and sources of vulnerability, relating to past and current life experiences and to his or her particular personality, which contribute to difficulties in listening to certain kinds of material from certain kinds of patients. Despite what may seem like oversimplified examples, this truth must be kept in mind. Yet it is a tradition in psychiatry to make such liabilities assets—to use them to aid in empathic understanding of the patient.

A final word needs to be said about training and maintenance of psychotherapeutic skill. Not so very long ago, psychiatric residents received far more extensive training in the understanding of character pathology and in the conduct of long-term psychotherapy. Additionally, these trainees routinely sought a personal psychoanalytic experience, even if they did not undertake psychoanalytic training. These trends no longer continue. It is the present author's viewpoint that the psychiatric physician requires a great deal of self-knowledge and the skill to routinely probe inwardly in the course of conducting psychotherapy. To develop and maintain these skills, a personal experience in analysis or analytic therapy, followed by ongoing supervision by senior clinicians skilled in psychotherapy, is essential. Peer supervision is another excellent aid. In the end, the psychiatrist will listen best if he or she understands as both patient and therapist how much can be learned about how human beings think and feel when a conflicted, troubled person engages in psychotherapy. Such understanding is effective because the clinician will maintain curiosity about his or her experiences in the therapeutic dyad.

References

Arlow JA: The genesis of interpretation. J Am Psychoanal Assoc 27(suppl):193–206, 1979

Beiser H: An example of self-analysis. J Am Psychoanal Assoc 32:3–12, 1984

Calder K: An analyst's self-analysis. J Am Psychoanal Assoc 28:5–20, 1980

Camp N: The Vietnam War and the ethics of combat psychiatry. Am J Psychiatry 150:1000–1010, 1993

Freud S: Thoughts for the times on war and death (1915), in Standard Edition of the Complete Psychological Works of Sigmund Freud, Vol 14. Translated by Strachey J. London, Hogarth Press, 1957, pp 273–302

Freud S: Introduction to Psycho-analysis and the War Neuroses (1919), in The Standard Edition of the Complete Psychological Works of Sigmund Freud, Vol 17. Translated by Strachey J. London, Hogarth Press, 1955, pp 205–215

Gardner MR: Self Inquiry. Hillsdale, NJ, Analytic Press, 1983

Jacobs T: The Use of the Self: Countertransference and Communication in the Analytic Situation. Madison, CT, International Universities Press, 1991

Kern J: Countertransference and spontaneous screens: an analyst studies his own visual images. J Am Psychoanal Assoc 26:21–47, 1978

Lindy JD: Vietnam: A Casebook. New York, Brunner/Mazel, 1988

McCarroll JE, Ursano RJ, Wright KM, et al: Handling bodies after violent death: strategies for coping. Am J Orthopsychiatry 63:209–214, 1993

McLaughlin J: The sleepy analyst: some observations on states of consciousness in the analyst at work. J Am Psychoanal Assoc 23:363–382, 1975

McLaughlin J: Transference, psychic reality, and countertransference. Psychoanal Q 50:639–664, 1981

McLaughlin J: The analyst's insights. Psychoanal Q 57:370–389, 1988

Schwaber E: Psychoanalytic listening and psychic reality. International Review of Psycho-Analysis 10:379–392, 1983

Schwaber E: Reconstruction and perceptual experience: further thoughts on psychoanalytic listening. J Am Psychoanal Assoc 34:911–932, 1986

Silverman M: Countertransference and the myth of the perfectly analyzed analyst. Psychoanal Q 54:175–199, 1985

Sonnenberg SM: Introduction: the trauma of war, in The Trauma of War: Stress and Recovery in Viet Nam Veterans. Edited by Sonnenberg SM, Blank AS Jr, Talbott JA. Washington, DC, American Psychiatric Press, 1985, pp 1–12

Sonnenberg SM: The analyst's self-analysis and its impact on clinical work: a comment on the sources and importance of personal insights. J Am Psychoanal Assoc 39:687–704, 1991

Sonnenberg SM: Self-analysis, applied analysis, and analytic fieldwork: a discussion of methodology in psychoanalytic interdisciplinary research. Psychoanalytic Study of Society 18:443–463, 1993a

Sonnenberg SM: To write or not to write: a note on self-analysis and the resistance to self-analysis, in Self-Analysis: Critical Inquiries, Personal Visions. Edited by Barron JW. Hillsdale, NJ, Analytic Press, 1993b, pp 241–259

Ursano RJ, McCarroll JE: The nature of a traumatic stressor: handling dead bodies. J Nerv Ment Dis 178:396–398, 1990

Winnik H: Contribution to symposium on psychic traumatization through social catastrophe. Int J Psychoanal 49:298–301, 1968

Return, Readjustment, and Reintegration: The Three R's of Family Reunion

John M. Mateczun, M.D., M.P.H., J.D.
Elizabeth K. Holmes, Ph.D.

Homer began his epic poem *The Odyssey* by telling the muse of poetry he wished to convey the story of a lonely man who had wandered the world for years attempting to return home after the Trojan War. In the poem we learn that Odysseus, the king of his land, was forced by powers beyond his control to endure many hardships before his attempt to return home was finally successful.

Homer was a keen observer of behavior and used great craftsmanship in authoring this compilation of myth and history, which is truly magnificent in its understanding of human nature. Joseph Campbell (1973) reminds us that myths speak to us, in picture language, of powers of the psyche that need to be recognized and integrated in our lives and that are common to mankind. We can glean insight into the processes of family reunion by examining the story of this prototypic sailor/soldier attempting to journey home and reunite with his family.

The story begins with Athene, goddess of wisdom and daughter of Zeus, presenting a plan to the gods to get Odysseus home. All of the other kings who survived the Trojan War have returned home. Agamemnon, the leader of the victorious forces, returned home and was murdered by his wife and her lover on his return. Throughout the poem, Agamemnon's unsuccessful reunion with his wife is contrasted with the story of Odysseus's reunion with his wife, the faithful Penelope.

Odysseus, whose entire crew has been lost during the journey home, is held by Calypso, who hopes to make him her husband. Calypso offers Odysseus immortality if he will become her husband—surely a temptation for this veteran of 10 years of war in a foreign land. Poseidon, ruler of the sea through which Odysseus must return home, desires revenge against Odysseus for blinding one of his sons, the Cyclops.

Athene visits the home of Odysseus. She finds that his house has been overrun by a group of men who are ostensibly courting Penelope but who are also wasting the household resources in a series of parties. Penelope does not know whether Odysseus is alive or dead. Athene talks to Odysseus's son, Telemachus, and advises him to learn what he can about the fate of his father. She exhorts Telemachus to face up to his responsibilities if he learns that his father is dead.

The first chapters of *The Odyssey* relate the story of Telemachus's search for his father and his own developing maturity. Telemachus begins his journey by expressing great anger to his mother's suitors. He then leaves home without telling his mother that he is going, rationalizing that she will only worry if she learns of his departure. When Penelope learns of his leaving, she becomes dejected. She remains locked in her room, where she cries and refuses to eat. In the meantime, Telemachus meets some of his father's friends and fellow veterans, who give him information about his father and many valuable gifts. Meanwhile, his mother's suitors plot to kill Telemachus.

Odysseus finally appears in the story, sitting on a beach, yearning for his family and weeping. Calypso bows to the will of Zeus and allows Odysseus to leave. Poseidon, however, sees Odysseus sailing home and stirs up a savage storm. He is driven into another land, where he is discovered by a princess after washing ashore. He reveals his true identity to the people there and begins telling a large assembly the long tale of his attempt to return home.

Odysseus tells them that in his journey he had sailed to the edge of the world after being informed by Circe, an enchantress, that he would have to visit Hades before he could return home. While in Hades, Odysseus talked with a seer who warned him of the various dangers that awaited him on his journey. The seer told Odysseus that he would arrive at his home unknown and friendless and that he would have problems reestablishing his position as master of the house. He was also told that he would have to regain the favor of Poseidon. If he were able to overcome these obstacles, the seer prophesied, Odysseus would have a long and peaceful life.

While Odysseus was visiting the souls near Hades, he unexpectedly spoke with his mother, who had died after he left for the Trojan War. He also spoke with members of his crew who had died. Odysseus became overwhelmed with emotion and rushed away.

After hearing his story, the listeners help Odysseus to return home. Upon arrival at home, Odysseus does not try to establish his old position immediately. Instead, he disguises himself in order to learn what is happening in his own household. In one of the most poignant scenes in the story, Odysseus discovers an old and toothless dog who is sick and near death at the gateway of his palace. The dog has not been cared for and lies in filth. It is Argus, his favorite dog, who has waited, ignored, for 20 years. Only Argus recognizes the disguised Odysseus. Argus raises his head to whimper and then dies.

Odysseus finally identifies himself and, with his son's help, kills those who have manifested such bad behavior. He sends for Penelope, who still does not recognize him. Telemachus scolds his mother for this failure, but Odysseus sends him away. Odysseus then speaks of things that only he and Penelope know. Penelope realizes that it is he for whom she had waited 20 years. Only then does Odysseus change into his royal garments. He and Penelope spend their first night together making love and telling each other of things that had happened while they were apart. The goddess Athene goes so far as to delay the sunrise to give them more time together.

This, however, is not the conclusion of the poem. The next day Odysseus takes his son and goes to visit his father, Laertes. His father greets him with great joy. When they are confronted by a group who are out to avenge those that Odysseus and Telemachus had killed, Laertes kills the father of those who had tormented Penelope. Ultimately, Athene intervenes in the conflict, establishing peace between the factions, and Odysseus is able to return to his reign as king.

This timeless story serves as a reminder that there are pitfalls on the path to a successful reunion. It also illustrates parts of the processes of return, readjustment, and reintegration that we will term the "three R's of reunion" (Table 14–1).

The Concepts of Family and Return

It is perhaps mostly through stories such as *The Odyssey* and stories' modern analogues, movies, that reunion problems of veterans and their families have been brought into the public consciousness. Movies such as *Coming Home, The Deer Hunter,* and *Apocalypse Now* depict the dilemmas of reunion in a powerful fashion.

Table 14–1.   The three R's of reunion

Return
  Rituals of homecoming

Readjustment
  Regression
  Recognition of change

Reintegration
  Communication
  Negotiation
  Consensus

There is relatively little systematic research on the specific theme of reunion. The literature generally shows a similarity in the difficulties faced by individuals and families. Both these similarities and these differences must be examined to arrive at rational recommendations for programs and interventions.

Any "union" that involves people entails two human beings who are growing and changing and who, after separation, may not fit neatly back together again as a couple. This should come as no surprise, since couples may not even stay together neatly without any separation!

Without a departure, there can be no return. There is a considerable literature on the process of separation and its attendant losses, as is discussed in some of the preceding chapters of this volume. There is a loss of companionship, the loss of sexual union, the loss of a partner in decision making and child discipline, the loss of social opportunities, and the loss of a partner in sharing day-to-day burdens. For a child, there is the functional loss of a parent. In the case of military families during war, there is also the constant background dread that these losses may become permanent if the servicemember is killed. Feelings of sadness, loneliness, fear, and anger are normal responses to these losses.

Concerns of family members become concerns for deployed personnel who are unable to take any active role in problem resolution. The consequent worry affects their ability to carry out their mission and in some cases may render servicemembers ineffective. Recognizing the importance of families, the services have set up programs to help spouses and families adapt to the separation. These programs often offer training on issues such as legal and financial planning and basic life skills. In addition, some military programs offer support groups, information, and other support services to diminish the stress of separation.

In "healthy" individuals, stress, itself, stimulates adaptation. Little is known about what constitutes a "healthy" relationship or "healthy" family. Similar to the individual in his or her growth and development, families, too, are theorized to experience developmental stages and "tasks." In a military population there are families in all stages of development. Because the military is composed primarily of younger people, both servicemembers and their families often are in the earlier stages of individual and family development and maturation.

Healthy individuals are the foundation of healthy couples, and healthy couples are the foundation of healthy families. It is helpful to consider families along several dimensions that typify health (Kaslow 1982). These dimensions include a "systems orientation" in which the healthy couple or family believe themselves to be an entity with trust and mutual respect and with shared paths, goals, and values, in which the following are present:

- "Boundary issues" are handled such that appropriately separate identities are maintained, privacy is allowed, and adult sexual needs are met.
- "Contextual issues" are handled through open communication, with desires and expectations conveyed and consistent communication.
- "Power" in the structure is egalitarian and mutually supportive, and equity, individuality, and happiness are valued more than being "right" or maintaining control.
- "Affective issues" allow for a wide range of emotions, including the expression of anger, optimism, good-natured teasing, and a sensing of the absurdity of life.
- "Negotiation" takes place, allowing joint "wins" rather than compromise that includes some "loss" on all parts or conciliation that is experienced as a "loss" by the conciliator.
- A "transcendental" value system exists in which there are a clear and shared belief system, a kinship with the world, a belief that the family members matter, and an abiding sense of meaning and purpose.

Clearly, the presence of such family attributes will be the result of many maturational processes and will be present in families and couples to varying degrees. The fewer maturing experiences the individual or family have had, the less likely it is that these capabilities will be present. Irrespective of the maturational stage of individuals or families, they must adapt to the losses during separation and reach a new equilibrium.

The Return of Prisoners of War

As discussed in greater detail in Chapter 17 of this volume, there are lessons to be learned from families and servicemembers who have endured some of the longest separations. Hunter (1984) reviewed the experiences of prisoners of war (POWs) from Southeast Asia and their families. Wives who had children or working wives who were more active and socially oriented coped better. Those at highest risk for poor adaptation were immature, extremely dependent wives, foreign-born wives, and wives who were isolated within a civilian community.

Many anxieties and stresses of family separation were relieved by adequate preparation. Open communication about the possibility of the POW's return aided adaptation. The data suggest that family adjustment during separation will influence the adjustment of the family and the POW upon return.

One year after reunion the wives reported that the most crucial factor in good marital adjustment was spousal agreement on their husband's future career plans. Spousal agreement on family roles and values was also important. Wives' levels of self-esteem affected the relationship: those with higher self-esteem reported better adjustment. Wives described other issues that were important for successful reunion. These included spousal agreement on the amount of affection shown and on sexual matters. For both POWs and wives, *agreement* on roles proved more important in explaining adjustment than who actually performed which roles.

Generally, how well children coped during the POW's absence was a direct reflection of how well the mothers were coping with the separation. Upon the POW's return, the greater the discrepancy in parental perception on family roles and tasks, the worse the father-child relationship.

At 2 years after reunion, the major problems noted were parent-child relationships (24%), the marital relationship (19%), personal adjustment of the family members (19%), and occupational adjustment (12%).

At 4 years after reunion, the divorce rate for the POWs was 32%, about three times the rate of matched control subjects (11%–12%) who had been deployed during the Vietnam conflict. The POW families remained more "matrifocal" than control families. The rank order of major problems was the same for both POW families and control subject families (i.e., parent-child, personal, marital, and occupational adjustment).

At 5 years after reunion, families that had stayed together had renegotiated and stabilized family roles fairly well and were well integrated. By the end of the 7-year study, family roles were stable, families were future oriented, and future plans were more a matter of concern than current problems.

Hunter believed that the reunion period could be more stressful than the separation. He recommended that communication skills training and family counseling be offered to reunited families. The longer the separation, the more time it would take for the family to reach homeostasis. For POW families separated for 5 years or longer, homeostasis generally was achieved within 2 to 3 years.

The Three R's of Family Reunion

The Return

The *return* is that stage of reunion that entails the actual physical reunion of those who have been separated. The return is stressful because it requires change. For example, problems that were routinely encountered as crews and families returned from ship's deployments led Navy chaplains in the 1970s to institute a program for returning personnel that has since been continued in various forms by most of the armed services. After Operation Desert Storm, every returning Navy ship had mandatory reunion briefing. Some of the other uniformed services offered similar programs. In addition, briefings at home were held by many family support groups and organizations but were unevenly attended.

Originally, chaplains met with sailors' wives and families and discussed their concerns and apprehensions about the sailors' homecoming. Common concerns included wondering how much the husband or parent had changed, how the husband would view the way finances had been handled, how the husband would view the way the children had been reared in his absence, how newly gained independence would be viewed, and, for children, whether or how punishment or rules would change after the father's return.

After meeting with the families, the chaplain or other representative then went to the ship, which was still at sea. The chaplain explored with the crew members their concerns and then shared with them the general concerns of the wives and children. The chaplain then met with the families again to share with them the concerns of those at sea and to help prepare a homecoming celebration.

Rituals are an important part of the return. The function of ritual is to give form to human life (Campbell 1973). Ritual can act as a guide to behavior and is a powerful catalyst for change. Ritual plays an important role in facilitating grief in the aftermath of combat; it is especially important for those who are wounded in combat and who are still hospitalized and in the process of adapting (Mateczun and Holmes-Johnson 1985).

Homecoming rituals can heighten emotional states and facilitate the expression of feelings. These rituals signify the importance of events and, as noted above, can help individuals and families by acting as a guide. A ship or unit may have rituals that signify the end of the deployment. Families and friends who are preparing for homecomings usually meet and discuss the upcoming changes, as well as review the events that occurred during separation. This process facilitates closure for those remaining ashore. Often, large community celebrations of welcome and thanks are planned.

The greetings of veterans of Desert Storm as they returned home are good examples of the use of ritual. There were informal greetings, such as that by the community members in Maine, who turned out to greet veterans while their aircraft refueled. More formal rituals, such as parades and the dedication of monuments, signified to veterans and families an acknowledgment of the sacrifices and the importance of what had been accomplished. Return celebrations held at unit levels helped to recognize families and give thanks to them for the sacrifices and contributions they had made. These celebrations stand in stark contrast to the return of veterans during the Vietnam War.

Sex is an important part of return for those who have had a sexual relationship, and many couples have developed rituals that they use for these occasions. Such rituals vary from an urgent visit to a motel to elaborate romantic vacations.

One of the most important functions of these homecoming rituals is to remind returning warriors that they are no longer at war and must begin to readjust to life at home. The warrior must leave behind the mental state that was used for survival, grieve whatever losses have been suffered, or to readjust to the life they once knew. Even the manners of the field and of shipboard life must be left behind lest the warrior ask a bemused family to "pass the f——g salt" at the dinner table.

Readjustment

The new habits of daily life are most noticeable to those who have been apart. It is as if families and couples recognize each other but have a sense that the other is not really who he or she says he or she is—that the other is somehow "disguised" and not who he or she was thought to be.

In fact, some of the most common clinical difficulties seen during this period result exactly because someone turns out not to behave or to have behaved as the partner thought they would or would have. An increase in patients with suicidal ideation and patients with suicide-related behaviors is encountered in the wake of return. For most of these patients, the suicidal ideation or suicide-related behaviors are associated with issues of "fidelity" or "loyalty," when returning servicemembers find that their spouses have not been "faithful" sexually or have been financially irresponsible, or in some other way behaved differently than "expected." This increase in incidence of suicidal ideation and suicide-related behaviors is also true among spouses who find that the returning warrior has not met some crucial expectation that the spouse had of the relationship.

Fears of having been replaced in the heart of loved ones or having been betrayed sometimes become realities. When this occurs, it is usually the precipitant of acute problems in the re-adjustment period. These occasions are painful, and in some cases they are lethal. This can be a particularly dangerous period for those who have developed no support systems upon which to rely. Most military families live distant from families of origin and may not have access to such support. Some people also have extraordinary feelings of dependency focused entirely upon the family. With support, most often from peers or someone with more life experience, and sometimes from professionals, these occasions of betrayal and loneliness are not lethal. Clinical help is usually necessary for those who have had clinical problems that predated the crisis.

Regression in family functioning while under the stresses of readjustment is not uncommon. Less mature patterns of communication, behavior, or roles may be seen. Such regression seems to happen in virtually all families and should be viewed as part of the natural process of readjustment.

It is sage advice for everyone during this period to "size up" the situation before taking any action. Time is an ally. It takes time to remove oneself from one context and put oneself in another. The returning individual must first recognize those habits and frames of mind that must be "killed" so that he or she can reveal his or her "true" self again in family relationships. Returning individuals must understand that partners and family may not "see" them as they believe themselves to be. Partner and family usually expect to "see" the person that was there before separation. However, over the course of the separation, each family member will have changed. The essence of readjustment lies in the recognition of these changes and the allocation of time for equilibration.

Case Example: Readjustment Difficulties

Petty Officer Jones, a 23-year-old sailor who worked in the boiler room aboard ships, had been on active duty in the Navy for 4 years and had been married for 3 years. He lived with his wife, 2-year-old son, and 1-year-old daughter near the Navy base, which was several hundred miles from either family of origin. For the past 3 years he had been deployed aboard a ship at sea for 18 months, including deployment in support of Operation Desert Storm, from which he was returning.

During his deployment he had received regular letters from his wife that reported what he had come to expect as the usual problems during deployment. On the day of his return his family greeted him at the pier. Later that day his wife told him that she intended to obtain a divorce and marry another man. She asked him to leave the house and live aboard ship. He visited several bars and became intoxicated and morose. He returned to ship, where he impulsively ingested 20 "muscle relaxants" that had previously been prescribed, thinking that he would rather be dead than endure the emotional pain that he was suffering. He then told a shipmate what he had done. His shipmate informed the watch personnel, who arranged transportation to the local naval hospital, where Petty Officer Jones was evaluated and admitted to the intensive care unit (ICU) with diagnoses of "suicide attempt, acute alcohol intoxication, barbiturate ingestion [from the 'muscle relaxants']." The psychiatry resident who had the watch early that morning reviewed the chart, tried to interview the still intoxicated patient, and made some evaluation of suicide risk while pondering the diagnostic dilemmas engendered by translating Petty Officer Jones's behavior into the diagnostic criteria of DSM-III-R [American Psychiatric Association 1987]. Ultimately, she decided to provisionally diagnose an adjustment disorder, not otherwise specified, specifying the "moderate" acute stressor of marital separation on Axis IV.

Petty Officer Jones was observed in the ICU, with no difficulty being noted, and transfer was arranged the next day to the psychiatry service. Although distressed, the patient denied any suicidal ideation. The resident thought that the patient was also "hungover" but was unable to find any diagnostic criteria that applied. Over the next 3 days, Petty Officer Jones was provided with crisis intervention, during which he was able to identify and articulate his mixed feelings of sadness and anger; supported in communicating with his wife, who refused to take part in his treatment or participate in any future marital therapy; aided in formulating a strategy for dealing with his children; and referred to resources such as legal counseling. The resident thought that the patient had some "dependent" personality traits and noted that the situation was quite similar to experiences that Petty Officer Jones had had in childhood. He was discharged from the hospital and placed in a support group, where he did well.

Reintegration

The term *union* implies a state with considerations beyond the self—that is, beyond "selfish" considerations. A union is more than the sum of its parts and also results in each of the partners giving up some things. Such is also the case for reunion. Once changes are recognized, they must either be integrated into the family structure or set aside. Failure to integrate or set aside changes that have occurred will foreclose the possibility of reunion.

It is worthwhile to remember that during a parent's deployment, children usually will have changed more than adults because of the pace of their natural development. Changes in children will often be dramatic to the returning parent. In addition to the obvious physical changes, there have likely been equally dramatic psychological, emotional, and spiritual changes that may take more time for a parent to recognize.

Case Example: Reunion With Children and Spouse

Sergeant Mary Johnson, a 28-year-old reservist from the Midwest who had been activated during the Gulf War, was seen by the psychiatry service in conjunction with evaluation for somatic complaints. A mother of three children, she had deployed to the Gulf on Christmas Eve, shortly after her mother had suffered a stroke. During her deployment she worked predominantly in warehouses in Dhahran. After an initial lag period, she received mail from her family throughout her stay in Southwest Asia.

Sergeant Johnson recalled that her trip home from Southwest Asia was "the most beautiful thing I've ever experienced except for my marriage and having my children." A computer programmer, she returned to her civilian job 6 weeks after getting home. Sergeant Johnson described having had some initial difficulty in thinking through computer programs, but she gradually returned to her previous level of functioning. She said that her two older children had done "okay" during her absence but that her 8-year-old son had had a difficult time. He developed a bald spot on the top of his head that doctors said was related to stress. He had had problems concentrating at school and had to repeat the same grade the following year. Sergeant Johnson said that by the time she returned home, her husband was "just about at the end of his rope" because of the stress associated with caring for the children and the house, coupled with his concern and worry for her safety.

Sergeant Johnson described the onset of irritability upon her return: "Things that shouldn't bother me, I'm letting bother me. My husband put a parking sticker on my car. He put it on crooked, in the wrong place, and on a dirty window; I got a ticket for it." Sergeant Johnson said that she had liked the independence and freedom she experienced during deployment and chafed at resuming her peacetime roles: "When I first got back I didn't want to be around my family, I felt like they were going to smother me." She noted that she had not completely settled in to the old routine: "Everything seems so dull. I miss all the people I was over there with so much. Sometimes I get depressed missing it." Sergeant Johnson denied symptoms of depression other than irritability. She participated in routine debriefings and family orientations on reunion issues. Her son's anxiety resolved and his schoolwork improved.

The losses of separation are easier to identify than the losses of reunion. Whereas most expect to experience losses at separation, few anticipate losses during reunion. However, some roles, habits, and thoughts acquired during separation must now be set aside and new ones integrated or the reunion will not be successful. Individuals must accommodate to a new structure or the structure will fail. As in the example above, even such simple things as eating habits must be reexamined.

Negotiation plays a central role in successful reintegration. Negotiation connotes an active process of communication. Without dialogue there will be no integration. As the military family matures, it is important that skill in negotiation be developed. Most military families can acquire this skill through contact with various military agencies and programs. Negotiation differs from compromise and concession. In compromise, all parties may see themselves as "losing" something. Concession is marked by the acquiescence of one party and the "victory" of the other.

Change must be negotiated and integrated—change that has occurred in the individuals that make up the family, changes that have occurred between family members, and changes that may be demanded from outside the family such as a change of duty station that requires the family to move. Attempts to maintain the former status quo, the old union, do not acknowledge such changes. The result of such attempts will, to a greater or lesser degree, be a dysfunctional union. Such failures that come to attention most frequently reflect a family "heritage" that individuals have brought from families of origin and, most frequently, the "rules" of communication that they learned.

It is not the *structure* of the family itself or who *actually* performs any specific role in the family, but, rather, the *agreement* among family members on relationships that will effect a successful reunion. Children, having their own unique needs, will most often model and reflect the mechanisms that their parents use in this process of reintegration.

Special Cases of Reunion

Some reunions present special challenges (Table 14–2). Such is the case for the combat wounded. When the servicemember is seriously injured and there is severe residual impairment, it is common for friends and family members to wonder privately if everyone would have been "better off" had the servicemember been killed outright. Indeed, this is also a common reaction of the wounded themselves. The physical changes associated with combat injuries can be dramatic, and adaptation may require extensive rehabilitation. Being dependent on others for routine matters of daily life may seem intolerable to formerly healthy servicemembers. In turn, having someone dependent for such

Table 14–2.   Special reunions

Combat wounded
    Wish to have died
    Dependency
    Rehabilitation
    Denial

Nontraditional relationships
    No authorized access to services
    Fear of discovery

Extended families
    Parents of adults
    Parents as veterans
    Consensus

needs may seem intolerable to the family. When possible, involvement of family members in rehabilitation is useful. Once again, as in the case of readjustment, time is an ally. The initial wish for death usually abates after the first year, to such an extent that there may even be denial that one could ever have harbored such thoughts.

There are relationships separate from marriage that may require consideration. Such relationships can often be dealt with as though the partners were married but may create "systems" problems within the military. A fiancée or fiancé may well have an established relationship but no authorized access to services, including therapy or military health insurance, which require the legal status of a dependent. For partners who have a relationship not recognized legally, such as homosexual servicemembers, seeking therapeutic help may often appear to dictate that the military system be avoided or the individual will run the risk of "discovery."

The military, itself, is often seen as a monolithic entity by civilians, servicemembers, and therapists. Ridenour (1984) related that a common theme in therapy may be the members' desire that the military change, but not the individual. Blame and responsibility are often projected upon the military. With such patients, two challenges for the therapist are to not become allied with the projections, whatever the therapist's personal position about the military, and to not become a "controlling foster parent," even if that is eagerly sought by the patient (Ridenour 1984).

In reunion, most of the focus is on the nuclear family. However, as the story of Odysseus suggests, the extended family—and, in particular, parents—are crucial to a completed reunion. The returning warrior must "go to" the parents. Parents have likely had many interactions with the veteran's spouse and children. A parent's joy upon the soldier's return and guidance in how to deal with problems can be real boons. Much of what the veteran's parents have to offer will depend on their own maturation and integration of changes in the past. Veterans may also have a role in helping the children of fellow veterans; telling the children about the parent's experiences may help the children better understand the changes in a parent.

A therapy group for active-duty members with symptoms of posttraumatic stress disorder (PTSD) revealed common themes. The servicemembers came from different age groups and experienced dissimilar traumas, ranging from Vietnam War combat to shipboard disasters. One striking similarity that emerged was that almost all had come from military families and had fathers that had been in combat. Interestingly, their fathers had usually stayed in the military after their combat, as did these veterans. Difficulties that they experienced in attaining intimacy with their own children reflected what had happened between them and their own fathers.

For some, the service itself may be seen as a parent. There are those who enter the service to leave behind families of origin that may have been abusive, alcoholic, or destructive. Such young people may not have any specific relationships to which they will reunite, yet they still need to recognize changes in themselves in order to readapt to their communities. The model that they emulate will likely be the noncommissioned officer superior to them in the chain of command whom they respect.

One common myth repeated by many is that the best way "to forget" so that readaptation will occur is to "get drunk." Although drinking will certainly cause memory problems if used in sufficient amounts for sufficient time, however, it impedes rather than facilitates effective readaptation.

The veteran must also readapt to the military, itself, upon return. For many, readaptation to the restrictions and routine of garrison life may be difficult after the experiences they have gone through. In contrast to reunion with friends and family, it is not possible for the veteran to negotiate with the military. However, communication can considerably ease the transition.

There are two themes in *The Odyssey* that are most instructive for those in helping professions who attempt to effect or set the background for a positive reunion. Foremost is the telling of the story. Everyone must be able to tell his or her personal story, not just a "sea story" or a "war story." The person must relate the story from his or her viewpoint, including his or her emotional responses, rather than tell it as though it happened to someone else. The second theme is the use of expectancy. When the expectation that reunion will be successful is communicated (although it may take the nearly 20 years that Odysseus wandered the earth), it is more likely that the reunion will, in fact, be successful. Therapists will be greatly aided by giving the expectation that reunion, despite some turbulence, will ultimately be successful. In a co-therapist context, therapists and co-therapists can model successful adaptive processes for members, couples, and families in treatment.

Case Example: Consulting With Large Organizations

A training hospital that had nearly half of its staff deploy to Operation Desert Storm requested a consultant to identify organizational concerns related to reintegration and to recommend a program of action. The consultant noted that the hospital personnel affected comprised several groups. Those that had deployed had gone primarily to one unit, but many had gone to other mobilization assignments as well. Reserve personnel had to augment the staff, and those active-duty hospital personnel who "stayed behind" had different concerns. Generally all personnel had unrealistic expectations of the length of time that should be necessary to "fit back in" to the reintegrated hospital.

Numerous personal, family, occupational, and organizational concerns were evident. Cross-sectional interviews were held that revealed a wide spectrum of these concerns. Affective symptoms of anger, guilt, and anxiety were endorsed by personnel. Some noted an increase in compulsive behaviors such as cleaning, spending, and drinking. Many described ruminating about their careers and relationships. Occupational concerns included job assignment, peer support, decreased productivity, and career planning. A host of organizational or "system" issues were noted: the perception of unequal recognition for deployed and stay-behind staff, and "boundary" problems in reestablishing formal relationships that had been relaxed during deployment (e.g., being on a first-name basis regardless of rank).

The families of deployed personnel complained of difficulties in sharing responsibility, fears of infidelity, reclaiming more active parenting roles, and financial problems.

The consultant recommended a 1-year program of education and, when necessary, intervention regarding the reintegration process. A plan was suggested that would start with a program for mental health personnel who would then aid in implementing the following actions:

1. Brief the command personnel on the reintegration process and on findings from the consultation and program objectives.
2. Produce a videotape as an educational aid that highlights individual responses to the readjustment process and uses a cross section of people with experiences to which others could relate.
3. Produce a handout in which normal and abnormal responses are outlined, to be made available at every clinic and inpatient nursing station.
4. Conduct department work-site education/intervention programs with small-group sessions including intervention assessment and postintervention evaluations.
5. Identify special "at-risk" groups, such as those that had deployed to different assignments, and offer programs.
6. Identify reservists and mail educational information to them including that on the availability of Veterans Administration programs.
7. Identify individuals, such as Vietnam War veterans, who are more at risk for reactivation of PTSD symptomatology and offer individual services.
8. Use command public affairs to help with positive media exposure.
9. Establish prevention measures for possible future deployments, including a presentation on psychological aspects of the deployment cycle as part of the hospital orientation.
10. Promulgate lessons learned for the benefit of personnel in the future.

Military Programs

When one is conceptualizing coordinated programs to facilitate reunion, the fact that "healthy" individuals, couples, and families adapt to separation and reunion most effectively (but not without problems) leads to certain conclusions. Preparation is key. Deployment may come without notice, and just as warriors train so as to be ready, a family that prepares will be more ready to face the uncertainties ahead.

Family Readiness Programs

An understanding of basic life skills that are necessary for simple survival leads to programs that assist in legal planning (e.g., a will, powers of attorney), financial planning (e.g., budgeting, designation of who will pay the bills), child care planning (e.g., designation of who will take care of the kids, consideration of how they will get to school and where they will get health care), and other basic necessities. Classes that result in skills in child rearing and communication are often seen as "therapy" instead of basic readiness for deployment.

Support Structures

Resources such as the "key wives" programs (hopefully "key spouse" programs in the future) and unit "ombudsmen" can be critical for effective communication—particularly for families of units that deploy together. The ability of people in these contexts to mobilize resources for individuals can be phenomenal. It should be recognized, however, that most spouses work, take care of children, and assume other responsibilities and that an expectation that any one spouse, even a commanding officer's, can and should be able to do all things for all people is unfair and untenable.

Spiritual Support

Chaplains are a resource that can be utilized for support in general. The spiritual guidance and comfort they have offered military members and their families have always been of great importance. In a secular world the aspect of spirituality in individuals' lives can easily be overlooked in planning. Churches where families worship have traditionally provided crucial social and spiritual support.

Family Advocacy Programs

Family advocacy programs, sponsored by the military, are designed to provide assessment, referral for counseling, and tracking of spouse and child abuse. The installation's family advocacy program should be contacted whenever spouse or child abuse is suspected.

Family Resource and Service Centers

Family resource and service centers, also sponsored by the military, provide resources for various skills training, counseling, and referral. The personnel typically are experts on military life and military systems.

Military Mental Health Professionals

Each of the services has uniformed mental health professionals who can be accessed through the medical treatment system. Professionals come from the disciplines of social work, psychiatric nursing, clinical psychology, and psychiatry.

Other Organizations

Many national organizations provide programs and support. For example, the Navy–Marine Corps Relief Society offers financial support in crises, and the National Military Family Association lobbies effectively on matters affecting military families. Organizations such as the Red Cross and the USO may also provide programs and services. Community or local programs are sometimes offered; for example, during Operations Desert Shield and Desert Storm, many professionals offered pro bono services to military family members in their community.

In planning for reunion, there may be private organizations that offer specific programs. A *reunion support series* (Perez and Embry 1991), consisting of six booklets providing information targeted at military personnel, spouses/significant others, and children, and for friends, relatives, schools, and communities, was independently distributed during the Gulf War.

The armed services lack any unified, consistent structure for coordinating human services support, either during deployment or in preparation for reunion. There are, in fact, competing models and professional "turfs" for how such services and support should be conceptualized and provided. Anyone wanting to put together a comprehensive program must face these challenges. Preventive services and programs generally are "hard to sell," especially during times of downsizing. As a result, programs generally are put together during a crisis and are reactive rather than proactive. Continual emphasis must be placed on family programs lest they be forgotten until the next war.

References

American Psychiatric Association: Diagnostic and Statistical Manual of Mental Disorders, 3rd Edition, Revised. Washington, DC, American Psychiatric Association, 1987

Campbell J: Myths to Live By. New York, Bantam Books, 1973

Hunter EJ: Treating the military captive's family, in The Military Family. Edited by Kaslow FW, Ridenour RI. New York, Guilford, 1984, pp 167–195

Kaslow FW: Portrait of the healthy couple. Marital Therapy 5:519–528, 1982

Mateczun JM, Holmes-Johnson EK: The psychiatric care of the combat injured, in Proceedings of the Fourth User's Workshop on Combat Stress (Consultation Report 85-002). Edited by Manglesdorf AB, King JM, O'Brien DE, et al. Fort Sam Houston, TX, U.S. Army Health Services, 1985, pp 180–195

Perez J, Embry D: The Reunion Support Series, Vols 1–6, Quality Time. Tucson, AZ, Project ME, 1991

Ridenour RI: The military, service families, and the therapist, in The Military Family. Edited by Kaslow FW, Ridenour RI. New York, Guilford, 1984, pp 1–17

15 The Care of Those Returned: Psychiatric Illnesses of War

Ronald J. Koshes, M.D.

Bill had been married for 17 years. Almost as long as his military career. After returning from his tour in Southwest Asia, Bill, a highly decorated, senior noncommissioned officer, began staying out late, drinking excessively, arguing with his wife, and finally began using cocaine. For the latter offenses, he was removed from the Army despite his long and distinguished military career. Now divorced, Bill is looking for a job. He is tormented by nightmares of seeing dead Arab soldiers and uses alcohol daily to help him sleep.

At an Army community hospital during Operation Desert Storm, a slow and steady rise in the referral of soldiers of higher enlisted rank with problems of alcohol and/or drug use was noted. The incidence of domestic violence and problems with children also increased. Disciplinary actions against soldiers for insubordination, showing up late to work, and failure to report to work also appeared to rise; there was a general sense of poor morale. Some soldiers needed to be hospitalized. For some returning personnel, the stress of returning home to failed or failing marriages or of readjusting to garrison life and an army that had begun downsizing was too much.

Some soldiers sought treatment while in the Persian Gulf. Chaplains, social workers, psychologists, and behavioral science technicians were there in support of troops. At a primary intervention level, briefings were given in the theater concerning managing anxiety about family and friends back home. Some evacuation hospitals housed psychiatric patients, and a number of patients were evacuated home because of psychiatric reasons.

Often, the treating physician during this time asked, "Is the increase in problems related to Operation Desert Storm? Are these soldiers manifesting the delayed stress reactions of deployment and exposure to war?" In this chapter I explore these questions. First, I review the basic principles of the management of stress reactions in the combat setting, with an emphasis on the need for continuation of care to prevent long-term effects. I then review treatment modalities for managing returning soldiers, focusing on an inpatient setting, and indicate directions for further research.

Historical Overview of Psychological Injury and Readjustment

Although each war has taught military psychiatrists something new about the management of combat-related injuries, treatment doctrines have held to the notion that soldiers are to be treated nearest the site of injury, as quickly as possible, with the expectation that the soldier will return to his or her unit as soon as possible. This doctrine has been clearly stated by several authors as the simple mnemonic PIES (proximity, immediacy, expectancy, and simplicity) (Artiss 1963). Depending on the type of war, certain psychiatric illnesses are expected. Massive and sporadic stress will increase the incidence of combat stress reactions and may prevent return to duty (Marlowe 1986; Noy 1987). In rapidly progressing, high-intensity ground wars, there are likely to be more anxiety and hysterical conversion-related disorders. Those individuals in slow-moving, low-intensity battle situations are likely to suffer more from substance abuse problems and depression (Crocq et al. 1985; Jones 1985). At the close of the war, there can be an increase in problems such as alcohol and drug abuse and family abuse and in disciplinary actions. This increase appears to be related to readjustment to garrison life and reunions with families (Brill and Kupper 1966; Rothberg et al. 1994). Some of the problems, both acute and long-term, that have been associated with combat are listed in Table 15–1.

How veterans of war fare in comparison with civilians and with those soldiers who do not deploy is an important question. The experience of war is likely to be a unique experience. During war there is group bonding, license to kill, and denial of mortality or, alternatively, an intense fear of mortality. In many instances, a suspension of critical, analytical, and rational thinking may occur.

Those soldiers returning from Vietnam suffered higher rates of alcoholism, drug abuse, and suicide than did their civilian or military peers (Borus 1974; Centers for Disease Control 1989; Hoiberg 1980; Rahe 1988). World War II soldiers separated for "psychoneurosis" in 1944 showed a 20% excess mortality over the period 1946 to 1966 (Baker 1984). Overall, there was a nine-fold increase in the suicide rate for World War II veterans (Pokorny 1967). In a sample of Vietnam veterans, Figley (1978)

Table 15–1.   Types of psychiatric disorders seen in veterans of war

Acute reactions
  Depression
  Conversion disorders
  Brief reactive psychoses
  Adjustment disorders
  Substance abuse, dependence, intoxication, and withdrawal

Chronic reactions
  Posttraumatic stress disorder
  Marital and family problems
  Impulse control problems
  Substance abuse and dependence

---

found that combatants had impaired interpersonal adjustment but that this was not a sustained effect. He characterized the maladjustment as "more verbal fights, more frequent violent fantasies, violent dreams, and getting 'high' more often" (p. 109). Figley noted that the combatant group had fewer close friends and lower morale than the noncombatants. Many veterans with combat stress reactions recover and do well: "Time heals all wounds" (Horowitz and Solomon 1975).

Treatment of Battle Fatigue

The risk associated with untreated battle fatigue is the disintegration of a unit's effectiveness in accomplishing its mission. As mentioned earlier, the basic tenets of treating combat fatigue rely on mental health professionals and unit personnel who are committed to the principles of treating closely, quickly, simply, and with the expectation that the soldier will return to duty. Underlying this approach is the value that the unit commander places on his or her soldiers and the investment the soldier has in the unit (Gifford et al. 1992). Factors found to be protective against psychiatric casualties in the 1982 war in Lebanon were 1) confidence in one's own skills as a soldier, 2) belief in the legitimacy of the war, 3) trust in one's weapons, 4) confidence in one's comrades, and 5) trust in one's commander. Unit cohesion was also positively correlated with postcombat adjustment and health indicators. The more cohesive the unit, the fewer symptoms its members reported on various postcombat surveys (Belenky 1987).

If diagnosed with combat exhaustion or combat fatigue, the soldier is treated in or close to the unit and returned to duty. When a soldier is so impaired that he or she cannot function effectively in the unit, the soldier is evacuated outside of the combat area. If the dysfunction involves severe psychosis or a severe conversion reaction, the soldier usually cannot be returned to duty even with the most intensive types of treatments and, therefore, must be evacuated.

There may be embellishment of symptoms and an incentive to remain in the sick role. Psychological factors such as secondary gain can play a role in soldiers with physical problems who are sent to the rear. For example, in the assault on Okinawa and in the Korean War, as battle injuries increased, so did sick call rates. As the time spent in sick call increased, the chances for return to duty approached zero (Blood and Ganker 1993).

Returning Home

When a soldier can no longer function in the theater of war, he or she is evacuated—usually to a medical treatment facility to the United States. The system of evacuation can be unpredictable, despite the intense work of coordinators. Some authors have observed that evacuations can be affected by staffing in theater (Garland 1993).

The evacuation process, itself, is uncomfortable. Often soldiers are on cramped, cold, noisy, long, and dark evacuation flights. Generally, an attempt is made to return soldiers to the hospital closest to their unit or to their home. The overall process is characterized by waiting and uncertainty; the soldier can feel out of touch, totally disconnected from his or her unit, family, and friends. In a time of war, the efficiency required by medical personnel and the need for these personnel to avoid burnout may limit the soldier's access to warm human interactions or friendliness. He or she may learn that the easiest way to get attention is to emphasize the medical or psychiatric problem.

Treatment

Specific treatments of combat stress reactions, such as conversion disorders, depression, anxiety, and posttraumatic stress disorder (PTSD), are grounded in certain theoretical constructs. Traumatic experiences in war can then be understood in various models, each of which suggests a rich repertoire of interventions (Abse 1984).

Caring for soldiers with war-related injuries is a difficult task. First, for the providers, there is the fear of being overwhelmed with casualties. This fear can generate a level of anxiety that can permeate the organization and lead to dysfunction. When patients finally arrive, staff may feel angry because the patients are not "sick enough," presenting with character problems as well as stress illnesses and often having had several weeks to recover before arriving at the tertiary-care hospital. In Operation Desert Storm, the casualties were far fewer than had been anticipated and planned for.

Transference and countertransference problems in the provision of treatment for returned Desert Storm soldiers were important to address (Table 15–2). A risk of burnout is associated with caring for veterans of combat. The highly emotionally charged content of their stories and problems often compels listeners to become personally involved. Those at greatest risk of countertransference difficulties are usually the technicians. These paraprofessionals spend the greatest amount of time with the patients and generally have less formal education about these therapeutic challenges. Identification with the young soldiers and their trauma is a countertransference reaction seen especially in young, inexperienced staff. Other common staff countertransference reactions include the projection of rage onto patients and a tendency to infantilize patients. For some

---

Table 15–2.   Challenges of transference and counter-transference

Transference
  Staff project unacceptable aggressive impulses onto patients.
  Staff infantilize patients.

Countertransference
  Ward staff overly identify with patients.
  Staff question morality of their roles.

---

staff members, work with these patients can stimulate moral questions and prompt a reexamination of their association with the military.

Debriefing groups for staff provide an important avenue for assisting hospital personnel in meeting the challenges of working with patients with war-related casualties. Empathic listening plays an important role in preventing staff burnout. The creation of comfortable working conditions and the provision of a quiet break room also help prevent burnout.

Specific Treatments

It is important that treatment for veterans be carried out in a secure setting, as was done for those of previous wars. Most of the work to be done involves the telling of stories about the war—about the experience of going to battle. The creation of an environment in which patients feel that they can talk candidly, and without repercussion, about commanding officers, military operations, and other military or political personnel facilitates the work. The general therapeutic goal is to help the soldiers integrate the traumatic material of war into their total life experiences (Koshes and Rowe 1992).

Debriefings best occur in a group setting. The opportunity to have one's experiences validated by others who have been through similar circumstances plays a central therapeutic role. Group debriefings also diminish stigmatization and overpsychologizing of symptoms. Hearing of others' painful combat experiences often diminishes obsessive thoughts and decreases the intensity and personal relevance of traumatic memories. Group settings reduce isolation and provide reunions with comrades (Koshes et al. 1995).

Other modes of therapy are also useful in treating patients with traumatic combat experiences. Especially helpful may be group, individual, and family therapy aimed at facilitating the expression of fears and frustrations. These therapies also assist the individual with reintegration into his or her military unit, family, and social network. Behavioral therapies and hypnosis can be of benefit in decreasing avoidant behaviors and panic associated with PTSD. Amytal interviews have proved beneficial in reducing morbidity associated with conversion reactions (Blank 1982; Borus 1973; Defazio 1984).

Pharmacological therapies are targeted for specific symptoms of combat stress reactions (van der Kolk 1983). The use of short-acting benzodiazepines has been advocated in the treatment of battle fatigue to reduce anxiety, induce sleep, and promote rapid return of soldiers to the battlefield. Conversely, in a combat setting, antipsychotic medications (e.g., haloperidol or chlorpromazine) should be avoided if return to the field is imminent, because of their slowing of important self-protective responses. Additionally, it has been speculated that the use of these antipsychotic agents may ultimately worsen PTSD symptoms. The putative mechanism for this effect is the blunted affect associated with these medications that diminishes the individual's ability to process the emotionally charged traumatic materials adequately.

For the individual returned from war who may be suffering from PTSD, other medications such as anxiolytics or antidepressant medications may be required (Davidson et al. 1990; Feldman 1987; Fesler 1991; Frank et al. 1988; Kinzie and Leung 1989; March 1992; Nagy et al. 1993; Shay 1992; Silver et al. 1990; Turchan et al. 1992). These medications are usually prescribed to target specific symptoms of PTSD. Recently, electroencephalogram (EEG) findings (Peniston and Kulkosky 1991) have implicated a kindling phenomenon and suggest a role for the use of anticonvulsant medications in treatment of PTSD (Wolf et al. 1988).

Assessment and Diagnosis

Diagnostic issues relating to combat and the resultant "labeling" of patients represent dilemmas for the mental health professional. Many soldiers will satisfy the diagnostic criteria for a DSM-IV (American Psychiatric Association 1994) diagnosis, and yet the potential negative effects of labeling a soldier as psychiatrically ill must be carefully weighed. Labeling a person with an illness can reinforce the "sick" role and delay or prevent the soldier's return to the unit or to a useful role in military or civilian life. Most of the combat casualties who suffer from battle exhaustion have a severe adjustment disorder that is acute. A few will have psychotic reactions, whereas others will manifest significant anxiety components in their presentation. A good clinical interview that assesses degree of symptomatology is most important with this population (Scurfield and Blank 1985).

Development of Treatment Plans

Once a soldier has been identified as having a combat-related disorder, the treatment setting becomes an important consideration. Ideally, a military environment is maintained to minimize regression into a patient role and to avoid stigmatizing the soldier as having a severe mental illness rather than a reaction to combat. Rehabilitative units for combat fatigue separate soldiers with typically less severe psychiatric diagnoses from medically ill patients and retain a military atmosphere through the use of uniforms, assignment of duties, inspections, and so forth. Regardless of the setting, the goal of the treatment must be clear and supported by the treatment team. Characteristics of an effective inpatient treatment setting for veterans of war with combat-related psychiatric illness are presented in Table 15–3.

Usually, the main treatment goals are the reduction of morbidity and the reintegration of the soldier into some useful military function. In the case of delayed combat reactions, such as PTSD, depression, and substance abuse, the treatment goals will also include changing the behaviors of the individual. The following case example illustrates a common presentation for a soldier referred to a mental health clinic following the

Table 15–3.   Characteristics of an effective inpatient treatment setting for veterans of war

- Reinforcement of the fact that the experience of the soldier in combat is valid and important
- Encouragement of the use of community-validated experiences
- Emphasis on the fact that psychiatric pathology is different from war-related stress disorders
- Valuing of independence over dependence
- Close resemblance to an active-duty military unit
- Adherence to military protocol

Persian Gulf War. Although the soldier's exposure to combat-related traumas was minimal, the effects of deployment were significant.

Case Example 1

History of present illness: Sergeant McHenry, a 26-year-old male active-duty soldier, was referred by Command for a mental status evaluation as required for a misconduct separation. He was being discharged from the Army because of poor duty performance and repeated incidents of sleeping while on guard duty.

At the time of the evaluation, Sergeant McHenry reported feeling depressed for several weeks because of financial and marital problems. He described two incidents in which he became physically violent toward his wife, prompting her to leave him. He wanted marital therapy, but his wife told him that "it is too late." Sergeant McHenry focused primarily on his feelings about the marital situation and did not seem appropriately concerned about his imminent discharge from the Army.

Sergeant McHenry stated that he had been married for only a few months before being deployed to Saudi Arabia. He reported that while he was in the Persian Gulf, he longed to be with his wife and became increasingly negligent of his duties. He received two Article 15's (i.e., disciplinary actions) for sleeping on guard duty and several counseling statements for poor job performance. He was also barred from reenlistment and demoted from Sergeant to Private First Class. Sergeant McHenry's commander felt that his problems were related to his experiences in Saudi Arabia and to being deployed away from his wife.

The soldier did not report any symptoms associated with his war experience. However, he noted that upon his return from the war, he no longer felt it was important to take care of his responsibilities and got himself in serious financial trouble. He also admitted being inattentive to his wife and placing unreasonable demands on her. Sergeant McHenry stated that he became easily irritated and had become physically violent on a couple of occasions.

At the time of his evaluation, Sergeant McHenry had served in the Army for more than 8 years, with overseas tours in Germany and Korea. He had no record of any problems before his deployment to Saudi Arabia. Since the onset of his marital and financial problems, Sergeant McHenry's performance had deteriorated and his self-esteem had reached an all-time low. He blamed the Army for causing his divorce and attributed his financial problems to the deployment.

Mental status examination: At the time of the first visit, the patient looked fatigued. He was oriented to time, place, person, and situation. His thought process was normal, and there were no hallucinations, delusions, or paranoia. Insight and judgment were questionable as evidenced by his inability to recognize his contribution to his problems and his tendency to repeat behaviors that continued to create problems for him. His mood was depressed and his affect was appropriate. He reported vague suicidal thoughts but denied suicidal intent. The most serious symptom reported was his inability to sleep. His appetite was fine. He reported feeling tired all the time and lacking motivation to do anything.

Intervention: The soldier was given Benadryl to help his sleeping difficulty; stronger medication was avoided because there was some potential for suicidal behavior. Sergeant McHenry responded well to psychotherapy focused on helping him better cope with the anger associated with his deployment, and his separation and eventual divorce from his wife. He began to look at his situation with more hope. He formulated a plan to begin paying his bills and was looking into civilian employment opportunities by the time that therapy terminated.

Careful treatment planning is essential to successful work with combat stress casualties. The guidelines in Table 15–4 pertain to the treatment planning process.

Specific dysfunctional behaviors are identified, such as increased use of alcohol; inability to control temper; anxiety symptoms related to novel circumstances; lack of self-esteem in the marital relationship; and sleep and appetite disturbances. Each member of the treatment team is responsible for specific interventions and monitors the progress of treatment. For instance, an initial hospital treatment plan for the soldier whose case history began this chapter is described below.

Case Summary

Sergeant First Class William Bentley is a 44-year-old male who describes a 14-month history of sleep and appetite disturbance, increased use of alcohol, communication problems with his wife, and a recent judicial action for his use of cocaine that has resulted in his separation from the Army. He endorses symptoms of PTSD to include anxiety, in-

---

Table 15–4.   Essentials of treatment planning

- Be specific in the identification of functional problems.
- Prioritize problems.
- Define problems as immediate and long-term.
- Make objectives specific, measurable, and timed.
- Set goals that are achievable.
- Involve the patient in his or her own treatment planning.
- Make available to all staff and the patient a written document in which the treatment plan is described.

---

creased startle response, avoidance, and flashbacks of his tour of duty in Saudi Arabia.

Areas that must be addressed by the treatment plan include sleep and eating problems when under stress, difficulty communicating with his wife, abrupt transition from military to civilian life, and aftercare. His inability to control use of alcohol (and cocaine), and the PTSD symptoms, are also targets for intervention.

Specific interventions are delegated to various members of the treatment team. After completing the assessment of the patient, the psychiatrist must first determine the best setting for treatment—that is, whether SFC Bentley should be hospitalized or treated as an outpatient. The indications for antidepressant and/or antianxiety agents should also be addressed. If medications are warranted, specific targets for medication and possible side effects should be delineated. The psychiatrist should also consider what talking therapy would be most beneficial. For SFC Bentley, individual and group psychotherapy were helpful in facilitating his expression of fear and frustration associated with leaving the Army.

The nursing staff played an important role in monitoring the patient's sleep and appetite, educating the patient about his medications, and conducting individual counseling to facilitate verbal expression. Activities therapies were also employed; the patient was enrolled in groups that focused on the development of self-esteem and communication skills. He was also introduced to leisure activities that provided alternatives to alcohol (and cocaine) use.

The social work service arranged for outpatient psychiatric treatment and counseling for the patient's alcohol and cocaine problems. The social work service also scheduled family meetings to improve communication skills.

The goals and objectives for this patient included target dates and were specific and measurable. For example, goals were set to ensure that the patient slept 8 hours per night and ate three meals per day within 7 days of hospitalization. Communication skills were enhanced through defining a goal of two episodes of conversation with his wife for

30 minutes or more that were not conflict-ridden, to be accomplished before discharge.

The patient was actively encouraged to prepare for his separation from the Army. His treatment plan specified that he describe two alternative career paths before discharge.

In conjunction with the social work service's discharge planning, the patient was tasked with identifying follow-up appointments with both an alcohol/drug counselor and an outpatient psychotherapist before discharge. He was also to identify three alternative ways to cope with stress other than alcohol use.

Quantifiable goals were also delineated for the patient's PTSD symptomatology: episodes of intrusive thoughts, flashbacks, avoidance behavior, and anxiety were to be diminished by 75%.

Complications

Complications in the recovery of psychiatric casualties of war may be related to the availability and organization of services as well as to the individual's psychopathology. Soldiers returning from war are often processed back to their original units or homes in large numbers. Because a large amount of information needs to be covered in a short period of time, soldiers with individual issues or concerns may not fully understand the process of which they are a part. Often, the large influx of returning soldiers strains the resources of the medical care system. Thus, health care providers may be harried and may demonstrate less friendliness and concern for patients. Referrals for additional medical or psychiatric care may be made hurriedly without the usual time needed for preparing and assessing the patient. Also, because soldiers are eager to reunite with families, some may downplay any problems they are having in order to hasten the discharge process. Moreover, some soldiers believe that referrals for mental health consultation may harm their careers. In one study, only 11% of Air Force personnel who had been referred for a mental health consultation were on active duty 6 years later (Retzlaff and Deatherage 1993).

Reintegration

The medical evaluation of soldiers serves a duty both to the ill or impaired patient and to the organization. The psychiatrist must address the question of whether the soldier is capable of returning to duty. When the military psychiatrist is answering this question, his or her dual agency to the interests of the military organization and to the individual may conflict. In frontline evaluations, if the soldier is impaired such that his or her return to duty would endanger his or her life or the lives of others in the unit, then the soldier should be evacuated to the rear for further treatment and disposition. Some soldiers will be found to have psychiatric conditions that render them medically unfit for further military service, and their cases will be forwarded for disability evaluation.

The disability system is a rather complex and time-consuming process that determines the individual's level of dysfunction, the presence of preexisting conditions, and the degree to which active-duty service affected the condition. On the basis of an evaluation of these data, a determination is made of whether the soldier is entitled to compensation by the government. Health care access, as well as other education, monetary, and housing benefits, is also affected by this determination.

Follow-up in the disability system can be difficult to carry out. Some veterans contend with care providers who are not familiar with the nuances of treating postcombat disorders. Moreover, some practitioners doubt the existence of PTSD as a unique clinical entity, feeling instead that dysfunction is caused by personality disorders, alcoholism, or other deep-seated psychological trauma.

During the post–Vietnam War era, follow-up studies of the general health and functioning of these veterans were difficult. Studies demonstrated higher rates of suicide, alcoholism, and drug abuse in veterans of the Vietnam War. The most difficult time for veterans appeared to be within the first 3 years after the war. More recent data have shown that rates of dysfunctional behavior following deployments and redeployments from military operations can cause an increase in problems with alcohol, drugs, spouse abuse, and child abuse (Rothberg et al. 1994). Many of these behaviors would otherwise be labeled sociopathic and indicative of a personality disorder. In the context of military exercises, however, these maladaptive behaviors are likely part of a "release phenomenon" seen when soldiers return home from war (Brill and Kupper 1966).

Unique Factors in the Persian Gulf War

When the reserve forces were mobilized during Operations Desert Storm/Shield, many reservists had to quickly make a transition from civilian to military life. Some reservists were unprepared to do this, as were some units. It was discovered that some individuals had medical problems that rendered them nondeployable. This was especially problematic when it was the unit commander or senior noncommissioned officer who could not be part of the deployment because of medical problems. Because of personnel shortages created by disability or family emergencies, some units were rounded out with soldiers belonging to different commands. The incorporation of these new members posed special challenges because of the importance of unit cohesion in combat. The following case example illustrates some of the special challenges confronting deploying reservists.

Case Example 2

History of present illness: Sergeant Jill Schmidt had been in the Army Reserves for nearly 10 years. As a petroleum supply specialist, she served a combat support role.

Sergeant Schmidt had no history of psychiatric treatment before joining the Army. The patient's desire to join the Army stemmed from a belief that she would be judged on her ability to get a job done and not on her educational background and family upbringing, nor on gender. Sergeant Schmidt was unmarried and gave no indication that she dated. She was well accepted by the unit, organizing several of the usual holiday events.

Her tour in Southwest Asia began in October 1990 when she deployed with her unit to the Kuwait border in support of ground combat forces. Once the border was crossed in the ground war, Sergeant Schmidt's unit was rapidly deployed and followed the ground forces into the lower half of Iraq. While there, Sergeant Schmidt reported witnessing dozens of dead Iraqi soldiers in various stages of decomposition and states of mutilation. By her report, the onset of her symptoms coincided with deployment and had been exacerbated by witnessing the destruction during the ground war.

When she returned home, Sergeant Schmidt found it difficult to adjust to unit life. She felt that her chain of command was unsympathetic to her requests for time off. Duties, which previously had been carried out without question, were now experienced by her as senseless and unproductive. The soldier began using alcohol more frequently and showing up for work later each day. Her military bearing declined considerably; she gained weight and failed the physical training test, placing her at risk for administrative separation. After numerous efforts at kindness and understanding, her commander's patience wore thin, and disciplinary action was considered. Sergeant Schmidt became acutely depressed, complaining of vivid nightmares and irritability. She was referred for psychiatric evaluation.

Course of treatment: Sergeant Schmidt began weekly psychotherapy and was placed on antidepressant medication for treatment of the neurovegetative signs and symptoms of depression. As she began talking more about the experience of war and seeing the dead soldiers, Sergeant Schmidt showed initial improvement at work. She did not volunteer information about her personal life and evaded questions concerning significant personal relationships. Sergeant Schmidt showed moderate anxiety when asked about her support system outside of work; her therapist approached this issue carefully because of what appeared to be affective instability.

Gradually, the soldier began to talk less about her experiences in Southwest Asia, but her symptoms did not resolve entirely. In fact, after a 3-month period of psychotherapy, it appeared that she was "cured" of her traumatic war experiences, yet continued to have problems at her unit: showing up for work late and being disobedient to her chain of command.

An amobarbital interview was performed to allow Sergeant Schmidt to express some of her fears and frustrations regarding her deployment and further explore the nature of her trauma. What became clear in the interview is that this soldier had experienced a trauma after her return from the war. Sergeant Schmidt had been living with another person in an intimate relationship for approximately 4 years. Shortly before the beginning of the ground war, she received a letter that indicated that her friend had left her. She remembered feeling full of rage and unable to adequately express those feelings. Sergeant Schmidt reported feeling full of rage at the men who had sexually abused and raped her in the past and that thoughts of killing them surfaced in her mind. She was from a physically abusive family. She had been sexually abused by a cousin at age 7 years and later raped when she was 16 years old. She related an incident of traveling on the road into Iraq and seeing a dead soldier who reminded her of the man who had raped her; unshaven and dark skinned with a black mustache. The patient had developed an acceptable way of dealing with the rage of her lost relationship by focusing on the death and destruction that was a real experience of the war. The unconscious guilt present over the wish fulfillment of death was too much for her to deal with in a conscious fashion, and, hence, the symptoms of PTSD arose.

Her therapy progressed in a rather straightforward fashion from that point on. Sergeant Schmidt talked about her losses and decreased her use of alcohol. She became more cooperative with command and began to reconstruct an acceptable social support network.

Conclusions

Psychiatric dysfunction resulting from war may not show up until years after the conflict has ended. The afflicted person usually does not suffer from severe character pathology or other primary psychological dysfunction. Rather, the war veteran is likely to have experienced profound events that may have been only partially processed. Dysfunction often occurs slowly and with an insidious onset. Problems with the law and with family, and substance abuse and dependence, may occur in those individuals who have not properly processed their experience of war. In turn, these veterans' problems affect families, significant relationships, and communities. The military history becomes of paramount importance in dealing with any psychiatric patient who may have been exposed to combat or been part of a deployment. Gaining an understanding of the history of the exposure, the affective experience, and the level of past functioning guides the clinician in choosing an appropriate therapeutic approach.

References

Abse DW: Brief historical overview of the concepts of war neurosis and of associated treatment methods, in Psychotherapy of the Combat Veteran. Edited by Schwartz HJ. New York, SP Medical & Scientific, 1984

American Psychiatric Association: Diagnostic and Statistical Manual of Mental Disorders, 4th Edition. Washington, DC, American Psychiatric Association, 1994

Artiss KL: Human behavior under stress—from combat to social psychiatry. Mil Med 128:1011–1015, 1963

Baker JE: Monitoring of suicidal behavior among patients in the VA health care system. Psychiatric Annals 14:272–275, 1984

Belenky GL: Psychiatric casualties: the Israeli experience. Psychiatric Annals 17:528–531, 1987

Blank AS Jr: Apocalypse terminable and interminable: Operation Outreach for Vietnam veterans. Hosp Community Psychiatry 33:913–918, 1982

Blood CG, Ganker ED: The relationship between battle intensity and disease rates among Marine Corps infantry units. Mil Med 158:340–344, 1993

Borus JF: Reentry, III: facilitating healthy readjustment in Vietnam veterans. Psychiatry 36:428–439, 1973

Borus JF: Incidence of maladjustment in Vietnam returnees. Arch Gen Psychiatry 30:554–557, 1974

Brill NQ, Kupper HI: Problems of adjustment in return to civilian life, in Neuropsychiatry in World War II, Vol I: Zone of Interior. Edited by Glass AJ, Bernucci RJ. Washington, DC, U.S. Government Printing Office, 1966, pp 721–733

Centers for Disease Control: Vietnam Experience Study: Health Status of Vietnam Veterans, Vol IV: Psychological and Neuropsychological Evaluations. Atlanta, GA, Centers for Disease Control, 1989

Crocq L, Crocq MA, Barrois C, et al: Low-intensity combat psychiatric casualties, in Psychiatry: The State of the Art, Vol 6. Edited by Pichot P, Berner P, Wolf R, et al. New York, Plenum, 1985, pp 545–550

Davidson JRT, Kudler HS, Smith R, et al: Treatment of posttraumatic stress disorder with amitriptyline and placebo. Arch Gen Psychiatry 47:259–266, 1990

Defazio VJ: Psychoanalytic psychotherapy and the Vietnam veteran, in Psychotherapy of the Combat Veteran. Edited by Schwartz HJ. New York, SP Medical & Scientific, 1984, pp 23–46

Feldman TB: Alprazolam in the treatment of posttraumatic stress disorder (letter). J Clin Psychiatry 48:216–217, 1987

Fesler FA: Valproate in combat-related post-traumatic stress disorder. J Clin Psychiatry 52:361–364, 1991

Figley CR: Symptoms of delayed combat stress among a college sample of Vietnam veterans. Mil Med 143:107–110, 1978

Frank JB, Kosten TR, Giller EL Jr, et al: A randomized clinical trial of phenelzine and imipramine for posttraumatic stress disorder. Am J Psychiatry 145:1289–1291, 1988

Garland FN: Combat stress control in the post-war theater: mental health consultation during the redeployment phase of Operation Desert Storm. Mil Med 158:334–338, 1993

Gifford RK, Marlowe DH, Wright KM, et al: Unit cohesion in Operation Desert Shield/Storm. Journal of the U.S. Army Medical Department, November/December 1992, pp 11–13

Hoiberg A: Military effectiveness of Navy men during and after Vietnam. Armed Forces & Society 6:232–246, 1980

Horowitz MJ, Solomon GF: A prediction of delayed stress response syndromes in Vietnam veterans. Journal of Social Issues 31(4):67–80, 1975

Jones FD: Lessons of war for psychiatry, in Psychiatry: The State of the Art, Vol 6. Edited by Pichot P, Berner P, Wolf R, et al. New York, Plenum, 1985, pp 515–519

Kinzie JD, Leung P: Clonidine in Cambodian patients with posttraumatic stress disorder. J Nerv Ment Dis 177:546–550, 1989

Koshes RJ, Rowe BA: Psychiatric debriefing following Operation Desert Shield/Storm. Journal of the U.S. Army Medical Department, November/December 1992, pp 14–17

Koshes RJ, Young SA, Stokes JW: Debriefing following combat, in War Psychiatry: Textbook of Military Medicine. Edited by Jones FD, Sparacino LR, Wilcox VL, et al. Washington, DC, Office of the Surgeon General, U.S. Department of the Army and the Borden Institute, 1995, pp 271–290

March JS: Fluoxetine and fluvoxamine in PTSD (letter). Am J Psychiatry 149:413, 1992

Marlowe D: The human dimension of battle and combat breakdown, in Military Psychiatry: A Comparative Perspective. Edited by Gabriel RA. New York, Greenwood Press, 1986, pp 7–24

Nagy LM, Morgan CA, Southwick SM, et al: Open prospective trial of fluoxetine for posttraumatic stress disorder. J Clin Psychopharmacol 13:107–113, 1993

Noy S: Battle intensity and the length of stay on the battlefield as determinants of the type of evacuation. Mil Med 152:601–607, 1987

Peniston EG, Kulkosky PJ: Alpha-theta brainwave neuro-feed-back for Vietnam veterans with combat-related post-traumatic stress disorder. Medical Psychotherapy 4:1–14, 1991

Pokorny AD: Suicide in war veterans: rates and methods. J Nerv Ment Dis 144:224–229, 1967

Rahe RH: Acute versus chronic psychological reactions to combat. Mil Med 153:365–372, 1988

Retzlaff R, Deatherage T: Air Force mental health consultation: a six-year retention follow-up. Mil Med 158:338–340, 1993

Rothberg JM, Koshes RJ, Shanahan J, et al: Desert Shield deployment and social problems on a U.S. Army combat support post. Mil Med 159:246–248, 1994

Scurfield RM, Blank AS Jr: A guide to obtaining a military history from Vietnam veterans, in The Trauma of War: Stress and Recovery in Viet Nam Veterans. Edited by Sonnenberg SM, Blank AS Jr, Talbott JA. Washington, DC, American Psychiatric Press, 1985, pp 263–291

Shay J: Fluoxetine reduces explosiveness and elevates mood of Vietnam combat vets with PTSD. Journal of Traumatic Stress 5:97–101, 1992

Silver JM, Sandberg DP, Hales RE: New approaches in the pharmacotherapy of posttraumatic stress disorder. J Clin Psychiatry 51:33–38, 1990

Turchan S, Holmes VF, Wasserman CS: Do tricyclic antidepressants have a protective effect in posttraumatic stress disorder? New York State Journal of Medicine 92:400–402, 1992

van der Kolk BA: Psychopharmacological issues in posttraumatic stress disorder. Hosp Community Psychiatry 34:683–692, 1983

Wolf ME, Alavi A, Mosnaim AD: Posttraumatic stress disorder in Vietnam veterans: clinical and EEG findings: possible therapeutic effects of carbamazepine. Biol Psychiatry 23:642–644, 1988

16 Psychiatric Intervention With Medical and Surgical Patients of War

Harold J. Wain, Ph.D.
John T. Jaccard, M.D.

War, disaster, illness, and injury conjure up many emotions and perceptions. The meanings of these events are predicated on one's previous experience, culture, religion, expectations, conditioning, personality style, and so forth. When confronted with these events, most individuals ask, "How will this disaster impact upon me? on my family? on my livelihood?" Some persons have experienced the trauma of war directly as a result of being injured or having some disruption in their emotional experience. The returning veteran who is injured is in this group. How to treat and foster the recovery of this group of veterans is central to the return home.

To create a treatment strategy for Operations Desert Shield/Storm veterans who had been air evacuated to a stateside hospital, we, the present authors, integrated our backgrounds and training (both of us had experienced Vietnam in different capacities). We recognized that the caregiver who is anticipating working with the repercussions of traumatic events must first plan to minimize the impact of the war trauma on the patient and ensure and facilitate appropriate medical treatment. Physicians and others responsible for evaluating and treating victims

415

of war trauma and other disaster victims must be alert to both the physiological components and the psychological aspects of injuries and disaster. In this chapter we address some of the theoretical and pragmatic concepts that we have developed over our careers and that contributed to the consultation-liaison psychiatry program at Walter Reed Army Medical Center (WRAMC) during Desert Shield/Storm. These concepts served to organize the treatment interventions for the returning Gulf War veteran in the hospital (Table 16–1).

The Experience and Metaphor of Trauma

War, injury, and other disasters threaten ego integrity and can constitute a narcissistic injury that can cause chronic medical and psychic trauma (Figley 1985; Rangell 1976; Wilkinson 1983). The soldier who is injured in war feels out of control and demoralized; his or her psychological homeostasis is disrupted. One consequence of disaster and trauma is the possibility of posttraumatic stress disorder (PTSD) (van der Kolk 1984; Williams 1980). This disorder prevents the resolution of the trauma, as dissociated material intrudes into the individual's consciousness as he or she relives events of the past trauma. The patient may experience periods of intrusive thoughts or dreams followed by periods of numbing and, eventually, social withdrawal from societal standards and involvements.

Table 16–1.   Goals of the consultation-liaison service

Support the medical treatment.

Support the medical staff.

Support the patient.

Use interventions that are syntonic with the patient's personality style.

Recognize and reinforce patient's adaptive defense mechanisms.

Maintain a flexible evaluation and treatment approach.

Meet the patient "where he or she is."

Since the Vietnam War, the significance of posttraumatic stress syndromes and the complications of trauma have become prominent in the literature. The implications of the psychological sequelae of trauma inflicted through war and during natural disasters have been well documented in the literature since World War II (Grinker and Spiegel 1945; Kardiner 1941, 1947; Glass 1969; Horowitz 1976). Although in this chapter we emphasize PTSD as a consequence of trauma, there are many other psychological sequelae that can occur.

Trauma as a concomitant of war and/or disaster is not a new concept. Kaiser (1968) described the work of Brody, who, in 1837, spoke of the sequelae of war and its impact. Trauma has also been a prominent element in psychoanalysis. It was a central theme in Freud's concept of the individual's psychodynamics (Breuer and Freud 1893–1895/1955). Freud originally advocated that trauma only occurred in certain stages of development. He later revised this perspective to suggest that a traumatic event can reoccur throughout one's life. Freud (1917 [1916–1917]/1963) described trauma as an overwhelming stimulus that was too powerful to be worked through in a normal way and as a conflict that was so overwhelming that it disrupted one's homeostasis.

From the perspective elaborated by Freud, trauma results in regressive behavior based on the individual's inability to cope with the overwhelming traumatic stimuli that one faces. Some analysts (e.g., Furst 1967) suggest that individuals facing a trauma may have to use mental mechanisms more typical of the time before formation of the ego in order to deal with the overwhelming stimuli. As a result, habitual adaptive mechanisms and defenses are no longer able to function as effectively as they had in the past (Furst 1967).

Much has been learned from the experience of those who have dealt with both psychological and medical trauma. The rapid restoration of homeostasis and the maintenance of the adaptive capacities of the individual are primary (Glass 1954). Interestingly, an analysis of Vietnam War casualties by Figley (1978) suggested that compared with previous wars, there were fewer psychiatric casualties from the Vietnam War era, at least traditional combat casualties. (The American Civil War, our bloodiest, probably had the greatest psychological impact.) Many suggest that the personnel policies that were implemented during the Vietnam War were the result of psychiatry's past experiences with posttraumatic symptoms. Thus, tours of duty were short (365 days, except for the Marines, who stayed 13 months), and R&R (rest and relaxation) was prescribed, allowing personnel to withdraw to places where personal safety was, for all practical purposes, ensured. Also, more sophisticated combat psychiatry was introduced. A policy of ensuring that soldiers would not be exposed to prolonged periods of shelling and bombardment was advocated. The principles of treating the soldiers close to their unit, of giving them the support they needed, and of relying on group and unit dynamics to facilitate cohesiveness were also present. Compared with Korea and World Wars I and II, these were revolutionary policies.

From this perspective, one wonders why, upon the return home of Vietnam War veterans, posttraumatic symptoms became so prominent. Many factors may have contributed to this overall phenomenon. Perhaps one of the most pivotal determinants was that soldiers were deployed individually and returned similarly, rather than in a unit. Each individual faced the scorn of the American public upon returning home, without the help of any unit support. The returning soldier faced life without a group to belong to.

During World War II and other wars, there had been heroic attempts at helping the individual make the adjustment to returning home. Movies of the time suggested that the returning soldiers were heroes (Wechter 1944). Wounded individuals were honored, receiving their own "red badge of courage." These supports were severely lacking during and after the Vietnam War. The soldier was scorned. America was in conflict. In lieu of being in a safe environment, the returning soldier was again embattled in a land where the enemy could be anyone. Rather than being viewed as a hero, the soldier was ostracized and isolated.

Bourne (1970) suggested that the number of psychiatric casualties in the Vietnam War were fewer than in previous wars because of the use of drugs while in combat during this era. His perception was that many soldiers medicated themselves through the use of drugs. The drugs allowed these soldiers to distance themselves from the combat and, at times, from who they were. Their critical judgment could be suspended, and they could distance themselves from the conflict they were experiencing (i.e., about whether their mission was effective or, in some cases, even justified). Many felt that only by using drugs would they be able to endure and survive the Vietnam conflict.

The fact that the Vietnam War was seen as a clandestine war changed many soldiers' perceptions and feelings. There was no clear enemy. Those who were allies during the day might be enemies at night. For many soldiers the image of Vietnam was the ambush or hidden mines. The inability of the soldier to understand the language or mode of behavior of the enemy or of some of the allies contributed to the level of frustration that many felt. This may also have contributed to the sense of helplessness that many American soldiers had in terms of fighting and identifying the enemy. Many times friends were hurt by the unseen enemy and survivor guilt developed (Lifton 1972, 1973a, 1973b). Many soldiers felt rage that later was displaced onto others. The dehumanization of the war and its actors may have resulted, in part, from the soldier's code, "Serve your country"; however, who and what one is serving is not clear. As a result, a lack of trust quickly developed in those deployed to Vietnam, because individuals did not know who was their ally and who was not. Without trust and with loneliness and isolation being common, the whole environment can become traumatic and an individual may become hostile, defenses may build up, and displacement may later occur. In this setting it makes sense that after leaving the war area, other problems may emerge (Horowitz and Solomon 1975).

In general, it appears that the experience of trauma leaves one feeling unsure of one's environment. It is a threat to self integrity. One's sense of vulnerability is heightened. People learn not to trust others, and their self-esteem decreases. Their ability to monitor themselves and maintain appropriate vigilance is compromised. Trauma thus serves as an overall narcissistic injury.

In this way, trauma can recall for the trauma victim a time of regressive functioning and a psychological return to the past. It pushes the victim's personality structure and defenses to the limit, somewhat akin to what occurs when one is undergoing a prolonged medical trauma. Being pushed to such limits may facilitate inappropriate regression. Healthy adaptation is regression in the service of the ego; the individual, though compromised, can adapt. In contrast, pathological adaptation is marked by regression to an earlier stage of development without the capacity to use adult defenses. Thus, pathological regression is not adaptive to the present situation. Latent feelings of rage, anger, and frustration may be present following the trauma. In addition, trauma may exacerbate and promote previous pathology.

Illness

In addition to understanding the experience of trauma, the consultation-liaison staff must understand the significance and meaning of illness in order to be able to respond effectively to the veteran who is injured in war. The patient with medical illness often experiences the illness as a loss of control. Restoration of control for the patient by returning the body to homeostasis is one of the goals of the physician and the patient. A variety of treatments may be required: pharmacotherapy, surgery, physical therapy, and psychotherapy and other behavioral treatments. Again, regardless of the treatment, one of the goals is to help patients regain control over themselves.

Although not a substitute for clinical competence, the establishment of a positive relationship with the patient may facilitate and expedite the regaining of homeostasis. The patient is in a vulnerable position and needs the support and guidance of a caring figure. Medical illness can tax one's adaptive functions.

Personality styles that in the past may have been effective in coping are now compromised. In turn, patients may respond in a less-than-optimal manner. Medical illness is one of the greatest stressors. The patient's response to his or her illness may interfere with developing a productive working relationship with the medical care team. Transference (and countertransference) issues may become prominent.

Illness can also be experienced as a threat to one's narcissistic integrity. The threat of possible death, or loss of a body part, may leave one feeling vulnerable, helpless, and dependent. The patient may also develop a fear of or discomfort with strangers because of his or her sense of becoming dependent upon the many unknown people around him or her. Added to these threats is the anxiety of leaving loved ones and the safety of one's home, which contributes to the feeling of dislocation and helplessness. These feelings and vulnerabilities can lead to seemingly adolescent-like or childlike conflicts with the staff. In general, regression and dependency are prominent.

The stress and anxiety of an illness may trigger the "psychological immune system" to respond with the patient's usual psychological defense mechanisms. Some defense mechanisms will facilitate adaptation and recovery, whereas others may cause more disruption. The patient uses defense mechanisms in an attempt to adapt and control anxieties. As the individual struggles to resolve the underlying conflict, defenses may be put into overdrive, resulting in further malfunctioning. The maladaptive psychological response is much like the physiological immune system's malfunctioning in an autoimmune disease. To cope with hospitalization and or chronic illness, the patient must be able to use defense mechanisms that can facilitate an effective response to illness. Regression in the service of the ego and effective denial can be appropriate responses. In contrast, pathological regression increases the patient's feelings of helplessness, dependency, and powerlessness. Pathological denial is evident in the patient's minimizing or exaggerating physical concerns or risks. Increased symptoms and pathological behavior can result.

Vietnam War Experiences

The experiences of the authors during the Vietnam War also helped form the intervention plan for the casualties of the Persian Gulf War. One of the authors was a psychologist at WRAMC during the Vietnam War era, while the other author served as an infantry officer in Vietnam. From these and other experiences, we learned that the primary goal in treating returned casualties was to ensure immediate and effective medical treatment and then to minimize the psychological effect of trauma on the patient. Individual attention to the personality structure and response style of each patient was necessary. Attempting to force all patients into any one mold was not productive and at times increased the patient's distress as well as that of the staff.

The volume of patients during the Vietnam conflict precluded ongoing individual treatment. Group interventions were most pragmatic. Most of the groups were supportive in nature and at times educational. The groups allowed the patients to recapture the feeling of belonging and to overcome the loneliness and isolation they felt. The groups also allowed the patients to deal with some of their concerns and conflicts as well as to gain a sense of direction.

Teaching the patients a means to master their conflicts and modeling stress reduction techniques were important interventions. Alertness to drug and alcohol problems was part of every evaluation. Before beginning group therapy, each patient was seen individually and debriefing principles were used, with the individual discussing war experiences and feelings of anger and frustration.

As at many hospitals, an organized psychiatry consultation-liaison service (Lipowski 1974) was not a part of the WRAMC Department of Psychiatry at the time of the Vietnam War. Outpatient psychiatry was responsible for consultation to the patients on the medical-surgical wards. Personnel from psychology, social work, and nursing were all part of the outpatient clinic.

During the Vietnam War era, we also learned that it was necessary to provide support for the health care workers who were working with war casualty patients. Working with the patient alone was not sufficient. Many of the nursing staff had served in Vietnam and had conflicts similar to those of the patients they were treating. In retrospect, many patients and staff felt alone and isolated on their return from Vietnam. This feeling was exacerbated in the Washington, D.C., area by the proximity of the many antiwar demonstrations and the feeling of alienation from the community the demonstrations caused.

It was important at WRAMC during the Vietnam War era to help the staff deal with their own frustrations and conflicts. Many of the medical staff had their own posttraumatic stress issues; others had problems handling the mutilated bodies of their patients. Other staff, returning from Vietnam, demonstrated the same lack of trust as did the soldiers. Anger and frustration were displaced to their present job from their previous assignment or their involvement with the war. Thus, preparation for the arrival of war casualties required treatment plans for the staff as well as for the patients.

The senior staff at WRAMC recognized the stress on the staff, the lack of esprit de corps, and the lack of communication. The chief nurse requested support groups for her staff. To maximize group cohesiveness, we used homogeneous groups. For example, those working in the same position (e.g., head nurses) were in one group. To gain acceptance from each group, we used the nursing supervisors' group as the model for other groups. Involvement of the senior group facilitated the junior staff's participation in their own group. At first, there was much suspiciousness, apprehension, fear, and lack of trust. The group facilitators were seen as informers for the chief nurse. Trust developed only after the promise of confidentiality was proven over time.

In general, individuals were initially reluctant to participate in the groups. Although people showed up for the groups and participated, many of them did so apparently because it was known that the chief nurse supported these groups and the participants felt an obligation to partake. Over time, however, by making the initial focus task oriented and demonstrating respect for each individual, the co-leaders came to be accepted by the group members. Empathy, listening, respect, concreteness, and pragmatism were the leading interventions (Table 16–2).

After working with the nursing supervisors' group, we worked with their assistants, then with the ward masters, and then with head nurses and nurses on the ward. In the groups, the staff focused on task-oriented problem solving and ways of enhancing their empathic communication with others. Stress reduction techniques were also taught. These ingredients became the springboard for dealing with other personal issues. However, the sanctity of the workplace was adhered to, and self-disclosure that might disrupt the working relationship was generally handled individually outside the groups. As trust and acceptance increased, the group handled more personal issues. The principles of military psychiatry were central. Goal-directed behavioral interventions, increased communication, and an alertness to the conflicts of others were core objectives. Stress reduction techniques, including relaxation training, hypnotic intervention, and cognitive reframing, were also part of our interventions.

After the successful completion of the intervention with these groups, we received increasing requests to build the esprit

Table 16–2. Goals of co-leaders of support groups for hospital staff who are working with victims of trauma

Increase esprit de corps.

Increase communication and sensitivity toward others.

Increase trust.

Debrief.

Provide support.

Educate.

Teach stress reduction techniques.

Teach cognitive reframing approaches.

de corps of other wards, of staff groups, among nurses, and so forth. (Interestingly, we noted that as the nurses who participated in these initial groups were promoted to higher ranks, reassigned, and then returned to WRAMC, they requested the groups in order to build their unit's morale.)

Patient support groups were conducted based on the goals of debriefing (Table 16–3). This approach allowed each patient to share his or her experiences, and whatever conflicts he or she felt, without value judgments. Debriefing allowed some patients to manage their stress, frustration, and anger without the additional burden of a psychiatric label. Forming an alliance with the patient, establishing a sense of trust, and facilitating the patients' connection with one another were thought to be important goals for the group leaders. The ability of the group leaders to communicate in an empathic, respectful, and concrete manner was very important and considered to be a key ingredient of a successful outcome in these work groups. Some of the other key ingredients were warmth, self-disclosure, and the ability to confront in a manner that allowed the individual to recognize the incongruities in his or her story so that he or she could grow from the confrontation. Cognitive reframing, relaxation techniques, and methods of mastering conflicts were also part of the interventions.

Table 16–3.   Goals of co-leaders of patient support groups for hospital staff

Build trust.
Provide support.
Debrief.
Establish a safe environment.
Facilitate a sense of belonging and connection.
Educate.
Increase communication skills.
Teach stress reduction techniques.
Teach cognitive reframing approaches.

Operations Desert Shield and Desert Storm

When the buildup of troops for Operation Desert Shield began, we organized our treatment plan around those elements we believed were important to delivering the psychological/psychiatric support necessary for wounded soldiers who would come to WRAMC. A high number of casualties were expected. Planning was initiated with concern and anxious expectation. We first had to ascertain which staff would be available, who would be involved, and how their training might need to be supplemented. Based on a review of our backgrounds and experiences, we decided to build a program that would maximize the experiences at WRAMC that had been helpful during the Vietnam War era as well as during other battles, natural disasters, and traumatic events. Our program needed to be sensitive to the needs of the patients and the staff treating them. Alertness to the possible use of alcohol or drugs by soldiers as a way of treating themselves was high. Knowing theoretical models and clinical approaches would be useless unless the staff applying them were supported, well trained, understood, and appreciated. We focused on the importance of group dynamics and unit cohesiveness as well as the need to make each individual recognize that he or she had played a role and had earned his or her "red badge of courage."

During the troop buildup in the fall of 1991, the directors of the mental health resources at WRAMC met in ongoing meetings to coordinate treatment approaches. The commanding general appointed the chairman of the Department of Psychiatry as the one responsible for this work group. The chairman appointed the chief of the psychiatry liaison service as the head of the task force. Members from psychiatry, child and adolescent psychiatry, psychology, social work, chaplains, nursing, and occupational therapy were on the task force. The goal of the group was to provide mental health care to all Operation Desert Shield patients coming into the medical-surgical units. The consultation-liaison service consisted of one psychiatrist, one psychologist, two psychiatric fellows, two fourth-year residents, two psychiatric nurses, one social worker whose specialty was substance abuse, one psychology intern, and one biofeedback technician. We were told we would be given additional support, and eventually staff from the reserves joined us. These additional staff consisted of two psychiatrists, two psychologists, and four psychiatric nurses (Table 16–4).

Plans were drawn up to train the new staff and refresh the regular staff in skills of debriefing and support groups, knowledge of dissociative states and posttraumatic stress, and the skills of consultation. Workshops were developed to train the staff in the important therapeutic principles of psychiatric illness and psychological responses to medical disease and the principles of casualty and staff care learned during Vietnam. In particular, we emphasized an understanding of the meaning of being a patient, the impact of war trauma, and the potential problems of treating dissociative disorders. We reviewed with the staff the anguish a patient feels when war traumas are real,

---

Table 16–4. Consultation-liaison service staff at Walter Reed Army Medical Center before, during, and after Operation Desert Storm

---

Staff before Operation Desert Storm
  1 Psychiatrist
  1 Psychologist
  2 Psychiatry fellows
  2 Psychiatry residents
  2 Psychiatric nurses
  1 Social worker
  1 Psychology intern
  1 Biofeedback technician

Staff added during and after Operation Desert Storm
  2 Reserve psychiatrists
  2 Reserve psychologists
  4 Reserve psychiatric nurses

---

alive, forceful, and recent. Potential transference and counter-transference issues were also part of the training. The staff's need to be empathic, genuine, and respectful along with the goal to develop a working relationship with the patients and the medical-surgical staff was also emphasized.

Clinically, we formed two teams, each planned to operate 10 hours with a 2-hour overlap. Daily meetings with each service (medicine, surgery, etc.) and every nursing shift were planned. During our review of patients, we would ensure that appropriate individuals were involved with the patient. We planned to make rounds with the medical and surgical staff on their patients to provide "curbside" consultation and to facilitate discussion of psychiatric care issues.

Importantly, these functions were all to be carried out in addition to the normal daily table and walk rounds that we characteristically conduct on patients referred to our service. The potential for overwhelming casualties was high, and the expectation at that time included a large number of casualties being processed through WRAMC and referred on to other hospitals, including civilian hospitals activated under the Nations Emergency Medical Preparedness plans and by the Veterans Administration.

The consultation-liaison service's table rounds would facilitate our ability to plan appropriate clinical interventions and ensure that patients would be followed. The two authors were to serve as consultants and supervisors to the teams.

A general format was instituted to ensure that each patient received a thorough evaluation (Table 16–5). Debriefing every patient was to be a major part of our initial intake. Debriefing every casualty, regardless of psychiatric status, would make the debriefing process routine and would help staff avoid turning every patient into a psychiatric casualty. At the same time, we would be able to monitor each patient, offer him or her education and support, and be available to him or her to treat more complex issues when and if appropriate.

A consult was to be sent to the consultation-liaison service on each casualty that arrived. The nurse members of the consul-

Table 16–5.   Stages of patient evaluation at Walter Reed Army Medical Center

Receive consult.

Debrief.

Support.

Initiate administration of research questionnaire.

Clinically evaluate.

Convene staffing conference.

Communicate with primary physician and ward staff.

Provide individual intervention.

Provide group intervention.

Provide continued follow-up of patient and document his or her progress.

tation-liaison team were primarily responsible for the debriefings. Another staff member would then follow up with a traditional clinical interview.

We had hoped to standardize the evaluation and, as part of the clinical interview, have everyone use the same questionnaires, as well as the Hamilton Depression Scale (Hamilton 1960) and Anxiety Index (Hamilton 1959), a new somatoform screening test, and the Hypnotic Induction Profile (H. Spiegel 1973). The latter tool was to help ascertain which patients could benefit most rapidly from hypnotic intervention. It could also be used to help understand dissociative responses in some of the patients. Headquarters was to let us know when patients would be arriving. As a part of and an adjunct to the debriefing process, questionnaires were provided and developed based on a collaborative research project with the Department of Psychiatry of the Uniformed Services University of the Health Sciences (USUHS) and the Department of Military Psychiatry at Walter Reed Army Institute of Research (WRAIR). Research meetings and plans with members of the USUHS and WRAIR faculties were held weekly during the fall of 1991. The research project was an attempt to understand and define what variables may have contributed to the soldiers' injuries, response, and recovery. It was planned that by obtaining detailed information on these patients, we would enhance our lessons learned and learn more about handling trauma victims of both military and civilian disasters.

A major goal of our intervention plan was to decrease the posttraumatic stress symptoms associated with medical treatment and/or prevent medical intervention from precipitating psychological symptoms such as the recall of traumatic war events (e.g., the recovery room being perceived as an abusive situation similar to when the soldier was a captive of the Iraqis).

For dissociative responses and disorders, we taught the staff interventions to increase the patient's sense of control and to teach the patient techniques of effectively distancing himself or herself from the trauma while eventually integrating the dissociative material. The staff learned about potential abreactive material associated with war trauma and ways to desensitize themselves to the potential intensity of the affect of the patient.

A major component of PTSD is the effect of dissociative material on the patient's stream of consciousness. The ultimate intent was to have the patient able to integrate his or her dissociative behavior into normal consciousness. The patient's feeling of being overwhelmed needed to be decreased, and the patient needed support and education.

The treatment goal was to teach the patient to interpret his or her trauma in a more constructive manner and to prevent the experience from becoming overwhelming. In accord with this plan, the treatment plan included the following (Table 16–6):

1. To provide or help the patient find a safe environment.
2. To console the patient.
3. To help the patient confront and recognize what had occurred.
4. To help the patient consolidate into his or her life narrative what occurred so that the problem becomes manageable.
5. To help the patient cognitively reframe his or her traumatic experience in the context of his or her experience and the experience of the unit to which he or she belongs.

Table 16–6.   Treatment goals for trauma patients

Establish a safe environment.
Establish a supportive environment.
Console patient.
Condense information.
Assist patient in cognitively reframing events.
Support patient in confronting and recognizing problems.
Teach patient control and mastery techniques.
Integrate dissociative component into consciousness (when
   appropriate).

6. To teach the patient that he or she can be in control.
7. To help the patient move toward integrating the experience
   without being overwhelmed.

Hypnotic and cognitive techniques were at the forefront of
treatment of dissociative disorders (D. Spiegel 1985; D. Spiegel
et al. 1988; Wain 1993). Beginning, advanced, and refresher
courses in these techniques were developed for the staff.

The staff were taught how to lead support groups similar to
those that were successfully employed during the Vietnam War
era. The staff were also taught the value of task-oriented support
groups. Again, the roles of empathy, genuineness, respect, and
goal-directed behavior were highlighted.

The War

When the conflict began, many of our plans were ready to be
initiated. Because of the medical evacuation system, however,
the first patient did not actually arrive until the conflict was
nearly over. Initially, we focused on working with the nursing
staff, decreasing their stress and anticipation of the war. The essence of the famous World War II quotation—that the greatest
fear is fear itself—was a good descriptor of this stage of war at
the hospital. One must remember the huge number of casualties that were expected and the possibilities of chemical and

biological warfare casualties to recapture the fear and worries of being overwhelmed that were felt by the hospital staff.

The wards responded to a general offer made by the consultation-liaison service. Support groups, with a consultation-liaison nurse and one other staff person or resident as co-leaders, were begun. Fears of the staff included fear of dealing with casualties and fear of touching injured bodies. Staff members' anxiety over whether they themselves might be sent overseas was common.

Other concerns that were commonly felt by staff throughout the hospital included how to integrate the newly arrived reservists into ward and staff functioning. Some of the permanent staff had concerns that the reservists were usurpers who would replace them when they left for Saudi Arabia. Such concerns created many conflicts for the endogenous staff. Though the reservists were supposed to have training that was equal to that of the active component, many of the reservists' skills were not on par with those of their counterparts. Finding ways of integrating the reservists into the normal schedule became difficult for some departments. Many of the active-duty medical staff also perceived the reservists as separate. The reservists' concern about being called up and not being used effectively was also present. Many of the physicians and nurses called up for active duty were frustrated and angry that their lives were disrupted, especially when there was a paucity of work to be done. Even after the war was over and many of the troops were on their way home, reservists were not given specific dates of discharge. This uncertainty led to many conflicts for this group, because they wanted to return to their own vocational endeavors. The consultation-liaison staff provided support and brief intervention for these anxieties of the hospital staff. The continued search for appropriate activities for the reservists was also necessary. Frequently, consultation with supervisors of the reservists was necessary to help mediate the frustrations.

Over the course of the Persian Gulf conflict, the psychiatry consultation service saw approximately 175 injured service-members whose injuries were part of Operation Desert Storm and occurred during the troop buildup. The injuries included all of those expected as a result of war trauma: head injuries, shrapnel wounds, amputations, gunshot wounds, burns, and so forth. Several of the injuries were accidentally caused by faulty equipment, carelessness, and so forth. These injuries resulting from accidental causes were initially seen by the hospital staff as "different," and the staff felt more conflict associated with these patients' care. After intervention from our service, the staff were more accepting of these patients.

Most of the injured soldiers had no psychiatric disorder. It was important to reassure the patients of this. Some patients, when they received a psychiatric consult, were concerned that perhaps they also were experiencing a psychiatric problem that they were not aware of. Others felt that the consult was an invalidation of their medical condition. Reassurance about these issues was usually effective. A brief supportive statement that our intervention was routine was very welcomed.

Many administrators and lay staff had developed a belief that all returnees might have PTSD. This was not the case, and it was very important to change this perspective to avoid making psychiatric patients out of nonpatients. This task became a major focus of our service as part of the organizational consultation efforts.

Many of the soldiers who did not have their unit's support appeared to have more difficulty in their recuperation. When a unit determined that a soldier was responsible for his or her own injury or had been singled out for special rewards even though he or she was, the group thought, responsible for his or her injuries, the soldier often did not get much support from his or her group. Our goal was to provide the support that they needed to tolerate their medical treatment.

Case Example 1

The patient, a male reservist in his 30s, was referred by Orthopedics after he had been evacuated to WRAMC. He had suffered several fractures and fragment wounds. During his deployment and hospitalization, he had received recognition by nonmilitary leaders. This special status contributed to his unit members' rejecting him and withdrawing support. This caused much frustration and anguish for the patient. We offered support, which helped him use effective defenses needed to cope with the medical treatment he was receiving. An attempt at reconciliation between the unit and the patient was eventually undertaken. Unit support continued to be necessary to facilitate the recuperative process.

Several patients were depressed on their return and they received the appropriate psychotherapy and pharmacology. Fewer than 10% of the patients we saw had PTSD symptoms. Individuals received treatment in the hospital and follow-up as outpatients.

Case Example 2

The patient, a female in her 30s, had been injured in a SCUD attack. She initially seemed to cope well. She showed no psychiatric symptoms and complied well with treatments. As she became less concerned about physical problems, significant insomnia, anxiety, depression, and dependent behavior emerged. Despite participation in individual supportive psychotherapy and group therapy, the patient developed the full syndrome of PTSD. As other unit members left the hospital, she felt more lonely and developed a pathological dependence on her therapist and the medical center. Through extensive insight-oriented therapy, she was able to recall a past episode of rape and significant verbal abuse as a child. These appeared to have increased her sense of vulnerability to the trauma in the Persian Gulf. Her symptoms of insomnia responded to trazodone. Her PTSD was treated with continued individual and group therapy.

Transferring patients' psychiatric care to regional centers upon discharge was sometimes problematic. At times, patients' difficulties in obtaining follow-up mental health appointments prompted the patient's new primary care provider to obtain telephone consultation with the WRAMC C/L service, rather than to work with local resources as had been arranged.

Case Example 3

The patient, a female in her 20s, had incurred a hand injury during a missile attack. Before the war she had been a reservist. She was moved from her unit to another to fill a space. She appeared to have not developed a sense of cohesion with this new unit before deployment. She had a history of good performance and was known as a task-oriented individual. Although her injury did not have a significant effect on her Army job, it was a serious impediment to her civilian job. She had posttraumatic stress symptoms, but these resolved with support. Individual and group support helped her to regain her previous goal-directed orientation. She sought reasonable compensation for her injury and was given supporting statements to transfer duties at her civilian job to a position for which the sequelae of her injury were not a major impediment. Phone contact with her and her husband after discharge provided support for the couple to reestablish their marital relationship and the patient's ability to function once again as an effective mother.

Some patients had atypical pain responses following some minor injuries. At times, their pain presentation provided entrée into the medical-psychiatric system. Some patients presented with somatic complaints without any anatomical correlate. These symptoms were eventually identified and treated as conversion disorders. A few patients, when relieved of the conversion symptom, developed PTSD symptoms.

Case Example 4

The patient, an active-duty male in his 20s, was referred for evaluation of his syncopal episodes. Neurology and cardiology workups were within normal limits. After his psychiatric evaluation, a diagnosis of conversion disorder was made. After participating in insight-oriented psychotherapy and learning hypnotic techniques, the patient was able to control his syncopal episodes. After the resolution of his physical symptoms, nightmares of a family who had been burned during the war in the Persian Gulf and whom he had seen afterward became intensified. Upon further exploration with hypnotic techniques, he was able to describe his feelings for his close friend who was killed during an attack. Through the treatment, he was able to regain control over the terror he experienced and was returned to duty with psychiatric follow-up at his duty station. [This patient's case demonstrated Lifton's (1973a) concept of "survivor guilt."]

As expected, another small group of individuals who were admitted to the hospital at the time of the war distorted where they had received their injuries. For example, some of these patients would suggest that they were injured in the desert, when, in fact, further evaluation revealed that they had never left the States. Two patients in particular were eventually transferred to our inpatient unit with factitious disorders. Other soldiers complained about the air evacuation system and the loneliness and fear they felt while waiting for transportation. The lack of disclosure as to where they were going also created discomfort for them.

Many patients described the inconvenience caused their families by their deployment and injury. At times, the massive television coverage that occurred helped bring the war closer to home for the families, but it also created a constant reminder of the danger that loved ones faced. The importance of family support to the injured soldier was a prominent ingredient in an effective treatment approach for many of the patients (Gruter 1981). Patients frequently received support from family members either over the telephone or in person.

Another group of patients who came to our attention were veterans and others who had experienced traumas in the past but had not received any psychiatric intervention. The conflict and the bombings brought back past traumas for individuals who had been in bunkers during World War II, who had been involved in Korea or Vietnam, or who had experienced other traumatic events. Some others reexperienced the traumas of being body handlers that they had experienced during previous conflicts. The traumas were experienced as if they had happened yesterday.

Case Example 5

The patient, a woman in her 50s, was referred by Orthopedics for low back pain following a motor vehicle accident. Her referral coincided with the beginning of the bombing in Desert Storm. Percocet had been prescribed to help decrease her pain. Problems with insomnia had also recently developed. After evaluation, she was diagnosed as having psychological factors affecting her physical condition. She was also noted to be a good hypnotic subject. Hypnotic techniques were used to control her pain, and she was able to decrease her use of Percocet. However, the insomnia remained, and she reported she was having nightmares and reoccurring intrusive thoughts. The thoughts were related to her childhood experience in Europe, when she had been confined in a shelter during World War II. The nightmares had been absent for more than 40 years. By learning and using cognitive reframing and hypnotic techniques, the patient gained control over her nightmares. The recent threat of her accident and Desert Storm had become so overwhelming that a regression to her childhood trauma had occurred [see Lidz 1946].

We also interviewed the returning Army prisoners of war (POWs). (For discussion of principles of interviewing returning POWs, see Segal 1974 and Stenger 1985). They were separated from the other service POWs, and each had his or her own experience. The concepts of unit cohesiveness and group support could not be offered the POWs because of the politics of the situation and the transiency of their stay at WRAMC. The one patient who stayed for a period of time was able to receive the same treatment approach that the other wounded soldiers received.

After the Conflict

Our service continues to see individuals who served in Operations Desert Shield\Storm and who may now be manifesting some latent responses. Several have recently had gastrointestinal problems without any specific or concrete diagnoses after several repeated evaluations. These patients are evaluated and treated with the same sensitivity that we utilized during the actual conflict period. Some of the postconflict patients did not feel themselves to be a part of the team that was victorious and had the public support. We became their advocates and continue to follow them. Patients continue to present with atypical symptoms, and some suggest that it was their involvement in Desert Shield/Storm that may have caused their problem. We continue to evaluate whether the present conditions are related to or are a result of these individuals' having endured any psychic trauma because of their participation in Desert Storm.

Case Example 6

The patient, a male in his late 20s, was referred by Surgery because of ongoing problems with pain and depression. The patient had had surgery for a nerve entrapment. After group therapy, hypnosis, and brief insight-oriented treatment, he was able to gain control over the pain and his depression decreased. However, he continued to complain about vague abdominal distress and fatigue. The patient's complaints were similar to those of others who returned from the Gulf and who complained of abdominal distress even after all gastrointestinal workups had been negative. He had also been refractory to previous antidepressants. This patient continues to be followed by Outpatient Psychiatry.

Conclusions

We saw many patients during and after the conflict. The capacity to be flexible in evaluations and treatment approaches has been a priceless attribute in working with these patients. Attempting to fit patients into a rigid treatment program or diagnostic formulation does not recognize the variety of health, illness, and coping strategies of the injured soldier and may sabotage any ongoing relationship. Being able to recognize and use a biopsychosocial approach (Engel 1977; Wain 1992) with these patients facilitates the understanding of the presenting problem and advances treatment. Although our entire treatment program, fortunately, could not be tested because of the rapid resolution of the conflict, our tenets were based on our past experiences and encompassed both theoretical and pragmatic approaches. Trauma can create an experience of being overwhelmed that leads to the loss of homeostasis and failure of previously adaptive coping mechanisms (Solnit and Krist 1967). The goals of our interventions were consistent with this adaptational viewpoint. Our plan was to help the patient find a safe place where support could be obtained and the patient could learn to master, rather than be overwhelmed by, stimuli. A variety of supportive, psychotherapeutic, and/or pharmacological techniques are useful in the restoration of this homeostasis.

The principles of consultation-liaison psychiatry (see, e.g., Lipowski 1974; Wain 1979) in may ways parallel the principles of military psychiatry (see, e.g., Glass 1969; Jones and Johnson 1975). Both sets of principles advocate consultation, rapid intervention, prevention, and return to previous level of functioning outside the hospital as soon as possible. The soldier who has been injured in battle, if possible, returns to the front after psychiatric symptoms related to the trauma are ameliorated; analogously, the patient who was originally admitted to the hospital for medical illness continues to receive more medical treatment in the hospital after the psychiatric symptoms associated with the illness are treated. The principles of consultation-liaison psychiatry were effectively implemented in our program. Our backgrounds and experiences in understanding the meaning of being a patient and the impact of trauma from both a theoretical and clinical level were invaluable in our being able to establish a mental health treatment delivery system.

References

Bourne PG: Men, Stress and Vietnam. Boston, MA, Little, Brown, 1970

Breuer J, Freud S: Studies on hysteria (1893–1895), in Standard Edition of the Complete Psychological Works of Sigmund Freud, Vol 2. Translated and edited by Strachey J. London, Hogarth Press, 1955, pp 1–319

Engel G: The need for a new medical model: a challenge for biomedicine. Science 196:129–136, 1977

Figley CR (ed): Stress Disorders Among Vietnam Veterans: Theory, Research, and Treatment. New York, Brunner/Mazel, 1978

Figley CR: Psychosocial adjustment among Vietnam veterans: an overview of the research, in Trauma and Its Wake: The Study of Treatment of Post-Traumatic Stress Disorder, Vol 1. Edited by Figley CR. New York, Brunner/Mazel, 1985, pp 57–70

Freud S: Introductory lectures on psycho-analysis, Part III (1917[1916–1917]), in Standard Edition of the Complete Psychological Works of Sigmund Freud, Vol 16. Translated and edited by Strachey J. London, Hogarth Press, 1963, pp 241–476

Furst S: Psychic Trauma. New York, Basic Books, 1967

Glass AJ: Psychotherapy in the combat zone. Am J Psychiatry 110:725–731, 1954

Glass AJ: Introduction, in The Psychology and Physiology of Stress. Edited by Bourne PG. New York, Academic Press, 1969, pp 14–30

Grinker RR, Spiegel JP: Men Under Stress. Philadelphia, PA, Blakiston, 1945

Gruter L: Families of a post-Vietnam stress syndrome. The Family Therapist 2:16–17, 1981

Hamilton M: The assessment of anxiety states by rating. Br J Med Psychol 32:50–55, 1959

Hamilton M: A rating scale for depression. J Neurol Neurosurg Psychiatry 23:56–62, 1960

Horowitz MJ: Stress Response Syndromes. New York, Jason Aronson, 1976

Horowitz MJ, Solomon GF: A prediction of delayed stress response syndromes in Vietnam veterans. Journal of Social Issues 31(4):67–80, 1975

Jones FD, Johnson AW: Medical psychiatric treatment policy and practice in Vietnam. Journal of Social Issues 31(4):49–65, 1975

Kaiser L: The Traumatic Neurosis. Philadelphia, PA, JB Lippincott, 1968

Kardiner A: The Traumatic Neuroses of War. New York, P Hoeber, 1941

Kardiner A: War Stress and Neurotic Illness. New York, P Hoeber, 1947

Lidz T: Nightmares and combat neuroses. Psychiatry 9:37–39, 1946

Lifton RJ: Questions of guilt. Partisan Review 39:514–530, 1972

Lifton RJ: Home From the War. New York, Simon & Schuster, 1973a

Lifton RJ: The sense of immortality: on death and the continuity of life. Am J Psychoanal 33:3–15, 1973b

Lipowski ZJ: Consultation liaison psychiatry. Am J Psychiatry 131:623–650, 1974

Rangell L: Discussion of the Buffalo Creek Disaster: the course of psychic trauma. Am J Psychiatry 133:313–316, 1976

Segal J: Long-term psychological and physical effects of the POW experience: a review of the literature (NHRC Publ No 74-2). San Diego, CA, Naval Health Research Center, 1974

Solnit AJ, Krist M: Trauma and infantile experiences, in Psychic Trauma. Edited by Furst S. New York, Basic Books, 1967, pp 175–220

Spiegel D: Vietnam grief work using hypnosis. Am J Clin Hypn 24:33–40, 1985

Spiegel D, Hunt TI, Dondershine H: Dissociation and hypnotizability in post-traumatic stress disorder. Am J Psychiatry 145:310–308, 1988

Spiegel H: Manual for Hypnotic Induction Profile: Eye-Roll Levitation Method, Revised Edition. New York, Soni Medica, 1973

Stenger CA: American prisoners of war in World War I, World War II, Korea, and Vietnam. Paper presented at the Veterans Administration and Military Health Services Conference on Follow-Up Care for Returning Prisoners of War, San Diego, CA, March 1985

van der Kolk BA: Post-Traumatic Stress Disorder: Psychological and Biological Sequelae. Washington, DC, American Psychiatric Press, 1984

Wain HJ: Hypnosis in consultation liaison service. Psychosomatics 20:670–687, 1979

Wain HJ: Pain as biopsychosocial entity and its significance for treatment with hypnosis. Psychiatric Medicine 10:101–118, 1992

Wain HJ: Medical hypnosis, in Medical-Psychiatric Practice, Vol 2. Edited by Stoudemire A, Fogel BS. Washington, DC, American Psychiatric Press, 1993, pp 39–66

Wechter D: When Johnny Comes Marching Home. Cambridge, MA, Houghton-Mifflin, 1944

Wilkinson CB: Aftermath of a disaster: the collapse of the Hyatt Regency Hotel skywalks. Am J Psychiatry 140:1134–1139, 1983

Williams T: Post-Traumatic Stress Disorder of the Vietnam Veteran. Cincinnati, OH, Disabled American Veterans, 1980

Robert J. Ursano, M.D.
James R. Rundell, M.D.
M. Richard Fragala, M.D.
Susan G. Larson, M.D.
John T. Jaccard, M.D.
Harold J. Wain, Ph.D.
George T. Brandt, M.D.
Brucinda L. Beach, Lic.S.W.–C.

Nearly all wars result in prisoners. Prisoners of war (POWs) usually experience the most extreme traumas of war. In addition, they often have complicated reentrys into their home country. The greater their trauma, the more likely that psychiatric illness will result (Ursano et al. 1987; Wheatley and Ursano 1982). The Persian Gulf War was no different from other wars in this regard. The study of coping during captivity, as well as of psychological health and pathology following repatriation, has implications for psychiatric planning for future wars and for the treatment of other stressor-related psychiatric illnesses. In this chapter we present the initial evaluations of the Persian Gulf War POWs and briefly review the literature on the psychiatric effects of the POW experience. The prison experience and the experience of repatriation and reintegration into the family are discussed.

Psychiatric Assessment of the Persian Gulf War Prisoners of War

The Persian Gulf War resulted in 21 American POWs: five Army, eight Air Force, three Navy, and five Marine Corps. Nearly all were fliers; two were women. Before the repatriation, extensive consultation occurred to consider the plans for the POWs' recovery, medical evaluation, reunion with families, and return home. As in all POW returns, the pressure to return the POWs home rapidly was great. Medical data, however, support a more gradual reintroduction and "depressurization" process, including medical assessment, provision of information on the changes in the family and the world while the POW was in captivity, and then reunion in a protected environment with limited media intrusion.

Both captivity and reunion with the family were recognized as stressful for the POW. The POWs of Operation Desert Storm were taken for their initial evaluation and reentry to the hospital ship USNS *Mercy*. There they received initial medical and psychiatric assessment and informal debriefings. They were then flown to Andrews Air Force Base in Washington, D.C., where they were reunited with their families and taken to one of the three military medical centers in the Washington area (Walter Reed Army Medical Center [WRAMC], National Naval Medical Center, and Malcolm Grow USAF Medical Center) for further medical evaluation. Usually they stayed there for several days before their first "overnight" outside the hospital. Orientations were held for the families, and time was arranged for the POWs to get reacquainted with their families while in the hospital, where mental health support staff were available.

The Persian Gulf War POWs had been held captive for 7 to 48 days (median = 37 days; mean = 33). Weight loss ranged from 0 to 30 pounds (median = 20 pounds; mean = 17 pounds). Roughly half of the POWs sustained significant injuries either when they were shot down or as part of the torture and maltreatment that they received. Of the 21 POWs, two received a psychiatric diagnosis on repatriation. One was diagnosed with PTSD and one with adjustment disorder with mixed emotional features. Because there was concern about overdiagnosis and the effects of labeling, it was important also to examine prominent psychiatric symptoms and interpersonal problems noted during the evaluation. In addition to the POWs who received the psychiatric diagnoses, two others were diagnosed as having a life circumstance problem, two were noted to have an exaggerated startle reaction without other features of PTSD, and one was noted to be socially aloof, although it could not be determined to what extent this was new or a characteristic aspect of the individual's personality style. (On reevaluation 6 months later, both the startle reaction and the social isolation had greatly diminished.) Thus, in this group, approximately 10% had a psychiatric diagnosis; when all psychiatric "issues" or symptoms are considered, this percentage increases to approximately 33%. These numbers are similar to those reported in Vietnam War–era U.S. Air Force POW fliers immediately after their repatriation (Ursano 1985; Ursano et al. 1981).

Case Example 1

This male flier was shot down in sight of his wingman and hoped that his squadron mates had seen him eject. He received a broken arm on ejection. He was very concerned about being shot coming down in his parachute and felt somewhat relieved when he landed on the ground. He evaded capture for several hours but eventually was located by a passing group of soldiers. He was placed in tight cuffs and his arms tied behind his back. At the first interrogation site he was repeatedly beaten about the head and had his broken arm probed by a stick as the captors asked about the plans for the next air attack. After several days, he finally reached a more permanent cell. Here he could often hear and see Allied bombings. He was terrified that his prison would be hit by a bomb and he would be entombed. During captivity he felt "edgy" and would pace his cell hundreds of times per day. It was extremely cold at night, and food was limited. He was interrogated several times while in prison. He was at times taken outside for a mock execution and believed his captors planned to eventually kill him. He reported fantasies of being at home and of his favorite fast food restaurant. When other POWs were placed in nearby cells, he felt some relief. When the war was over and his captors came to take him to the Red Cross exchange, he thought they were planning to execute him. Only when he saw the Red Cross uniforms did he believe that he was really going home.

The capture of two military women highlighted one of the major concerns about sending women into battle: what would happen to female POWs? Major Rhonda Cornum, a flight surgeon who was captured after her helicopter was shot down, has related her experiences in the war (Cornum 1992). The horror of helplessness in the face of a comrade's torture is eloquently described in the following passage:

Then the guards came for Troy [a fellow POW] and marched him into another room down the hall. After a few moments, I heard Iraqi voices yelling in English from the room, shouting questions about what we were doing in Iraq. I imagined Troy in the room surrounded by Iraqi soldiers, but he said nothing. Then came the sound of a loud slap as someone hit him across the face. They asked another question, and when Troy didn't answer, they slapped him hard. Again and again, shouted questions; silence as Troy refused to speak; and loud, stinging slaps. Shouting. Silence. Whap, the sound of a hand across Troy's face. I felt terrible, helpless, I remembered being molested on the truck, and how Troy had felt so frustrated because he couldn't protect me. Now I was the one who was unable to protect him. I had been helpless from the moment we were captured because of my injuries, but it was far worse for me to feel helpless for someone else, for someone I cared about. (Cornum 1992, p. 113)

As a mother and wife, Major Cornum's story also addresses the impact of these roles on her and her family.

In the remainder of this chapter we explore the immediate and long-term consequences of captivity. Special attention is given to the American experience following other wars of this century. Areas of special importance in understanding the Gulf War POW experiences are highlighted.

Captivity

There is no one POW experience. For example, the average duration of POW imprisonment during the Vietnam War was substantially longer than during World War II and the Korean War. Many POWs were held captive in Vietnam for 6 to 7 years. In contrast, the captivity of the Persian Gulf War POWs lasted days (range 7–48 days). The severity of captivity conditions also varies in each war. The World War II Pacific theater POW camps were much worse than the European theater prisons (Beebe 1975; Dent et al. 1989). During the Vietnam War, the POW experience was much more severe before 1969 than after that date. That year was a turning point of the war and the beginning of the Vietnamese recognition that POWs could be politically important. In the Gulf War some of the POWs experienced torture and many feared death from bombings by the Allies themselves.

It is important to remember that repatriated POWs are always a subset of those who were lost, captured, and imprisoned. They are the survivors. We know nothing about those that never return.

The types of stressors experienced by POWs depend on the cultural and socioeconomic status of the captors, the geography and climate of the country, endemic diseases, the circumstances of capture (aircrew ejection, large-group surrender, etc.), the political climate, and the degree of resistance offered by the POW (Ursano and Rundell 1990). The degree of stress caused by these experiences depends on the physical conditions, degree of maltreatment, interpersonal issues during captivity, and the individual's appraisal of events (Biderman 1967). The role of culture itself as a stressor is frequently overlooked (Biderman 1967). Exposure to a country with limited resources, different rules of interpersonal and group relations, and different day-to-day personal and work habits can be stressful, regardless of any intent to deprive or demean a captured soldier. For the Persian Gulf POW, the Iraqi culture included vastly different attitudes toward women and toward anyone who was thought to be Israeli or Jewish.

Ursano and his group (1987) reviewed debriefing reports and medical questionnaires completed by repatriated Vietnam War POWs immediately after release in order to describe and quantify the stress factors of the Vietnam War–era POW experience. One section of the medical questionnaire included questions on the methods used by the North Vietnamese to control the prisoner's behavior. Each question was answered on a four-point scale that ranged from "never" to "very often." Debriefing reports were coded for frequency and type of maltreatments. With a factor-analytic technique, seven stress factors were identified: 1) psychological maltreatment, 2) physical torture and maltreatment, 3) solitary confinement, 4) interrogation, 5) threats and denials of privileges, 6) high-resister status (i.e., resisted interrogation/interaction extremely), and 7) duration of maltreatment.

A neurasthenic appearance in POWs after prolonged captivity was described by Greenson in World War II POWs and by Strassman in Korean War POWs (Greenson 1949; Strassman et al. 1956; see also Eitinger 1961). Both noted an apathy syndrome that was felt to be adaptive in the POW environment. Withdrawal and detachment increased the chances of survival. Energy was conserved, and the POW was less likely to stand out and challenge the captors, eliciting threats and torture.

Ursano and colleagues (1986) found, based on Minnesota Multiphasic Personality Inventory (MMPI) measures, that withdrawal and detachment were related to successful coping only in the high but submaximum stress Vietnam War POW group (i.e., those captured after 1969). In the maximum stress group, withdrawal and apathy were also present but were not predictive of successful coping. In this maximum stress POW group, denial, repression, and suspiciousness were associated with better coping. This finding suggests that cognitive coping strategies may be important in maximum stress settings after withdrawal from the environment has been attempted. With the passage of time, withdrawal and neurasthenia may be less helpful and other strategies such as fantasizing and pondering family concerns more useful (Deaton 1975).

At the time of capture, POWs must gain quick emotional control, deal with fears of death, and attend to the tasks necessary for survival. Expectations of rescue fade quickly after removal from the capture site; usually the prisoner is bound and/or blindfolded. A sense of disbelief may result from the rapid sequence of events and the radical change in roles from combatant to captive. The POW is forced to adapt to less— a state of chronic deprivation and anxious expectation. Feelings of longing for freedom, wishes for sympathy, dissociation, and fantasizing about home or retaliation are common. Hypervigilance, alertness, and orientation to details such as the jingle of keys or voices outside one's cell are adaptive mechanisms to decrease surprise and increase anticipation and preparation for the unexpected. Exploitative interrogations, confessions, isolation, boredom, demoralization about the uncertainty of the situation, and the need to make decisions regarding resistance and compliance are parts of the day-to-day experience. All of these were reported by the POWs of Operation Desert Storm. The hypervigilant state can be replaced by apathy, dysphoria, and withdrawal if captivity continues long enough. Although such a condition was commonly reported in Vietnam War, Korean War, and World War II POWs, the short duration of the Persian Gulf War made this level of withdrawal less characteristic. When imprisoned for long periods, POWs often engage in self-developed physical fitness programs, group communication, resistance, humor, creativity through projects and fantasies (e.g., learning a language, collaboration, fantasizing about the future, planning escape or sabotage), and helping other POWs.

Adaptation to and Coping With Captivity

The POW experience is often terrifying and inhuman, and it is always filled with the unexpected (Chodoff 1976; Richlin 1977) (Table 17–1). Biological stressors can be extreme and vary with both the geographic location and the demeanor of the captors. Physiological stress and emotional duress were both significantly higher in POWs held captive in the Pacific theater during World War II than in POWs held in the European theater. Maltreatment is directly related to the extent to which an enemy country sees the POW as politically valuable. In Vietnam, after 1969, conditions improved and torture and maltreatment of the POWs decreased. This change corresponded to the period during which it became clear to North Vietnam that the POWs could be an important political tool.

Survival during the POW experience is most related to the degree of injury at the time of capture and the availability of food, shelter, and medical care. For example, 4% of Canadian POWs in World War II died in European prison camps and 27% in the much worse Pacific prisons (Weisaeth 1989). Ursano and colleagues

Table 17–1. Captivity stressors

Physical	Psychological
Crowding	Boredom
Diarrhea	Close, long-term interpersonal contact
Epidemic diseases	Confinement
Exhaustion	Danger
Forced labor	Family separation
Infectious organisms	Fear/terror
Injuries	Guilt
Medical experimentation	Humiliation
Nutritional deprivation	Isolation
Sleeplessness	Threats
Torture	Unpredictability
Weather extremes	
Wounds	

(1986) found no relationship between resistance stance, "marginal coping" during captivity, or feeling benefited from the POW experience after return, and postrepatriation psychopathology.

Coping with the POW experience includes the use of cognitive mechanisms and interpersonal/social, behavioral, and fantasy coping strategies (Table 17–2). One author's experience with many of the 12,000 surviving World War II Pacific theater POWs of the Japanese led him to conclude that there were numerous attributes that allowed these 12,000 men to survive (18,000 did not survive) (Nardini 1952). These attributes included strong motivation for life, good general intelligence, good constitution, emotional insensitivity or well-controlled and well-balanced sensitivity, preserved sense of humor, strong sense of obligation to others, controlled fantasy life, courage, successful resistance, opportunism, military experience, and luck.

The POW's personality also affects adaptation and coping. In the crew of the USS *Pueblo*, captured and held by North Korea in 1968, immaturity, passive-dependency, and obsessive-compulsiveness were associated with poor adjustment (Spaulding and Ford 1972). Ford and Spaulding (1973) examined crew members of the *Pueblo* just after their release. Men who did well during captivity often had personalities described as "healthy" or "schizoid." They used a wide variety of ego defenses, particularly faith, reality testing, denial, rationalization, and humor. Men who handled the stress poorly were frequently diagnosed as being passive-dependent and were more limited in the number of ego defenses they used.

Schizoid behavior and introversion have been reported to be more adaptive than obsessive-compulsive, passive-dependent, or immature behaviors (Ford and Spaulding 1973; Spaulding and Ford 1972). Passive-dependency has been singled out as a particularly maladaptive response (Ford and Spaulding 1973; Spaulding and Ford 1972). Induction of dependency is advantageous to camp leaders in imposing their will (Bettelheim 1958). The psychological state of the POW during captivity has been described as "dependency, debility, and dread," termed "DDD" (Farber and Harlow 1957). Identification of adaptive personality characteristics requires further study. Personality resiliency and the ability to tolerate passivity do appear to be positively related to optimal adaptation (Singer 1981; Ursano 1979, 1985).

Jones (1980) reviewed six books written by former POWs who had been held in North Vietnamese prison camps. He iden-

Table 17–2. Coping strategies of prisoners of war

Cognitive	Interpersonal/Social
Caring for another	Collaboration
Feeling closer to God	Well-controlled sensitivity with captors
Focusing on the good	Resistance
Loyalty to country/family/ POW group	Withdrawal
Motivation for life	Studying guards' habits and using the knowledge to gain favor
Survival for some purpose	Maintaining military structure
Rationalization	Buddy system
Denial	Chain of command
Obsessional thinking	Code of conduct
Intellectualization	Group activities
Humor	Group affiliation
Flexibility	Military experience
Will to live	Peer pressure
Realistic expectations	
Introversion	**Fantasy**
Passive-dependence	Dissociation
Psychological regression	Fantasies of retaliation
Acceptance of fate	Fatalism
Communication	Hope
Control of panic	Idealized expectations of postrelease life
Discipline	"Talking to family"
Maintaining self-respect	
Behavioral	
Physical fitness	
Rituals	
Self-development activities	
Repetitive behaviors	
Communication	

tified coping strategies that sustained the POWs during imprisonment. Each man had a personal and strongly held standard of behavior. Ideals that were commonly reported as sustaining were 1) loyalty to country (e.g., remembering their heritage, focusing on their patriotic duty to resist), 2) idealization of their family (e.g., hoping to return with a feeling of having been worthy of them), and 3) alliance with fellow prisoners (e.g., communications, mutual support, cooperative resistance).

Maintaining military bearing is also reported to be an important adaptive behavior (Coker 1974). During the Vietnam War, identification with military ideals unified POWs in spirit and in their determination. The chain of command formalized and solidified the prisoner society in the camps. The Military Code of Conduct, which was modified after the Vietnam War, reportedly provided important guidelines for the POWs.

Probably the single most important adaptive behavior in all POW situations is communication. During the Vietnam War, a tap code was developed using a 5×5 arrangement of the alphabet (the letter k was omitted). The row and column of a letter could then be communicated. Ingenious mechanisms were used to spread messages. Coughing, sweeping, and tapping were all important means of using the code.

Additionally, the ability to express one's rage in hidden forms—the now historic picture of the *Pueblo* crew demonstrating a common American gesture of contempt—often provides a release from pent-up rage and hostility. There is a fine line, however, between appropriate resistance and provocative resistance (e.g., resistance that unnecessarily increases torture and maltreatment). Such POWs with poor coping skills who resist provocatively feel they could never comply, even to trivial requests. These POWs risk bringing torture on themselves and their comrades.

Coping with solitary confinement is often necessary and was so for the Persian Gulf War POWs. Singer (1979) reviewed journalistic accounts written by former Vietnam War–era POWs who had spent a great deal of time in solitary confinement. Several mental phenomena were prominent: 1) a propensity to review one's life with remorse and guilt, 2) recall of the past in vivid detail, 3) recall of unused academic or intellectual training, 4) extraordinarily vivid dreams with prolonged recall upon awakening, 5) intense, vivid, long-enduring fantasies (sometimes lasting days), and 6) a splitting of attention and awareness.

The firmer a POW's resistance stance, the more time he or she may spend in isolation as captors try to limit the "spread" of resistance behavior. In Vietnam, the longer the POW's duration of isolation, the greater was the POW's risk of psychiatric illness (Hunter et al. 1976). Cause-and-effect relationships, however, are unclear. Resistant, higher-ranking, and older POWs spend more time in solitary confinement and are tortured more often because of their leadership and resistance activities. However, it may also be true that individuals whose personality allows them to survive prolonged solitary confinement are more likely to maintain persistent resistance.

It is difficult to separate out the unique contributions of any one stressor to the development of psychopathology in POWs. High social isolation correlates with greater captivity stress in general. Ursano and colleagues (1987) and Hunter (1978) both reported greater rates of psychopathology among those POWs who spent the greatest time in solitary confinement. Hunter examined 100 former Vietnam War POWs and concluded that no definitive statement could be made as to any specific psychiatric disorders resulting from social isolation. However, she did find that former POWs from Vietnam who had experienced prolonged periods of isolation had significantly more guilt, ambivalence, suggestibility, superego development, and need for achievement than other former POWs (Hunter 1975, 1976, 1987).

Resistance and Collaboration

Resistance is a coping strategy that at times is required because of military necessity. For most POWs, especially pilots, militarily important information is only of concern during the first few hours or days of captivity. During this time most POWs are concerned that they not disclose information that will hurt their fellow soldiers and fliers. After this time, issues of resistance are more related to captor demands for subservience, compliance, or political statements. In Vietnam War and Korean War POWs, high resistance was seen more often among older POWs who had been held captive longer; this group also experienced more solitary confinement and harsher treatment (Hunter et al. 1976; Segal 1956).

In the Persian Gulf War, prisoners who were thought to be Jewish were especially harshly treated. In future regional and ethnic wars, the contribution of ethnic hatred to maltreatment of POWs may be particularly high.

The Persian Gulf War was also the first time that United States female servicemembers were held prisoner. In the prison camp, being female does not protect one from, and may attract, maltreatment and degradation.

Ursano and colleagues (1986) identified high resisters in the pre-1969 (highest maltreatment) group of Vietnam U.S. Air Force POWs. The high resisters were older, were more senior in rank, were pilots, and had spent more days as a prisoner. The authors found that, based on MMPI data, the high resisters showed greater energy, were more outgoing and extroverted, and showed less repression, constraint, and denial. In addition, the high resisters were more likely to experience conflict with authority and to be more independent and less socially conforming. In general, therefore, the high resister tended to be independent, energetic, less likely to bind his energy through cognitive mechanisms, and less attached to the group. These findings are in agreement with those from the Korean War (Schein et al. 1957; Singer and Schein 1958).

The high resister may at times provoke mistreatment. For example, in Vietnam, POWs who resisted the Oriental custom of bowing were severely punished. In general, these individuals had difficulty adjusting to the need to be passive and compliant. Their rigidity sometimes made life more dangerous for their fellow prisoners as well. This was not a major issue during the Persian Gulf War because the number of POWs held together was limited and the duration of captivity was relatively short.

Schein (1956) examined 759 POWs shortly after repatriation from Korean prison camps. He compared men who 1) collaborated, 2) actively resisted, and 3) took a neutral course (i.e., were neither collaborators nor extreme resisters). (A discussion of what constitutes collaboration and of other related issues is presented below.) Both resisters and collaborators had significantly longer internments, had been in service longer, were older, and were more intelligent. Additionally, they showed more psychopathic deviance (Pd scale of the MMPI). Resisters and collaborators, however, did not differ significantly from one another. No differences among the groups were found in rank, civilian occupation, religion, location of home community, or number of parents present in the home.

Singer and Schein (1958), using projective psychological testing, studied collaboration and resistance after the Korean conflict. They reported the counterintuitive finding that resisters and collaborators were more alike than different in most personality dimensions. Both showed less capacity to remain uninvolved with the environment. The authors suggested that what distinguished resisters and collaborators was not individual personality variables but rather which group they chose to attach to.

Collaboration (and resistance) comprises a continuum of behaviors and is not an all-or-none phenomenon. POWs collaborate in varying degrees. Most commit trivial acts such as signing peace petitions. A small number may engage in more persistent behaviors such as writing, signing, and soliciting signatures for peace petitions, delivering anti-American lectures to fellow prisoners, or aiding in indoctrination programs (Schein et al. 1957). Those POWs who collaborate with the enemy do so in part to eliminate the threat of mistreatment and to receive the benefits of preferential treatment.

The concept of collaboration has limited utility except in extreme cases. Importantly, collaboration is in many ways "in the eyes of the beholder." During the Persian Gulf War, the media, supported by U.S. government announcements, rapidly clarified that POWs might say things that their captors had forced them to say and that these statements should not be taken as an indicator of a bad soldier but rather of the bad enemy. This management of the meaning of captivity was very helpful for the returning POWs and also for undermining the usefulness of torture-induced statements, thus aiding in protecting the POWs during captivity.

In Vietnam, all POWs were "broken." For most, this was a profoundly guilt-inducing experience. As a result of the recognition of every individual's breaking point, new strategies to resist interrogation were based on repetitive fallback positions and on giving minor, nonsignificant information when resistance was no longer possible. Part of the importance of the communication network and of the military organization in the POW camp was their ability to provide relief from guilt through knowledge that others had broken. The communication fostered the development of specific guidelines for the POW on how and when to resist.

Medical and Psychiatric Illness After Captivity

The first follow-ups of World War II POWs, by Cohen and Cooper (1954), found significantly greater mortality in Pacific theater POWs primarily from accidents and tuberculosis. No excess mortality was seen in the European group. Gastrointestinal disorders, psychological problems, ophthalmic changes, cardiac disorders, and the effects of malnutrition and tuberculosis were also noted. Similar increased mortality rates were reported in Australian Pacific theater POWs (Dent et al. 1989). A follow-up study by Nefzger (1959) of World War II and Korean War POWs showed that the early excess mortality was at that time decreasing in the Pacific theater group. However, Korean conflict POWs continued to show excess mortality.

In all of the follow-up studies of World War II POWs, the psychiatric signs and symptoms remained among the most persistent postliberation findings for both the Pacific theater and

European theater groups. Psychiatric responses to the POW experience include a number of disorders as well as less well defined personality changes (Rundell et al. 1989; Ursano 1981), as
discussed below.

Posttraumatic Stress Disorder

The diagnosis of posttraumatic stress disorder (PTSD) and accompanying intrusive and avoidant symptoms is well documented in former POWs from several theaters of war up to
50 years after release (Atkinson et al. 1984; Kluznik et al. 1986;
Laufer et al. 1985; Page 1992). In one study, 67% to 85% of surviving former World War II POWs were found to have met the
criteria for PTSD at some time since repatriation (Kluznik et al.
1986). The sample, however, may have been biased because the
subjects were solicited by mail and, therefore, their psychiatric
status may not be representative of former POWs who did not
respond to the mailing or former World War II POWs at large.
However, the results suggested that PTSD was common in this
group of POWs. White (1983) found that 85% of a group of
POWs from Japanese camps had suffered at least moderately severe PTSD. Japanese POW camp survivors have consistently
been reported to have PTSD symptoms more frequently than
other POW groups, and the symptoms have been more severe
(Page 1992; Speed et al. 1989). Speed and colleagues (1989)
found that the strongest predictors of PTSD were the proportion of body weight lost and the degree of torture. In perhaps
the best-designed follow-up, Page (1992) found that high rates
of PTSD persisted 50 years postrepatriation, particularly in Pacific theater POWs, when compared with a control group.

The MMPI has been used both clinically and for research on
former POWs. In a 1986 study comparing World War II POWs of
the Pacific theater with those of the European theater, the highest scale elevations were found in Pacific theater POWs on scales
hysteria (Hs), depression (D), hypochondriasis (Hy), psychas-
thenia (Pt), and schizophrenia (Sc) (Wheatley 1981). Both
groups had scale scores that were clearly distinguishable from

those of a well-chosen non-POW control group. There have been attempts to develop an MMPI subscale for PTSD, one that could be applied to POWs. This scale has been used for Vietnam War and World War II veterans. In one study it showed no difference in rates of PTSD among Japanese versus European POW veterans, although PTSD was diagnosed clinically more often in POWs from the Pacific theater (Query et al. 1986).

Adjustment Disorder

In a study of repatriated U.S. Air Force Vietnam War POWs, Ursano and colleagues (1981) found that adjustment disorders and marital/occupational problems occurred in 17.2% to 18.2% of the sample at repatriation and in 9.2% to 15.8% at 5-year follow-up. These were the most common psychiatric diagnoses. Hall and Malone (1976) closely followed six former POWs and their families for 3 years following their return from North Vietnam and found the greatest cognitive, social, work, emotional, and family difficulties during the first 2 years after return. These problems, in general, eventually resolved, and no major psychiatric illness occurred in any of these men.

Depression

Paykel's review of the literature in 1978 revealed that the presence of traumatic events increases subsequent lifetime risk for depression twofold and for suicide sixfold. Some studies suggest that the prevalence of depression may decline after the first few years following a traumatic event (Green et al. 1983). The prevalence of major depression in Pacific theater POWs remained higher than in a non-POW control group even 40 years after their release (Breslau and Davis 1986; Page et al. 1991). Studies of MMPI results in repatriated POWs reveal elevated depression scales (Klonoff et al. 1976a). Page and colleagues (1991), using a large national sample of World War II POWs (European and Pacific theaters), Korean War–era POWs, and non-POW comparison groups, found elevated depressive

symptomatology on the Center for Epidemiologic Studies–
Depression Scale five decades after repatriation. POWs who
were younger, who were less well educated, or who had received harsher treatment were more likely to report depression
(Page 1992).

Psychoactive Substance Use Disorders

Alcohol abuse appears to be more common in former POWs
than in demographically related groups (Beebe 1975; Cohen
and Cooper 1954). Studies that control for demographic, socioeconomic, and precaptivity psychiatric history, however, are
few. There are morbidity data and other evidence to suggest
that alcohol abuse is problematic in many former POWs and
should be carefully considered during medical and psychiatric
examinations. Kluznik and colleagues (1986) reported that 40
years after World War II, a postwar diagnosis of alcoholism was
present in 50 of 188 POWs from the Pacific theater who volunteered for medical and psychiatric examination. Of that group,
67% also had a history of PTSD; therefore, the alcoholism may
have been primary or secondary. Alcohol use can be a form of
self-medication (Birkheimer et al. 1985; Helzer et al. 1976) and
may suppress nightmares, diminish autonomic hyperactivity,
and foster more pleasant, nontraumatic fantasies (van der Kolk
1983). Alcohol excess frequently accompanies PTSD (in 41%–
80% of cases) (Breslau and Davis 1986; Sierles et al. 1983).

Anxiety Disorders

Before DSM-III (American Psychiatric Association 1980) and the
diagnostic category of PTSD, the most frequent diagnoses given
to psychiatrically ill former POWs were anxiety reaction, anxiety
state, and anxiety neurosis (Beebe 1975). Anxiety disorders
other than PTSD remain frequent in former World War II POWs
(Engdahl et al. 1991; Kluznik et al. 1986). In one study, 143 of
the 188 former POWs in the sample met the criteria for an anxiety disorder other than PTSD (Engdahl et al. 1991). Generalized

anxiety disorder was most frequently reported (103 of 188) in this group; there was a large degree of overlap with PTSD. In some studies, up to 95% of patients with PTSD met the criteria for at least one other DSM-III-R (American Psychiatric Association 1987) anxiety disorder (Query et al. 1986). Panic attacks and panic disorder have been reported in some studies to be frequent in persons exposed to trauma; however, the frequent occurrence of these attacks and this disorder in this population has not been universally found (Horowitz et al. 1980).

Personality Change

Personality changes resulting from the POW experience need not be pathological. Sledge and colleagues (1980) identified a distinct group of Vietnam POWs who felt they had benefited from their experience. In fact, those individuals who experienced the greatest stress during captivity were most likely to believe they gained psychologically from the experience. These POWs often report that their POW experience led to their redirecting their goals and priorities and moving toward psychological health (Ursano 1981; Van Putten and Yager 1984; Yager et al. 1984). Personality shifts may also be a part of the findings of particular MMPI profiles related to particular POW stressors (Sutker et al. 1991). Nonpathological personality change appears to be dependent on the nature and severity of the experience as well as the preexisting personality. As mentioned before, in World War II and Korean War POWs, a profound apathy syndrome was noticed (Greenson 1949; Strassman et al. 1956). In contrast, Vietnam War–era POWs studied by Ursano (1981) showed movement toward character rigidity, decreased interpersonal relatedness, heightened drive to achieve, and the experience of time pressure. Such changes are neither pathological nor beneficial in and of themselves. Sutker and colleagues (Sutker and Allain 1991; Sutker et al. 1990, 1991), in their study of Korean War POWs, found suspiciousness, apprehension, confusion, isolation, detachment, and hostility. Eberly and associates (1991) found persistent elevated negative affect in World

War II POWs 40 years postcaptivity, which the authors interpreted as an adaptational change to accommodate the captivity.

Ursano (1981) has discussed possible reasons for the different personality shifts in the POW context based on intrapsychic and adaptational shifts. Two types of change—apathy and rigidity/high energy (drive)/interpersonal distance—serve adaptive functions in a similar way. Which type of change develops may depend on the circumstances of imprisonment, such as the amount of physical torture, chronicity (Vietnam War–era POWs experienced longer imprisonments than did Korean POWs), level of deprivation, opportunity for active and passive expressions of aggression, and the types of threats experienced by the POW. These variables are in turn dependent upon the type of war, the socioeconomic conditions of the enemy, the political climate, and the culture of the captors.

From the intrapsychic perspective, conflict within the ego and within the superego can be seen as the result of heightened aggressive drives bound up during the captivity situation. Such drives are then discharged through the demanding punitive elements of the superego and/or the ambitious, hard-driving pursuit of goals and ideals embodied in the ego-ideal. The apathy syndrome seen in Korean War POWs may be partially explained as the result of the punitive superego's victory in this intra-superego conflict. In contrast, heightened aggressive drives can also be discharged in the service of the ego-ideal. In this case, determination, character rigidity, and interpersonal distance may be the result.

Predictors of Psychiatric Distress

Severity of Captivity

The severity of captivity is a result of both the duration of imprisonment and the degree of maltreatment and deprivation. The length of captivity alone is not a good measure of captivity severity. Pacific theater World War II POWs were exposed to significantly greater physical, environmental, and psychological stress than were European theater POWs. Only 40% of 30,000 POWs held by the Japanese survived the war (Nardini 1952). Disease and malnutrition were common (Beebe 1975; Nefzger 1959). Mortality, largely because of tuberculosis, was also higher just after repatriation in the Pacific theater group (Nefzger 1959). Accidents and liver cirrhosis remained significantly more common for many years. Beebe (1975) found a higher number of medical and psychiatric symptoms, greater disability, and more maladjustments in Pacific theater POWs than in European theater POWs. The former group continues to have higher hospital admission and illness rates. Higher rates of liver cirrhosis suggest a higher frequency of several hepatic diseases and alcoholism in the Pacific theater group (Klonoff et al. 1976b; Nefzger 1959). Page (1992) found continued high rates of psychiatric and medical morbidity in the Pacific theater group into the 1980s.

In Vietnam, POWs captured before 1969 had both longer captivity and substantially more deprivation, torture, and maltreatment than those captured in 1969 or after (Hunter 1978; Ursano et al. 1987). Ursano, Wheatley, and colleagues (Ursano et al. 1981; Wheatley and Ursano 1982) demonstrated a greater degree of psychiatric readjustment problems in repatriated U.S. Air Force POWs captured before 1969 than in those captured after 1969. Pre-1969 captives had a higher frequency of psychiatric diagnoses and abnormal MMPI scales. The overall MMPI profiles of the pre-1969 captives also deviated farther from the norm than did those of the post-1969 captives on the initial MMPI. The pre-1969 captives showed increased repression, a higher level of denial, greater suspicion, and more distrust. The post-1969 captives' second MMPI profile 5 years later was lower and looked more like the norm profiles established for air crew members; in contrast, the profiles of the pre-1969 captives had remained essentially unchanged.

Similar findings were reported by Benson and colleagues (J. W. Benson, D. L. Bizzell, P. F. O'Connel, unpublished manuscript, Naval Aerospace Medical Institute, 1979) in U.S. Navy and Army Vietnam War–era POWs. The authors divided POWs into four groups: 1) officers captured before 1969, 2) enlisted personnel captured before 1969, 3) officers captured after 1969, and 4) enlisted personnel captured after 1969. These groups were examined for differences in immediate and delayed posttraumatic psychopathology. The enlisted personnel exhibited significantly more postrepatriation psychopathology than did the commissioned personnel. Significant improvement was noted between the first- and the fifth-year follow-up only in officers captured after 1969. These results indicate that after controlling for officer-enlisted status, greater captivity stress, as measured by the duration and intensity of captivity, was associated with more negative psychiatric outcome in both groups and greater persistence of problems in the enlisted group. In another study, it was found that Vietnam War–era POWs who had been exposed to more prolonged isolation had higher rates of psychiatric disorder than did those who experienced more limited solitary confinement (van der Kolk 1984). This finding further indicates the importance of the severity of the captivity experience as a major predictor of psychiatric disturbance.

Several studies by Ursano have addressed the question of trauma as a cause of psychiatric illness. Ursano (1979, 1981) examined six repatriated Vietnam War POWs who had, coincidentally, been evaluated psychiatrically before their captivity. Using the precaptivity psychiatric data, he found that preexisting pathology or identifiable predispositions to psychiatric illness were neither necessary nor sufficient for the development of psychiatric illness after repatriation. Further data on the question of predisposition are provided by studies of captured Vietnam War–era U.S. Air Force fliers (Ursano 1981). Fliers are selected for their health and are screened for psychiatric illness before they are considered for flight school. Pre-1969 captives were demographically comparable to post-1969 captives and, in fact, might have been expected to show less illness because they were slightly older and more mature. It was found that, in fact, they had more psychiatric illness. Because this was found to correlate with the greater degree of stress experienced by this group, the data from this study further support the role of stress over predisposition in the development of psychopathology after severe trauma. Together, these data support the view that psychiatric illness may develop after the POW experience in the absence of preexisting illness or identifiable predispositions. Most PTSD theories have underestimated the role of adult personality growth and resiliency and overestimated the role of preexisting personality in determining the outcome of the POW experience (Singer 1981; Wheatley and Ursano 1982).

Readjustment

Repatriation and Reintegration

Most former POWs readjust well over time. However, it should be remembered that repatriation and reintegration are not synonymous with "recovery" in the sense of resolution of psychiatric signs and symptoms. The repatriated POW emerges from what is likely to be a prolonged period of emotional blunting, monotony, apathy, withdrawal, and deprivation, into a rapidly paced series of medical evaluations, family reunions, and public relations activities. The brief period of euphoria upon release is quickly replaced by a period of overstimulation. There may be an attempt to make up for things denied during captivity by activities such as overeating. Initially, released POWs are frequently compliant with the requests of the military and their physicians. But over several days to weeks, they usually begin to take a more active and independent stance (Newman 1944; Rahe and Genender 1983). There is a tendency for the repatriated POW to minimize potential psychological and psychosocial problems caused by his or her captivity.

In addition, most repatriated POWs, including those from the Persian Gulf War, have had little experience dealing with the media. The media is a substantial stressor that can have lifelong effects on the repatriated POW if, for example, a statement that the individual, later, wishes he or she "had never said" is broadcast around the world. It is very important both to shield the POW and his or her family from early intrusive media coverage and to offer training in the management of media requests. Based on lessons from the Vietnam War era and from hostage situations, such protection and training were routinely provided for those who might become POWs in the Persian Gulf War. Reminding POWs and their families that it is perfectly acceptable for them to say "No" can be a very important intervention.

After the tumultuous postrelease period, gradual readjustment and reintegration may continue throughout life. Reintegration occurs gradually, and the process is subject to reorganization with changing life circumstances.

Organizers in Adult Personality Development

Personality does not stop developing at the end of childhood or even adolescence (Colarusso and Nemiroff 1987). The fact that most neurophysiological and neuroanatomic development is finished before adulthood may provide some protection from radical departures in adult personality, but it is clear from animal studies that changes in neurophysiology and even neuroanatomy do occur during adulthood (Maclean 1986).

René Spitz (1965) discussed "organizers" of psychological development—that is, important experiences that structure feelings, thoughts, and behaviors of the present and thus influence future development and psychology. The oedipal phase and childhood traumatic events are two examples of such organizers. These organizing events are evident in psychotherapy when the therapist and patient identify organizing principles of past experience that are used to guide current behavior. It is useful to conceptualize adult traumas, such as being a POW, as a potential independent organizer of adult personality development (Ursano 1981). The trauma of POW experiences may induce psychopathology or personality growth or may resonate with themes already present from earlier organizing events or periods. Later, the symbolic recall of the POW events is the result of a current event activating this organizer. The recall serves as a symbolic vehicle to express the current conflicts and anxieties.

Family Issues

The effect of imprisonment and release on family members and the family system itself can be profound and enduring or minor and transient. One study of POW wives indicated that during the period of captivity, psychological and psychophysiological symptoms were common (Hall and Simmons 1973). Psychological issues included desertion, ambiguity of role, repressed anger, sexuality, censure, and social isolation. Separation anxiety, role distortion, and sleep disorders were common in the children. Male children were significantly more affected than female children.

McCubbin et al. (1975) interviewed families of 215 Army, Navy, and Marine Corps POWs approximately 1 year before the POWs' release. The families' normal patterns of coping with husband/father absence had been disrupted by the unprecedented and indeterminate length of captivity. The social acceptance, stability, and sense of continuity that are taken for granted in the intact family were lacking or severely taxed in the POW family.

Parental preoccupation and overprotectiveness are potential reasons for the occasional presence of higher degrees of overt psychopathology in children of persons exposed to trauma than in the original victim (Hunter 1988; Menninger 1959). In a study of the offspring of psychiatrically hospitalized concentration camp survivors, 70% had psychopathology severe enough to require hospitalization between the ages of 17 and 22, and 90%, before the age of 25 (Menninger 1959). A clinical sample of midteenage children of concentration camp survivors had more behavioral disturbances and less adequate coping behavior than a clinical control group (Axelrod et al. 1980). A study comparing current effects of long-term father absence during and after the Vietnam War (missing in action) and temporary absence (POW) revealed significant differences in the children. Both nervous symptoms and community relations were more impaired in the group of children whose fathers were missing in action (Dahl et al. 1977).

All of these studies suffer major methodological flaws but should serve as reminders of the potential impact of major life events as they are mediated through parents to children. Adolescents may be particularly sensitive to family tension. Their distress is often visible and can be disruptive for both the family and the community.

POW families who present for treatment are frequently in crisis. The resumption of precaptivity roles may be difficult for a mother who has successfully exercised both parental roles for several years, when the returned father has psychiatric symptoms and/or medical problems, and the children have become accustomed to having their mother to themselves. Adolescent males may be particularly vulnerable in such a setting. Treatment focuses on preserving family unity, enhancing the family system, and encouraging individual member development (McCubbin and Patterson 1982; McCubbin et al. 1982).

Conclusions

Prisoners of war suffer the most severe stressors of war. Repatriated POWs are a select group of survivors who have been able to adapt to captivity and maintain morale, hope, and health for months to years. The ability to communicate with other POWs during captivity is the most important coping strategy. The creative ways in which communication has been established and the content of what is communicated are the basis of many POW coping strategies.

Repatriation itself is a stressful event. The POW is faced with the outside world's view of his or her behavior and situation. He or she may face a changed world and certainly has much information to catch up on. Some events cannot be "caught up": the birth of a child, the death of a parent, a spouse who decided to seek a divorce, or the operational experience necessary to remain current in a profession. These are real losses to which the returning POW must accommodate. Most former POWs adjust well. For some, the experience serves as a personality-organizing focus that results in movement toward emotional growth and maturity; for others, no psychological change is evident; for still others, psychopathology develops. When psychiatric illness occurs following repatriation, the severity of the trauma and the status of social supports play a large role. Most psychopathology decreases with time, though recurrent, episodic, delayed, and chronic presentations of most of the reported posttraumatic psychiatric disorders are reported.

The stresses on the families of the POW are manifold, both during captivity and after repatriation. The family and the military community are critical elements in the recovery and readaptation of the POW.

Posttraumatic stress disorder, depression, and psychoactive substance use disorders are all seen in returned POWs. The coexistence of two or more of these is the rule. Determining which of the coexisting disorders is primary or secondary is usually less important than identifying and treating each. At repatriation, the Persian Gulf War POWs showed rates of psychiatric distress similar to those for Vietnam War–era POWs. The short duration of the Persian Gulf War and the relative health of fliers, who constituted the majority of POWs in that war, indicate that a good recovery could be expected.

References

American Psychiatric Association: Diagnostic and Statistical Manual of Mental Disorders, 3rd Edition. Washington, DC, American Psychiatric Association, 1980

American Psychiatric Association: Diagnostic and Statistical Manual of Mental Disorders, 3rd Edition, Revised. Washington, DC, American Psychiatric Association, 1987

Atkinson RM, Sparr LF, Sheff AG, et al: Diagnosis of posttraumatic stress disorder in Vietnam veterans: preliminary findings. Am J Psychiatry 141:694–696, 1984

Axelrod S, Schnipper OL, Rau JH: Hospitalized offspring of Holocaust survivors. Bull Menninger Clin 44:1–14, 1980

Beebe GW: Follow-up studies of World War II and Korean War prisoners, II: morbidity, disability, and maladjustments. Am J Epidemiol 101:400–422, 1975

Bettelheim B: Individuals and mass behavior in extreme situations, in Readings in Social Psychology. Edited by Maccoby EE, Newcomb TM, Hartley EL. New York, Henry Holt, 1958, pp 300–310

Biderman AD: Life and death in extreme captivity situations, in Psychological Stress: Issues in Research. Edited by Appley MH, Trumbull R. New York, Appleton-Century-Crofts, 1967, pp 242–277

Birkheimer LJ, Devane CL, Muniz CE: Posttraumatic stress disorder: characteristics and pharmacological response in the veteran population. Compr Psychiatry 26:304–310, 1985

Breslau N, Davis GC: Chronic stress and major depression. Arch Gen Psychiatry 43:309–314, 1986

Chodoff P: The German concentration camp as a psychological stress, in Human Adaptation: Coping With Life Crises. Edited by Moos RH. Lexington, MA, DC Heath, 1976, pp 337–349

Cohen BM, Cooper MZ: A Follow-Up Study of World War II Prisoners of War (Veterans Administration Medical Monograph). Washington, DC, U.S. Government Printing Office, 1954

Coker GT: Prisoners of war. U.S. Naval Institute Proceedings 100:41–48, 1974

Colarusso CA, Nemiroff RA: Clinical applications of adult developmental theory. Am J Psychiatry 144:1263–1270, 1987

Cornum R [as told to Copeland P]: She Went to War: The Rhonda Cornum Story. Novato, CA, Presidio Press, 1992

Dahl BB, McCubbin HI, Ross KL: Second generational effects of war-induced separations: comparing the adjustment of children in reunited and non-reunited families. Mil Med 141:146–151, 1977

Deaton JE: Coping strategies of Vietnam POWs in solitary confinement. Unpublished master's thesis, San Diego State University, San Diego, CA, 1975

Dent OF, Richardson B, Wilson S, et al: Postwar mortality among Australian World War II prisoners of the Japanese. Med J Aust 150:378–382, 1989

Eberly RE, Harkness AR, Engdahl BE: An adaptational view of trauma response as illustrated by the prisoner of war experience. Journal of Traumatic Stress 4:363–380, 1991

Eitinger L: Pathology of the concentration camp syndrome: preliminary report. Arch Gen Psychiatry 5:371–379, 1961

Engdahl BE, Page WF, Miller TW: Age, education, maltreatment, and social support as predictors of chronic depression in former prisoners of war. Soc Psychiatry Psychiatr Epidemiol 26:63–67, 1991

Farber IK, Harlow HF: Brainwashing, conditioning, and DDD (debility, dependency, and dread). Sociometry 20:272–285, 1957

Ford CV, Spaulding RC: The Pueblo incident: a comparison of factors related to coping with extreme stress. Arch Gen Psychiatry 29:340–343, 1973

Green BL, Grace MC, Lindy JD, et al: Levels of functional impairment following a civilian disaster: the Beverly Hills Supper Club fire. J Consult Clin Psychol 51:573–580, 1983

Greenson RR: The psychology of apathy. Psychoanal Q 18:290–302, 1949

Hall RCW, Malone PT: Psychiatric effects of prolonged Asian captivity: a two-year follow-up. Am J Psychiatry 133:786–790, 1976

Hall RCW, Simmons WC: The POW wife: a psychiatric appraisal. Arch Gen Psychiatry 29:690–694, 1973

Helzer JE, Robins LN, Davis DH: Depressive disorders in Vietnam returnees. J Nerv Ment Dis 163:177–185, 1976

Horowitz MJ, Wilner N, Kaltreider N, et al: Signs and symptoms of posttraumatic stress disorder. Arch Gen Psychiatry 37:85–92, 1980

Hunter EJ: Isolation as a Feature of the POW Experience: A Comparison of Men With Prolonged and Limited Solitary Confinement. San Diego, CA, Center for Prisoner of War Studies, Naval Health Research Center, 1975

Hunter EJ: The prisoner of war: coping with the stress of isolation, in Human Adaptation: Coping With Life Crises. Edited by Moos RH. Lexington, MA, DC Heath, 1976, pp 322–331

Hunter EJ: The Vietnam POW veteran: immediate and long-term effects of captivity, in Stress Disorders Among Vietnam Veterans. Edited by Figley CR. New York, Brunner/Mazel, 1978, pp 188–206

Hunter EJ: The psychological effects of being a prisoner of war: Vietnam veterans and their families, in Human Adaptation to Extreme Stress: From the Holocaust to Vietnam. Edited by Wilson J, Harel Z, Kahana B. New York, Plenum, 1987, pp 100–116

Hunter EJ: Long-term effects of parental wartime captivity on children: children of POW and MIA servicemen. Journal of Contemporary Psychology 18:312–328, 1988

Hunter EJ, Phelan JD, Mowery EC: Resistance posture and the Vietnam prisoner of war. Journal of Political and Military Sociology 4:295–308, 1976

Jones DR: What the POWs write about themselves. Aviat Space Environ Med 51:615–617, 1980

Klonoff H, Clark C, Horgan J, et al: The MMPI profile of prisoners of war. J Clin Psychol 32:623–627, 1976a

Klonoff H, McDougall G, Clark C, et al: The neuropsychological, psychiatric, and physical effects of prolonged and severe stress: 30 years later. J Nerv Ment Dis 163:246–253, 1976b

Kluznik JC, Speed N, VanValkenburg C, et al: Forty-year follow-up of United States prisoners of war. Am J Psychiatry 143:1443–1446, 1986

Laufer RS, Brett E, Gallops MS: Symptom patterns associated with posttraumatic stress disorder among Vietnam veterans exposed to war trauma. Am J Psychiatry 142:1304–1311, 1985

Maclean PD: Culminating developments in the evolution of the limbic system, in The Limbic System: Functional Organization and Clinical Disorders. Edited by Doane BK, Livingston KE. New York, Raven, 1986, pp 1–28

McCubbin HI, Patterson JM: Family adaptation to crises, in Family Stress, Coping, and Social Support. Edited by McCubbin HI, Cauble AE, Patterson JM. Springfield, IL, Charles C Thomas, 1982, pp 26–47

McCubbin HI, Hunter EJ, Dahl BB: Residuals of war: families of prisoners of war and servicemen missing in action. Journal of Social Issues 31:95–109, 1975

McCubbin HI, Cauble AE, Patterson JM (eds): Family Stress, Coping, and Social Support. Springfield, IL, Charles C Thomas, 1982

Menninger K: The academic lecture: hope. Am J Psychiatry 94:481–491, 1959

Nardini JE: Survival factors in American prisoners of war of the Japanese. Am J Psychiatry 92:241–248, 1952

Nefzger MD: Follow-up studies of World War II and Korean War prisoners. Am J Epidemiol 91:123–138, 1959

Newman FH: The prisoner of war mentality: its effect after repatriation. BMJ 1:8–10, 1944

Page WF: The Health of Former Prisoners of War. Washington, DC, National Academy Press, 1992

Page WF, Engdahl BE, Eberly RE: Prevalence and correlates of depressive symptoms among former prisoners of war. J Nerv Ment Dis 179:670–677, 1991

Paykel E: Contribution of life events to causation of psychiatric illness. Psychol Med 8:245–254, 1978

Query WT, Megran J, McDonald G: Applying posttraumatic stress disorder MMPI subscale to World War II POW veterans. J Clin Psychol 42:315–317, 1986

Rahe RH, Genender E: Adaptation to and recovery from captivity stress. Mil Med 148:577–585, 1983

Richlin M: Positive and negative residuals of prolonged stress, in Prolonged Separation: The Prisoner of War and His Family. Edited by Hunter EJ. San Diego, CA, Center for Prisoner of War Studies, Naval Health Research Center, 1977

Rundell JR, Ursano RJ, Holloway HC, et al: Psychiatric responses to trauma. Hosp Community Psychiatry 40:68–74, 1989

Schein EH: The Chinese indoctrination program for prisoners of war: a study of attempted "brainwashing." Psychiatry 19:149–172, 1956

Schein EH, Hill WF, Williams HL, et al: Distinguishing characteristics of collaborators and resisters among American prisoners of war. Journal of Abnormal and Social Psychology 55:197–201, 1957

Segal J: Factors related to the collaboration and resistance behavior of U.S. Army POWs in Korea (Department of the Army Technical Report 33). Washington, DC, U.S. Department of the Army, 1956

Sierles FS, Chen JJ, McFarland RE, et al: Posttraumatic stress disorder and concurrent psychiatric illness: a preliminary report. Am J Psychiatry 140:1177–1179, 1983

Singer MT: The Consequences of War Imprisonment Symposium, in Proceedings of the Twenty-Sixth Annual Conference of Air Force Behavioral Scientists. Edited by Levy RA. Brooks Air Force Base, TX, USAF School of Aerospace Medical Division (AFSC), 1979, pp 66–76

Singer MT: Vietnam prisoners of war, stress, and personality resiliency. Am J Psychiatry 138:345–346, 1981

Singer MT, Schein E: Projective test responses of prisoners of war following repatriation. Psychiatry 21:375–385, 1958

Sledge WH, Boydstun JA, Rabe AJ: Self-concept changes related to war captivity. Arch Gen Psychiatry 37:430–443, 1980

Spaulding RC, Ford CV: The Pueblo incident: psychological reactions to the stresses of imprisonment and repatriation. Am J Psychiatry 129:17–26, 1972

Speed N, Engdahl BE, Schwartz J, et al: Posttraumatic stress disorder as a consequence of the prisoner of war experience. J Nerv Ment Dis 177:147–153, 1989

Spitz R: The First Year of Life: Normal and Deviant Object Relations. New York, International Universities Press, 1965

Strassman AD, Thaler MB, Schein EH: A prisoner of war syndrome: apathy as a reaction to severe stress. Am J Psychiatry 112:998–1003, 1956

Sutker PB, Allain AN: MMPI profiles of veterans of World War II and Korea: comparisons of former POWs and combat survivors. Psychol Rep 68(1):279–284, 1991

Sutker PB, Winstead DK, Galina ZH, et al: Assessment of long-term psychosocial sequelae among POW survivors of the Korean conflict. J Pers Assess 54:170–180, 1990

Sutker PB, Winstead DK, Galina ZH, et al: Cognitive deficits and psychopathology among former prisoners of war and combat veterans of the Korean conflict. Am J Psychiatry 148:67–72, 1991

Ursano RJ: An analysis of precaptivity data, in Proceedings of the Twenty-Sixth Annual Conference of Air Force Behavioral Scientists. Edited by Levy RA. Brooks Air Force Base, TX, USAF School of Aerospace Medical Division (AFSC), 1979, pp 54–65

Ursano RJ: The Vietnam War era prisoner of war: precaptivity personality and the development of psychiatric illness. Am J Psychiatry 138:315–318, 1981

Ursano RJ: Vietnam era prisoners of war: studies of U.S. Air Force prisoners of war, in The Trauma of War: Stress and Recovery in Viet Nam Veterans. Edited by Sonnenberg SM, Blank AS Jr, Talbott JA. Washington, DC, American Psychiatric Press, 1985, pp 339–357

Ursano RJ, Rundell JR: The prisoner of war. Mil Med 155:176–180, 1990

Ursano RJ, Boydstun JA, Wheatley RD: Psychiatric illness in U.S. Air Force Vietnam prisoners of war: a five-year follow-up. Am J Psychiatry 138:310–314, 1981

Ursano RJ, Wheatley RD, Sledge WH, et al: Coping and recovery styles in the Vietnam era prisoner of war. J Nerv Ment Dis 174:707–714, 1986

Ursano RJ, Wheatley RD, Carlson EH, et al: The prisoner of war: stress, illness, and resiliency. Psychiatric Annals 17:532–535, 1987

van der Kolk BA: Psychopharmacological issues in posttraumatic stress disorder. Hosp Community Psychiatry 34:683–692, 1983

van der Kolk BA: Post-Traumatic Stress Disorder: Psychological and Biological Sequelae. Washington, DC, American Psychiatric Press, 1984

Van Putten T, Yager J: Posttraumatic stress disorder: emerging from the rhetoric. Arch Gen Psychiatry 41:411–413, 1984

Weisaeth L: Full documentation of appalling suffering of Canadian ex-POWs. WVF International Socio-Medical Information Center Newsletter 1(1):1–10, 1989

Wheatley RD: Intellectual, neuropsychological, and visuomotor assessments of repatriated Air Force SEA POWs, in Scientific Proceedings of the Aerospace Medical Association Annual Meeting, San Antonio, TX, May 1981

Wheatley RD, Ursano RJ: Serial personality evaluations of repatriated U.S. Air Force Southeast Asia POWs. Clinical Medicine 53:251–257, 1982

White NS: Posttraumatic stress disorder (letter). Hosp Community Psychiatry 34:1061–1062, 1983

Yager T, Laufer R, Gallops M: Some problems associated with war experience in men of the Vietnam generation. Arch Gen Psychiatry 41:327–333, 1984

18

From Soldier to Civilian: Acute Adjustment Patterns of Returned Persian Gulf Veterans

Jessica Wolfe, Ph.D.
Terence M. Keane, Ph.D.
Bruce L. Young, M.A.

A lthough prior research has demonstrated a clear association between wartime exposure and subsequent readjustment (Card 1983; Figley 1978, 1985; Green et al. 1989; Kulka et al. 1988, 1990; Rundell et al. 1989), surprisingly little is known about differences in soldiers' postwar psychological recovery or the factors that differentiate the acute readjustment period from later recovery phases.

This work was supported by research grants from the Department of Veterans Affairs Medical Research Service and the National Institute of Mental Health to Jessica Wolfe and Terence M. Keane. Additional funding was provided by a special Operation Desert Storm initiative through the Mental Health and Behavioral Sciences Service, Department of Veterans Affairs Central Office. We thank Drs. Paul Errera, Laurent Lehmann, and Robert Rosenheck for their invaluable support.

We gratefully acknowledge the statistical and methodological assistance of Avron Spiro III, Ph.D., Emmet Hikory, and especially Chaplain (LTC) William R. Mark, without whom this project would not have been possible.

To investigate soldiers' responses to deployment during Operation Desert Storm, we developed the Ft. Devens ODS Reunion Survey, a detailed self-report survey that was administered twice to a large sample of Persian Gulf War veterans who were deployed from New England. The data address the range of reported wartime stressors and a wide variety of soldiers' behavioral and psychological responses. Because of the way in which the data were gathered, the project offers clinicians and researchers some of the earliest and most systematically collected information on acute war stress and readjustment following modern warfare. The survey also provides the unique opportunity to compare the responses of male and female soldiers.

The data from this survey are especially useful because they potentially can help clinicians address questions that may be of interest in the evaluation and treatment of veterans of the Persian Gulf conflict. Some of these questions relate to distinctive characteristics of the Gulf War, such as consideration of the common types of wartime stressors from this deployment and whether these stressors differ from experiences typically described by veterans of other conflicts. Other questions deal more with clinical outcome. For example, what is the relationship between these deployment experiences and subsequent psychological and behavioral adjustment, specifically the development of traumatic stress disorders? What is the course of psychological reactions as they evolve over the first few months and years, and are different psychological interventions indicated? Finally, what, if any, is the relationship between special characteristics of the American Persian Gulf force—in particular, the broad inclusion of women in a wide variety of military occupational specialties—and subsequent readjustment? What can be said about differences between the experiences of men and women during this deployment, and is gender differentially linked to certain types of outcomes?

In this chapter we use data from our survey to help examine these questions. We explore patterns of readjustment as they relate to certain deployment stressors and investigating changes in soldiers' responses early in the return process and over the subsequent 2 years.

Background of the Survey

Initial media reports from the Persian Gulf War suggested that the time-limited nature and relatively low intensity of this war would yield negligible rates of psychological stress, at least as compared with the Vietnam War (Kulka et al. 1990). Anecdotal reports of soldiers almost immediately, however, strongly suggested the presence of discrete war-zone stressors (Wolfe et al. 1993a) and the corresponding impact of numerous aspects of the deployment process, ranging from marked concerns with domestic separation and job disruption to aftereffects of anticipating biological warfare and health problems. By surveying nearly 3,000 soldiers early in the return process, we hoped to systematically delineate stressors associated with this conflict and their relation to sociodemographic characteristics and outcome before there was any substantial confound from intervening homecoming or life events.

To date, nearly all studies of military personnel, with the exception of certain Israeli studies (e.g., Solomon and Mikulincer 1988), have been conducted years or decades after the completion of soldiers' military service. As a result, data from those studies could reflect substantial recall bias stemming from the effects of retrospective reporting and the probable impact of residual (or cumulative) distress on subjective appraisal of functioning (for discussion of these methodological issues, see Sutker et al. 1991). By administering the first phase of this survey before soldiers returned home, we hoped to diminish the effects of these reporting biases. In addition, the survey offered the unusual opportunity to examine any differential effects of wartime deployment based on gender, because the Persian Gulf War marked the first time that male and female U.S. service personnel served side by side in any significant number across a variety of units.

Survey Design

Administration

Early Phase (Time 1)

To enhance the validity and reliability of our data collection, we designed the reunion survey to be administered in several phases, with the earliest phase (Time 1) taking place within 5 days of the soldiers' return to this country, before soldiers returned home to their families and friends.

The initial phase of the survey was administered at Ft. Devens (Ayer, Massachusetts) to units as they returned to the base and underwent administrative processing. Approximately 60% to 70% of soldiers deployed through Ft. Devens were surveyed. The remainder were not available because of routine scheduling issues (e.g., administrative outprocessing by the base). No selection bias was apparent. During the evaluation, soldiers completed a series of detailed standardized and experimental questions dealing with their background, war-zone and deployment stressors (both traditional and novel), psychological outcome (including posttraumatic stress and general psychological symptomatology), coping, and overall well-being. All soldiers completed the paper-and-pencil survey with their unit. In this survey we specifically sought to improve on earlier studies of veterans' wartime experiences by including measures of both traditional and expanded dimensions of stressor exposure (e.g., assessment of domestic stress; unit accidents), based on the assumption that certain aspects of this deployment might constitute new and unusual stressors for military personnel. In addition, because knowledge about posttraumatic stress disorder (PTSD) has evolved significantly in the last decade, more precise measurement of stress reactions was also employed.

Based on previous research showing the utility of scaled combat exposure measures, we used a traditional, Likert-scaled combat instrument: a minimally modified version of the widely used Laufer Combat Scale (Gallops et al. 1981). We also incorporated a structured war-zone checklist instrument (Rosenheck 1992) that allowed more valid representation and broader endorsement of the diverse range of war-zone events that typified the Persian Gulf War environment (e.g., alert for biochemical attack).

The primary psychological and behavioral outcome measures included the well-standardized Mississippi Scale for Combat-Related PTSD (Keane et al. 1988), the Brief Symptom Inventory (Derogatis and Melisaratos 1983), a PTSD checklist derived from the existing cardinal DSM-III-R (American Psychiatric Association 1987) symptoms of PTSD, and the Coping Responses Inventory (Moos 1988). We also obtained data relating to a range of background and sociodemographic factors (e.g., age, race, marital and family status, education, substance use, occupation), as well as information on attitudes toward the deployment experience (e.g., individual and unit preparedness, family support).

First Follow-Up Phase (Time 2)

The first follow-up phase of the survey (Time 2) was completed in 1993 and offers a wealth of data from the period of roughly 18 to 20 months after initial deployment.[1] Included in this phase were most of the original questions and measures, particularly those that were likely to evidence any change. In addition, as veterans began to voice particular concerns after their return (e.g., deteriorations in health status), we revised the proposed Time 2 follow-up survey slightly to include a number of additional measures pertaining to family functioning, unit cohesion, health appraisal, and social and vocational adjustment. Incidences of intervening critical life stressors were also obtained, because these have been shown to relate in a number of situations to both the occurrence of previous stressor exposure and the mediation of subsequent psychological response (Breslau et al. 1991).

---

[1] A second follow-up phase is in progress (Time 3: 1994–1995).

By the time of the follow-up (Time 2), a number of units had disbanded and about 15% of respondents had left military service. Consequently, nearly half of the original units were resurveyed face-to-face at unit meetings that we attended to collect this information. To those units or individuals who could not be contacted in person, we mailed follow-up surveys with detailed letters describing the purpose and importance of the survey and providing general information on the nature of postwar readjustment and referral processes. These letters appeared to have helped in allaying concerns about how the data would be used and in handling misgivings about participating in a government-related project. For example, after a second letter from the research team, one veteran completed the survey, adding,

> Sorry for the delay in responding. . . . I am quite upset at how our unit was treated; I would give up my life for my country, and some of the blame is not ours. . . . War is not nice. . . . We did a damn good job and not everybody seems to know this.

Because the mail phase yielded an initial return rate of just over 68%, we also instituted a phone survey that was specifically designed to track original participants who had not responded by mail or who could not be located through their unit. This phase resulted in an additional response rate of 11%, bringing the total percentage of survey returns for Time 2 to 79.3%. This number provides a sufficiently high level of reliability for the purpose of comparing the results of Time 2 with those of Time 1.

Interested readers are referred to the paper by Wolfe and co-workers (1993a) for a more detailed description of the reunion survey's content and design.

Sample Composition and Veterans' Background Characteristics

For Time 1, the data we refer to in this chapter are based on the responses of 2,344 individuals. Substantially more men than women are represented: 2,136 men versus 208 women. Over-all, these individuals represent a majority subset of those who completed the initial survey. A remaining subset involves several Special Forces units whose data are not included here because of the substantially different nature of their background, training, and deployment experiences.

Although the units tested at Time 1 constitute only about 60% of the troops actually deployed to the Gulf from Ft. Devens, comparisons between our sample and data available for the Ft. Devens population overall suggest that our respondents are representative of the military population stationed at the base during that time. In addition, the sample we studied is moderately diverse, containing a number of ethnic minorities (7.6% African American, 3.6% Hispanic) and representing more than 46 different units with a wide range of military occupational specialties, from service support (e.g., quartermaster) to combat support (e.g., combat engineering). Active-duty, reserve, and National Guard components are represented. Additional demographics are listed in Table 18–1.

At the time of the follow-up (Time 2), the sample comprised 1,853 respondents, including 1,697 men and 162 women. This number of respondents represents a surprisingly high response rate (79.3%), considering the transient nature of much of the sample (i.e., military life often involves redeployment, numerous moves, and so forth). Comparisons between participants at Time 1 and nonparticipants at Time 2 on a number of demo-

Table 18–1.   Sample characteristics of Ft. Devens Operation Desert Storm Reunion Survey returnees

- More than 80% of the sample were Caucasian.
- Women were more likely to be unmarried than men.
- A greater percentage of women served as enlisted personnel rather than officers.
- Men were more likely to have had prior war-zone experience.
- The average age was 30 years, with men slightly older, on average.

graphic, exposure, and outcome variables did not show any significant differences.

Findings From the Survey

Initial Return (Time 1)

Exposure

The majority of respondents in our sample had low to moderate levels of traditionally defined combat exposure, and there were no significant differences in levels between men and women. Only 3% of either group would be designated as having heavy combat exposure based on prior wartime distinctions. On the expanded Operation Desert Storm exposure checklist, a measure designed to evaluate the distinctive experiences of the Persian Gulf war zone (e.g., hostile desert environment; exposure to biochemical attack; civilian death), levels of exposure were higher for men but remained comparable for men and women. For both sexes, the three most commonly endorsed stressors on the checklist were formal alert for chemical or biological attack, receipt of incoming fire from large arms, and witnessing death or disfigurement of enemy personnel (Table 18–2). These events were endorsed by one-half to three-quarters of all participants.

When veterans were given the opportunity to describe their single most stressful experience during deployment in an open-ended format, a slightly different finding emerged. Although combat stressors remained primary (48% men, 38% women), noncombat war-zone stressors (e.g., accidental unit death) were described as primary by nearly one-quarter of the sample (28% men, 24% women). Thus, interpretation of war-zone stress appears to require broadening to more adequately reflect the impact of nontraditional stressor events (and potentially gender) on psychological outcome. This need for a broader interpretation of war-zone stress is further supported by the fact that 25% of men and 20% of women in our sample reported domestic

Table 18–2. Deployment experiences of Ft. Devens Operation Desert Storm Reunion Survey returnees

- Combat exposure levels were moderately low overall.
- The three most common deployment stressors were (in order of most frequent reporting)
  —Formal biochemical alert
  —Receipt of incoming fire
  —Witnessing death or dismemberment of enemy
- 20% to 25% of respondents rated domestic crises as their primary stressor.
- For men and women, perceptions of combat and war-zone exposure increased significantly from initial return to 18-month follow-up.

stressors (e.g., dissolution of marriage, unexpected death of a loved one) as the primary source of trauma during their Gulf War service.

Psychological Outcome

PTSD symptomatology was measured by the Mississippi Scale for Combat-Related PTSD (Keane et al. 1988), a well-validated and reliable measure of war-stress symptomatology in veterans. Mean scores on immediate return were moderately low (mean = 62.3, SD = 13.5). These scores are well below the cutoff of 89 or higher that was used to identify wartime PTSD in a number of community-based samples of veterans from the Vietnam War era (Kulka et al. 1990). Nonetheless, scores for women were higher than those for men ($t[2,340] = 5.22$, $P < .001$) (Table 18–3). At Time 1, nearly 4% of men and 9% of women scored above the aforementioned cutoff ($\chi^2[1, N = 2,342] = 13.03$, $P < .001$. We have labeled this cutoff "presumptive PTSD" because more definitive diagnosis would require detailed, face-to-face diagnostic corroboration rather than exclusive reliance on symptom checklists.

Using a broader measure of general psychopathology, the General Severity Index of the Brief Symptom Inventory (Derogatis and Melisaratos 1983), we found that considerably higher

Table 18–3. Common responses of Ft. Devens Operation Desert Storm Reunion Survey returnees to Gulf War experiences

- Women significantly exceeded men on standard measures of posttraumatic stress disorder and general distress.
- Overall rates of clinical symptomatology increased two- to threefold at follow-up.
- Health complaints were prominent among returnees, particularly
  —General aches and pains
  —Headaches
  —Abnormal lack of energy

levels of distress were present: approximately 30% of soldiers scored in the clinically significant range. Once again, a greater proportion of women than men exceeded the cutoff; however, the difference was not statistically significant ($\chi^2[1, N = 2{,}337] = 1.24$). Thus, even though rates of presumptive PTSD appeared relatively low, considerable numbers of returnees described marked psychological distress in the early phase.

Examination of other characteristics associated with the presence of PTSD symptoms at initial return indicated that symptomatic returnees reported significantly more coping marked by cognitive avoidance ($t[106] = 8.62, P < .001$), resignation ($t[2{,}176] = 7.22, P < .001$), emotional discharge $t[2{,}181] = 13.08, P < .001$), total approach-based coping ($t[2{,}147] = 7.25, P < .001$), less unit cohesion ($t[71] = 4.58, P < .001$), and lower amounts of family cohesion ($t[56] = 2.55, P < .05$).

As expected from prior research (e.g., Keane et al. 1988; Kulka et al. 1990), there was a significant positive relationship between Operation Desert Storm war-zone exposure totals and Mississippi Scale for Combat-Related PTSD scores ($r[2{,}313] = .27, P < .001$).

Follow-Up Findings (Time 2)

A series of analyses focusing on individuals who responded to the survey at both times were performed to compare patterns of responses on stressor and outcome variables. We anticipated that, as in other populations (Baum 1990; Green et al. 1990; Prince-Embury and Rooney 1988), readjustment following war stress might follow along a variety of paths, ranging from enhanced sense of well-being to delayed symptom onset. We hypothesized that the clinical status of some individuals would change from Time 1 to Time 2. Furthermore, we predicted that overall rates of psychological distress would have increased by Time 2, based on the very early point at which the survey was initially administered and the probable buffering effects of the positive support that was widely available for returnees at the outset.

Exposure

Comparing the same subjects at both times, we found that self-reported combat exposure levels increased overall from Time 1 to Time 2. Proportional increments were similar for men and women.

Psychological Outcome

Like the exposure scores, measures of psychological outcome also demonstrated a significant overall increase for both presumptive PTSD (based on the Mississippi Scale for Combat-Related PTSD) and general distress (measured by the General Severity Index of the Brief Symptom Inventory). As at Time 1, female soldiers' symptom reports exceeded those of men in number of symptoms. At Time 2, 11% of male respondents had scores that exceeded the clinical cutoff for presumptive PTSD, which constitutes a $2\frac{1}{2}$-fold increase from Time 1, and 21% of female respondents had scores that exceeded the cutoff, an increase similar in magnitude to that for men between T1 and T2. More than 8% ($n = 120$) of men whose scores were below the PTSD cutoff at Time 1 had scores that surpassed the cutoff at follow-up, compared with nearly 15% ($n = 19$) of female respondents. Thus, a substantial number of individuals evidenced a negative change in the follow-up evaluation. Highly similar increments were found on the General Severity Index and related PTSD checklist measures.

Other Behavioral Indices

At Time 2, 32.4% of all the respondents (31.8% men, 40.1% women) reported that their health had changed for the worse since serving in Operation Desert Storm. As one respondent noted,

> I feel very uneasy over how sick I have become. I was not like this before. I was sick for several days in Saudi, and now it has been months. I have a rash that won't go away. I have aches, pains, my joints hurt; something is wrong! I'm scared the government isn't being honest about what could be wrong with us—even about the medications we took . . .

An analysis of health complaints showed that their prevalence varied across individuals. Men and women who had scores that exceeded the clinical cutoff for PTSD had significantly more health concerns than did individuals whose scores fell below the cutoff ($t[217] = 23.61$ $t[64] = 13.05$, respectively, both $P < .001$). Mean numbers of health problems in men and women whose scores exceeded the PTSD cutoff were nearly triple those of other soldiers (means = 13.8 and 15.7 for men and women, respectively, whose scores were above the cutoff vs. means = 5.7 and 6.7 for nonclinical men and women). The three most commonly endorsed health problems at Time 2 were general aches and pains, headaches, and a lack of energy (Table 18–3), all of which differed significantly by PTSD status ($\chi^2[1, N = 1,602) = 82.29$; $\chi^2[1, N = 1,601) = 62.15$; and $\chi^2[1, N = 1,601) = 113.90$, respectively; all $P < .001$); that is, soldiers with PTSD symptoms reported significantly more health complaints.

An examination of other characteristics associated with the presence of PTSD symptoms at Time 2 again indicated that symptomatology was significantly associated with more avoidant and resigned forms of coping ($t[1,514] = 7.54$ and $t[1,515] = 6.05$, respectively; both $P < .001$), poorer unit cohesion ($t[232] =$

5.99, $P < .001$), and less family cohesion ($t[170] = 7.26$, $P < .001$). As expected, the highly significant positive correlation between war-zone exposure and PTSD symptoms remained ($r[1,844] = .36$, $P < .001$).

To examine factors contributing to changes in clinical classification at Time 2 in more detail, we conducted a stepwise discriminant function analysis using predictors derived from preceding univariate analyses and a standard exploratory discriminant analysis. Men and women were combined for this procedure because the smaller female sample size precluded independent analyses. The obtained discriminant function was highly significant ($F[5,989] = 35.01$, $P < .001$, Wilks' $\lambda = .84$) and yielded a canonical correlation of .39, which accounted for 15% of the total variance. The analysis correctly classified more than 90% of subjects as PTSD positive or negative. A number of variables significantly predicted the emergence of PTSD at Time 2, including higher Operation Desert Storm (but not traditional) war-zone exposure; female gender; avoidant coping; less social support; and poorer family cohesion.

Interpretation of the Findings

Although rates of presumptive PTSD at Time 1 were modest in our sample, these rates increased substantially at the 18-month follow-up, to the point where they were more directly comparable to traumatic stress levels found both in veteran populations from other eras (see, e.g., Brill and Beebe 1955; Kulka et al. 1988, 1990) and in a number of civilian samples after catastrophic life events (see, e.g., Baum 1990; Green et al. 1990). Despite our initial predictions that the time-limited and circumscribed nature of this war would yield few adverse psychological consequences, the data presented here and elsewhere (e.g., Labbate and Snow 1992; Sutker et al. 1993; Wolfe et al. 1993a) confirm that total wartime exposure and exposure to particular stressor components (e.g., witnessing violence, severe injury, and death; anticipatory alert), as in other settings, are particularly aversive and affect the development of stress symptomatology in a noteworthy percentage of individuals (Green et al. 1989; Ursano and McCarroll 1990; Wolfe et al. 1993a; Yehuda et al. 1992). Although comments by some soldiers at follow-up revealed concern with perceived life threat associated with repeated military biochemical alert, the long-range impact of such events on recovery remains to be determined.

The emotional trauma described in the anecdotes and offhand comments appended to many surveys is especially striking. Particularly noteworthy are the strong similarities between the following remarks, from one of the respondents in our study, and those that often punctuate the memories of symptomatic Vietnam War veterans:

> I belonged to a hospital unit the whole time. . . . I saw and took care of many dead and wounded people, both military and civilian; children too. I have had nightmares of this time a lot. I would prefer to block it out and go on with my life. I don't know why—I can't.

Findings from returned soldiers are also consistent with several studies showing that acute stress levels often increase over time (Baum 1990; Prince-Embury and Rooney 1988; Sutker et al. 1993), whether as exacerbations of original stress reactions or in the form of delayed symptom onset. At present, the factors differentially associated with these alterations in both veteran and civilian populations are only partly understood and require substantially more study to determine their etiology (McFarlane 1992; D. Riggs, E. B. Foa, B. O. Rothbaum, et al., unpublished manuscript, 1993). Although supportive treatments may be especially effective during the early return period, the increases or chronicity of certain symptoms in our sample—for example, hyperarousal, sleep disturbance, and intrusive recollections—suggest preliminarily that more focused interventions such as cognitive-behavioral therapies and pharmacological agents are likely to be required in some instances.

In our sample we described a number of characteristics that

appeared to be associated with the observed temporal increases in PTSD, including avoidance-based coping and poor social support. Other investigators and clinicians have described a similar relationship between these variables and traumatic stress (e.g., Fairbank et al. 1991; Keane et al. 1985; Wolfe et al. 1993b). However, the relationship among these variables is not entirely clear. Impaired social functioning, diminished social cohesion, and poor coping, for example, may be epiphenomena of PTSD, reflecting the deleterious impact of PTSD symptoms on behavior rather than causal or etiological factors (Solomon and Mikulincer 1987). Regardless, these associated features are likely to cause difficulties for the treating clinician to the degree that they produce social withdrawal, treatment avoidance, or recurrent crises in daily living. Just as extended evaluations and the application of more sophisticated statistical models are needed scientifically to untangle chronological predictive and interactive effects, clinicians would be advised to monitor the effects of symptom interaction and exacerbation over the course of treatment (Table 18–4).

Our finding of an increase in perceived stressor levels at Time 2 warrants mention. Although exposure scores were significantly and positively related to symptom outcomes, we found a uniform increase in exposure reporting across the sample, extending in some cases to asymptomatic individuals. The study of the conditions under which reports and perceptions of stressor exposure vary is in its relative infancy. In one study involving a traumatic schoolyard shooting (Schwarz and Kowalski

Table 18–4. Suggestions for clinicians treating Operation Desert Storm returnees

- Recognize the broad spectrum of trauma, particularly sexual harassment of women during deployment.
- Assess the evolution of symptoms over time.
- Investigate contributions of premilitary and postmilitary stressors to psychological adjustment.
- Consider the broad range of health complaints and pursue appropriate referrals.

1991), the authors found that increments in the reporting of certain negative event characteristics (e.g., less proximity, greater life threat) were directly associated with PTSD symptoms. However, all subjects altered aspects of their recall during reevaluation. Thus, more investigation of the ways in which traumatic or stressful memories are encoded and retrieved is clearly indicated.

Based on data from a number of studies, the study of how pre- and postmilitary variables affect the course of adjustment over time is also critical (e.g., Vinokur et al. 1987). Although some evidence suggests that premilitary characteristics are of limited predictive value following intense combat (e.g., Foy and Card 1987), other studies have found that premilitary stresses exert independent, negative effects on postdeployment mental health (Vinokur et al. 1987), particularly under conditions involving stress that is of lower magnitude. As one returnee indicated,

> I think that some of my negative comments reflect the harshness of American life today. I'm supposed to be in early retirement and am working as a security person while trying to get a professional job! Lucky for me I have a great therapist. I am also trying to deal with the problem of low self-esteem and other issues that are still there from my childhood.

Other data substantiate the influence of certain sociodemographic characteristics. Hastings (1991) found that younger age at exposure adversely affected short-term outcome through lower psychosocial maturity and restricted vocational and psychosocial achievement. Green and co-workers (1990) similarly observed that lower levels of premilitary education and goal attainment had a negative effect on recovery for their sample of male Vietnam veterans. In older veterans, some adverse stressor effects seem to dissipate over the life span, particularly by mid- to late life, when a more solidly established sense of self and interpersonal relationships help to mitigate earlier traumatic experiences (Elder and Clipp 1988, 1989; Norman 1988). Norman (1988), in a study of female Vietnam veterans, has suggested that more positive life experiences take precedence with the passage of time, superseding the effects of preceding stressors (see also Solomon et al. 1991). We did not systematically explore cohort effects by age or developmental stage. Still, given previous research, clinicians might find it useful to explore age-related and developmental life-stage factors (e.g., vocational opportunities, availability and adequacy of social networks) in evaluating veterans' readjustment to wartime stress and in conducting disposition planning.

Our findings suggest preliminarily that female personnel were more symptomatic both at initial return and at follow-up. In men, some studies have shown that male soldiers' exposure to earlier war trauma (Solomon et al. 1990) and highly stressful childhood events (Vinokur et al. 1987) can intensify reactions to subsequent wartime events. A number of women in our sample had had prior military and wartime exposure, and it is possible that these events influenced their current symptom reporting. One difficulty in making this determination is that we did not systematically measure all preceding or concurrent stressors, for example, childhood sexual or physical abuse. Available data increasingly show that rates of childhood and adult sexual victimization are exceedingly high in women (Kilpatrick 1992; National Victim Center 1992), and prior exposure to these events could affect women's abilities to deal with subsequent episodes involving perceived or actual life threat (Resnick et al. 1992).

Other data we collected strongly suggest that sexual victimization (defined as sexual harassment, attempted sexual assault, and/or completed sexual assault) transpired during the Persian Gulf deployment at rates that exceed those estimated in the civilian population (Wolfe et al. 1992). More than half of our female respondents described incidents of sexual harassment that marked their service or that of a cohort. Many spoke directly and graphically of these experiences and of PTSD-like reactions to them, as did this recently discharged woman:

> I was raped by two [men] in our compound. There was not enough military police protection . . . they got away with it. I have been hospitalized twice and am in therapy due to nightmares and recurring flashbacks. . . . it has taken me over a year and I am not well yet. This should not have been allowed to happen . . .

Preliminary analyses of empirical data from these respondents indicate that, when combat exposure during the Gulf War is controlled, the rates of PTSD found in female soldiers in our sample who had experienced attempted or completed assault are significantly higher than those found in women who have been sexually assaulted but have no military war-zone experiences. Thus, the delineation of relevant stressor events cannot be overemphasized in either scientific or clinical efforts to understand the recovery process.

The high rates of health complaints at Time 2 were also noteworthy. Solomon and Mikulincer (1992) and others (e.g., Cohen and Williamson 1991) have shown that somatic complaints are significantly increased with high levels of traumatic stress. However, the relationship among somatic concerns, health status, and psychological distress, particularly traumatic stress, remains obscure (Cohen and Williamson 1991; J. Wolfe, P. Schnurr, P. J. Brown, J. Furey, unpublished manuscript, 1993). One possibility is that health reports are influenced by interoceptive cues stemming from the physiological and autonomic changes that accompany PTSD (Litz et al. 1992; Shalev et al. 1990; J. Wolfe, P. Schnurr, P. J. Brown, J. Furey, unpublished manuscript, 1993). Alternatively, high levels of stress and arousal may increase vulnerability to existing exogenous pathogens (for review, see Cohen and Williamson 1991), a hypothesis supported by findings of demonstrable changes in immunological status after exposure to severe stress (e.g., Kiecolt-Glaser and Glaser 1987). In some cases, practitioners may find that returnees present with a predominance of physical complaints. These concerns should be exhaustively evaluated in both medical and psychiatric contexts as long as diagnostic uncertainty exists and the interrelationship among these variables is equivocal.

Finally, the impact of postdeployment life events warrants mention. In our study, soldiers reported an average of 1.2 major life stressors since their return; for both men and women, the death of a friend or loved one was described as the most commonly occurring event. To date, at least one investigation has found an adverse impact of postwar stressors on veterans' adaptation (Miller et al. 1991). The way in which war stressors increase either exposure to or perceptions of subsequent critical life events, or, conversely, whether later events can retrigger previously well-managed stress reactions, will need careful evaluation as soldiers move ahead with their lives in civilian and military capacities.

References

American Psychiatric Association: Diagnostic and Statistical Manual of Mental Disorders, 3rd Edition, Revised. Washington, DC, American Psychiatric Association, 1987

Baum A: Stress, intrusive imagery, and chronic stress. Health Psychol 9:653–675, 1990

Breslau N, Davis GC, Andreski P, et al: Traumatic events and post-traumatic stress disorder in an urban population of young adults. Arch Gen Psychiatry 149:671–675, 1991

Brill NR, Beebe GW: A Follow-Up Study of War Neuroses (VA Medical Monograph). Washington, DC, Veterans Administration, 1955

Card JJ: Lives After Vietnam: The Personal Impact of Military Service. Lexington, MA, Lexington Press, 1983

Cohen S, Williamson GM: Stress and infectious disease in humans. Psychol Bull 109:5–24, 1991

Derogatis LR, Melisaratos N: The Brief Symptom Inventory: an introductory report. Psychol Med 13:595–605, 1983

Elder GH, Clipp EC: Wartime losses and social bonding: influences across 40 years in men's lives. Psychiatry 51:177–198, 1988

Elder GH, Clipp EC: Combat experience and emotional health: impairment and resilience in later life. J Pers 57:311–341, 1989

Fairbank JA, Hansen DJ, Fitterling JM: Patterns of appraisal and coping across different stressor conditions among former prisoners of war with and without posttraumatic stress disorder. J Consult Clin Psychol 59:274–281, 1991

Figley CR: Psychosocial adjustment among Vietnam veterans: an overview of the research, in Stress Disorders Among Vietnam Veterans: Theory, Research, and Treatment. Edited by Figley CR. New York, Brunner/Mazel, 1978, pp 57–70

Figley CR (ed): Trauma and Its Wake: The Study and Treatment of Post-Traumatic Stress Disorder. New York, Brunner/Mazel, 1985

Foy DW, Card JJ: Combat-related post-traumatic stress disorder etiology: replicated findings in a national sample of Vietnam-era men. J Clin Psychol 43:28–31, 1987

Gallops M, Laufer RS, Yager T: Revised Combat Scale, in Legacies of Vietnam: Comparative Adjustments of Veterans and Their Peers, Vol 3. Edited by Laufer RS, Yager T. Washington, DC, U.S. Government Printing Office, 1981, pp 444–448

Green BL, Lindy JD, Grace MC, et al: Multiple diagnosis in post-traumatic stress disorder: the role of war stressors. J Nerv Ment Dis 177:329–335, 1989

Green BL, Grace MC, Lindy JD, et al: Risk factors for PTSD and other diagnoses in a general sample of Vietnam veterans. Am J Psychiatry 147:729–733, 1990

Hastings TJ: The Stanford-Terman study revisited: postwar emotional health of World War II veterans. Military Psychology 3:201–214, 1991

Keane TM, Scott WO, Chavoya GA, et al: Social support in Vietnam veterans with posttraumatic stress disorder: a comparative analysis. J Consult Clin Psychol 53:95–102, 1985

Keane TM, Caddell JM, Taylor KL: Mississippi Scale for Combat-Related Posttraumatic Stress Disorder: three studies in reliability and validity. J Consult Clin Psychol 56:85–90, 1988

Kiecolt-Glaser JK, Glaser R: Psychosocial moderators of immune function. Annals of Behavioral Medicine 9:16–20, 1987

Kilpatrick D: On treatment and counseling needs of women veterans who were raped, otherwise sexually assaulted, or sexually harassed during military service. Presented prepared testimony to Senate Committee on Veterans Affairs, Washington, DC, June 1992

Kulka RA, Schlenger WE, Fairbank JA, et al: National Vietnam Veterans Readjustment Study (NVVRS): Description, Current Status, and Initial PTSD Prevalence Estimates. Washington, DC, Veterans Administration, 1988

Kulka RA, Schlenger WE, Fairbank JA, et al: Trauma and the Vietnam War Generation. New York, Brunner/Mazel, 1990

Labbate LA, Snow MP: Posttraumatic stress symptoms among soldiers exposed to combat in the Persian Gulf. Hosp Community Psychiatry 43:831–835, 1992

Litz BT, Keane TM, Fisher L, et al: Physical health complaints in combat-related post-traumatic stress disorder: a preliminary report. Journal of Traumatic Stress 5:131–141, 1992

McFarlane AC: Avoidance and intrusion in posttraumatic stress disorder. J Nerv Ment Dis 180:439–445, 1992

Miller TW, Martin W, Jay LL: Clinical issues in readaptation for Persian Gulf veterans. Psychiatric Annals 21:684–688, 1991

Moos RH: Coping Responses Inventory. Stanford, CA, Consulting Psychologists Press, 1988

National Victim Center: Rape in America: A Report to the Nation. Arlington, VA, National Victim Center, 1992

Norman EM: Post-traumatic stress disorder in military nurses who served in Vietnam during the war years 1965–1973. Mil Med 153:238–242, 1988

Prince-Embury S, Rooney JF: Psychological symptoms of residents in the aftermath of the Three Mile Island nuclear accident and restart. Journal of Social Psychology 128:779–790, 1988

Resnick HS, Kilpatrick DG, Best CL, et al: Vulnerability-stress factors in development of posttraumatic stress disorder. J Nerv Ment Dis 180:424–430, 1992

Rosenheck R: Overview of findings, in Returning Persian Gulf Troops: First Year Findings. Edited by Rosenheck R, Becnel H, Blank A Jr, et al. New Haven, CT, Department of Veterans Affairs, 1992, pp 3–18

Rundell JR, Ursano RJ, Holloway HC, et al: Psychiatric responses to trauma. Hosp Community Psychiatry 40:68–74, 1989

Schwarz ED, Kowalski JM: Malignant memories: PTSD in children and adults after a school shooting. J Am Acad Child Adolesc Psychiatry 30:936–944, 1991

Shalev A, Bleich A, Ursano RJ: Post-traumatic stress disorder: somatic comorbidity and effort tolerance. Psychosomatics 31:197–203, 1990

Solomon Z, Mikulincer M: Combat stress reactions, posttraumatic stress disorder, and social adjustment: a study of Israeli veterans. J Nerv Ment Dis 175:277–285, 1987

Solomon Z, Mikulincer M: Psychological sequelae of war: a two-year follow-up study of Israeli combat stress reaction casualties. J Nerv Ment Dis 176:264–269, 1988

Solomon Z, Mikulincer M: Aftermaths of combat stress reactions: a three-year study. Br J Clin Psychol 31:21–32, 1992

Solomon Z, Oppenheimer B, Elizur Y, et al: Trauma deepens trauma: the consequences of recurrent combat stress reaction. Isr J Psychiatry Relat Sci 27:233–241, 1990

Solomon Z, Benbenishty R, Mikulincer M: The contribution of wartime, pre-war, and post-war factors to self-efficacy: a longitudinal study of combat stress reaction. Journal of Traumatic Stress 4:345–361, 1991

Sutker P, Uddo-Crane M, Allain A: Clinical and research assessment of posttraumatic stress disorder: a conceptual overview. Psychological Assessment (J Consult Clin Psychol) 3:520–530, 1991

Sutker P, Uddo M, Brailey K, et al: War zone trauma and stress-related symptoms in Operation Desert Shield/Storm returnees. Journal of Social Issues 49:33–50, 1993

Ursano RJ, McCarroll JE: The nature of a traumatic stressor: handling dead bodies. J Nerv Ment Dis 178:396–398, 1990

Vinokur A, Caplan RD, Williams CC: Effects of recent and past stress on mental health: coping with unemployment among Vietnam veterans and nonveterans. Journal of Applied Social Psychology 17:710–730, 1987

Wolfe J, Young BL, Brown PJ: Self-reported sexual assault in female Gulf War veterans. Poster presentation at the annual meeting of the Association for Advancement of Behavior Therapy, Boston, MA, November 1992

Wolfe J, Brown PJ, Kelley JM: Reassessing war stress: exposure and the Gulf War. Journal of Social Issues 49:15–31, 1993a

Wolfe J, Keane TM, Kaloupek DG, et al: Patterns of positive readjustment in Vietnam combat veterans. Journal of Traumatic Stress 6:179–193, 1993b

Yehuda R, Southwick SM, Giller EL Jr: Exposure to atrocities and severity of chronic posttraumatic stress disorder in Vietnam combat veterans. Am J Psychiatry 149:333–336, 1992

19

Treatment of Veterans Severely Impaired by Posttraumatic Stress Disorder

Robert A. Rosenheck, M.D.
Alan Fontana, Ph.D.

Although the Persian Gulf War is now over, it is sure to live on in the memories of those who participated in it. Fortunately, most Persian Gulf veterans, after a period of readjustment, have resumed the threads of their lives and are continuing much as they had before their deployment to Southwest Asia. Others, however, as demonstrated in the chapters of this volume, are, and may remain, significantly distressed by their experiences. These veterans will continue to relive various war-zone experiences, ranging from the merely troublesome to the deeply traumatic, for weeks, months, or even years. What can we say about the long-term prospects for these veterans? What can we do to ameliorate their suffering?

Every war is unique to those who fought in it. Much has been made of the very real differences between the Gulf War and other 20th-century U.S. military actions. Nevertheless, amid important differences, many threads of commonality run through modern warfare generally (Fontana and Rosenheck 1993; Rosenheck and Fontana 1994), and the experiences of veterans of previous wars can be profitably recalled and reconsidered as we anticipate caring for Persian Gulf veterans in the years to come.

As reviewed in previous chapters, there is, regrettably, abundant evidence of the tenacity of war-related posttraumatic stress disorder (PTSD): from World War II (Archibald and Tuddenham 1965), the Korean conflict (Sutker et al. 1989), and the Vietnam War (Kulka et al. 1990b). Fifteen years after the last American soldier left Saigon, more than 15% of those who served in the Vietnam theater were found to be suffering from PTSD (Kulka et al. 1990b).

But even among those who suffer from PTSD, many veterans are able to sustain family life and work productively in spite of their symptoms, and more than a few find themselves moved by the inner pain and sorrow of their war experience to devote themselves, fully and wholesomely, to the care of their fellow veterans. In 1985, Steven Silver, a Vietnam War veteran psychologist working in the Department of Veterans Affairs (VA) medical center in Coatesville, Pennsylvania, noted an important change in what he called the mythos of the Vietnam veteran: a change from the outlaw mythos exemplified in movies such as *Taxi Driver* and *Rambo* to a generative mythos of the strong, sensitive, and caring survivor (Silver 1985). Many Vietnam veterans who suffer from PTSD have used their pain to propel their lives in creative and healing directions.

Our own analysis of data from the National Vietnam Veterans Readjustment Study (NVVRS) showed that among those diagnosed with PTSD who had never sought help (38% of all those currently suffering from PTSD), the majority (67%), when asked why they had not sought help, said they did not feel that their problems were serious enough to require special assistance and that they thought they would get better without help. Without minimizing the suffering of these veterans, for their pain is no doubt substantial, we seek here to contrast them with a group of veterans who also suffer from persistent PTSD but who are far more severely symptomatic and socially impaired (Friedman and Rosenheck, in press).

Clinical Characteristics of and Treatment for Severe and Persistent PTSD

The group of veterans with PTSD whose care is addressed in this chapter often suffer from comorbid conditions such as mood disorders and substance abuse, conditions that are compounded by suicidality in many cases (Table 19–1). As a result, these individuals make extensive use of health care services and sometimes also become involved with the criminal justice system. They are often unable to work because they are easily overwhelmed by storms of emotion and have difficulty responding to the demands of authority figures. For the same reasons, they find themselves severely socially isolated, having been abandoned or rejected by most of those who once loved them. This complex of problems may eventually result in exceptionally severe deficits in social adjustment such as extreme poverty, vagrancy, and homelessness. Impoverished and severely cut off from social support by war-related stresses, these veterans resemble other patients who suffer from disabling mental health problems. They are most likely to turn to public-sector providers of last resort for assistance, in many instances to programs offered by the VA.

In this chapter we present a portrait of this subgroup of veterans, an important minority within the larger minority who suffer from war-related PTSD. For these veterans, more than half of whom have suffered from PTSD for more than 20 years, as for other individuals disabled by severe psychiatric illnesses, vet-

Table 19–1. Characteristics of severely ill veterans who suffer from posttraumatic stress disorder

Severe and persistent symptoms	Legal system involvement
Comorbid disorders (e.g., depression, substance abuse)	Poor employment capacity
	Severe social isolation
Suicidality	Extreme poverty
Extensive use of health care services	Homelessness

eran and nonveteran alike, clinical care must be a delicate balance of limited expectations and realistic hopes. It is our belief that these veterans require specialized treatment embodying five general principles (Table 19–2):

1. *Long-term perspective.* Treatment of these veterans requires considerable patience because clinical improvement comes in small steps, often at long intervals. Expecting too much too soon may result in early termination.
2. *Attention to multiple domains.* Attention must be directed to multiple social adjustment domains as well as to conventional clinical problems. Needs for financial assistance, housing support, daily activity structure, and supported employment must be addressed at face value and not merely psychologized.
3. *Practical problem solving.* A practical problem-solving approach must complement an empathic, psychotherapeutic

---

Table 19–2.   Treatment principles for severely and persistently mentally ill veterans who suffer from posttraumatic stress disorder (PTSD)

Treatment must be viewed from a long-term perspective.
Clinical attention must be focused on multiple domains:
   —PTSD symptoms
   —Substance abuse
   —Social support
   —Structured daily activities
   —Financial assistance
   —Housing
   —Supported employment
A practical, problem-solving approach to the diverse domains should be used.
The clinician(s) should maintain flexibility.
   —Be available for intensive crisis intervention.
   —Tolerate periods of distancing or disengagement.
Continuity of care, providing dependability and consistency, should be ensured.

---

approach. Psychological understanding and practical assistance work synergistically with these patients, each one augmenting the effectiveness of the other.

4. *Flexibility.* Treatment must be responsive to fluctuating levels of need, with intermittent high-intensity treatment provided when crises arise, and periods of low-intensity or even interrupted treatment being accepted in less tumultuous times.

5. *Continuity of care.* Finally, through hard times and smooth times, through crises and periods of steady, if small, progress, these patients are best served through a consistent clinical presence that conveys to the patient that the clinician can be relied on to "do what can be done" in all situations.

An approach that embodies these principles, which, we must reiterate, is specifically indicated for severely and persistently ill veterans, marks a significant departure from the more acute, trauma-focused treatment usually recommended for patients with PTSD. In this chapter we provide a brief review of the treatment literature on combat-related PTSD and some new empirical data that we feel demonstrate both the existence of these war-veteran clients and their need for a treatment approach that is tailored to their unique circumstances.

Treatment Outcome Studies of Combat-Related PTSD

A recent review of more than 255 English-language reports on the treatment of PTSD (S. D. Solomon et al. 1992) reported only 7 randomized clinical trials involving combat veterans. In these studies, findings were mixed for various types of pharmacotherapy, with more improvement in anxiety and depressive symptoms than in specific symptoms of PTSD. Improvement was somewhat more consistently positive for systematic desensitization (Peniston 1986) and for exposure therapies (Cooper and Clum 1989; Keane et al. 1989b), although the number of subjects participating in these studies was small and, in most cases, more severe cases were excluded. Instances of exacerbation of symptoms were reported with exposure therapies, especially in veterans suffering from other disorders in addition to PTSD (Pittman et al. 1991). Although most of these studies were conducted at VA medical centers, comparison of symptom severity, social maladjustment, and functional disability with veterans who suffer from PTSD in the general population was not undertaken. As a result, we do not know how the samples in these studies compare with the general population of veterans suffering from PTSD. We do know, however, that treatment was not curative in most cases.

Several uncontrolled studies have addressed more typical samples of VA patients and have found notable but limited clinical improvement, especially in morale and social support (Boudewyns and Hyer 1990; Boudewyns et al. 1990; Fontana et al. 1993; Perconte 1989; Scurfield et al. 1990). Two of these studies, however, found evidence of symptom exacerbation after specialized inpatient or day treatment (Fontana et al. 1993; Perconte 1989). In most of these uncontrolled studies, however, the representativeness of the treatment populations was not systematically characterized, but it appears that these studies, too, noted limited response to the cogent and thoughtful treatment provided.

In the remainder of this chapter we explore the course of treatment of severely ill PTSD patients through a presentation of findings from a 1-year uncontrolled follow-up study of veterans receiving outpatient treatment in the VA's specialized PTSD Clinical Teams Program. First, we situate these patients in a larger context through a comparison of baseline clinical status and social adjustment characteristics with comparable information from a representative national sample of veterans suffering from combat-related PTSD but who have not sought VA mental health services. Second, we present the results of the follow-up study to examine 1) areas of clinical change, 2) the magnitude of change, and 3) potential moderators of change. Through this presentation, we hope to objectively characterize the clinical presentation and treatment course of a distinctly troubled and especially deserving group of veterans who are still struggling to make the long journey home. Fortunately, we can anticipate that only a small percentage of Persian Gulf veterans will find themselves in the circumstances of this group. But we must not forget that such veterans exist and that they often require a special type of treatment.

Department of Veterans Affairs PTSD Clinical Teams Program

The data presented here are derived from structured interviews conducted as part of the national evaluation of the VA PTSD Clinical Teams Program. Fifty-six PTSD clinical teams (PCTs) were established across the country by VA between 1989 and 1992 to provide treatment of PTSD to war-zone veterans in specialized clinical settings. Six of these teams, located in Boston, Jackson (Mississippi), Kansas City, New Orleans, Providence, and San Francisco, agreed to participate in an outcome study of the treatment of PTSD. Four of the six teams were led by nationally recognized experts in the treatment of PTSD. During 1990–1991, 554 male veterans of World War II, the Korean War, and the Vietnam War completed baseline assessment and agreed to be reinterviewed at 4-month intervals for 1 year.

Previous studies of factors associated with VA service use have shown that veterans who come to VA for health care services are more often minorities, poorer, more severely ill, and more functionally disabled than veterans who seek medical care from other sources (Rosenheck and Massari 1993). By legislative mandate, the federal government, and more specifically the VA, have a special responsibility for providing care to the most disadvantaged segment of the veteran population.

Previous studies have not, however, identified distinguishing characteristics of veterans who choose to use VA mental health services among those who suffer from PTSD. Data available from the NVVRS offer an opportunity for such a comparison.

The NVVRS was conducted on a national sample of veterans

of the Vietnam War era who were identified through computerized military personnel records. Details of sampling strategy and instrumentation can be found in the original report on the study (Kulka et al. 1989). Of greatest interest here is the fact that survey data allow characterization of a representative national sample of veterans who suffer from PTSD, with a well-validated cutoff score of 89 on the Mississippi Scale for Combat-Related PTSD (Keane et al. 1988).

The nationally weighted data for veterans in the NVVRS sample who had never used VA services (population estimate 494,186) and equivalent data from the Vietnam War veterans who participated in the PCT follow-up study ($N = 476$) are presented in Table 19–3. It is clear from this comparison that those who come to VA for help are at a considerable disadvantage, even when compared with other veterans suffering from PTSD. In addition to more frequently being black, being divorced, separated, or never married, and being considerably poorer, they are only half as likely to be employed, and approximately six times as likely to have made a suicide attempt in the past. In addition, they report almost twice as many indicators of alcoholism and score 25% higher in PTSD symptoms on the Mississippi Scale for Combat-Related PTSD. According to the NVVRS, only 20% of veterans who currently suffer from PTSD have ever sought mental health services from VA for their PTSD (Kulka et al. 1990). It appears that those who do seek help from VA for PTSD are quite different from other veterans suffering from PTSD, in that their problems are more severe and they appear to lack personal and social resources with which to cope with them. It is to the description of the treatment and clinical course of these veterans that we now turn.

Veterans Treated in the PTSD Clinical Teams Program: An Outcome Study

In the remainder of this chapter we examine immediate and subsequent change in adjustment over the course of the first

Table 19–3. Comparison of Vietnam War veterans suffering from posttraumatic stress disorder (PTSD) in the clinical sample seen by Department of Veterans Affairs (VA) PTSD clinical teams and veterans who had not used VA mental health services in the NVVRS

	PTSD clinical team: Vietnam veterans (*N* = 476)	NVVRS: no treatment at VA (*N* = 494,186)[a]
Age (years)	42.94	44.30
SD	3.22	4.26
Race		
White	71.2%	71.2%
Black	25.0%	18.3%
Hispanic	1.1%	5.4%
Other	2.7%	5.2%
Marital status		
Married	47.3%	66.8%
Widowed	1.1%	1.2%
Separated	9.2%	6.2%
Divorced	30.9%	18.0%
Never married	11.6%	7.9%
Employed	36.6%	73.7%
Education (years)	13.05	12.68
SD	2.36	2.39
Earned income	$5,755	$18,996
SD	$9,864	$12,545
Total income	$13,937	$19,985
SD	$13,344	$12,066
Combat–Legacies[b]	10.64	9.64
SD	2.84	3.38
Combat–Keane[c]	28.20	25.15
SD	8.96	10.35

(continued)

510 EMOTIONAL AFTERMATH OF THE PERSIAN GULF WAR

Table 19–3. Comparison of Vietnam War veterans suffering from posttraumatic stress disorder (PTSD) in the clinical sample seen by Department of Veterans Affairs (VA) PTSD clinical teams and veterans who had not used VA mental health services in the NVVRS *(continued)*

	PTSD clinical team: Vietnam veterans (N = 476)	**NVVRS: no treatment at VA (N = 494,186)[a]**
PTSD diagnosis	81.7%	20.7%
Mississippi Scale for Combat-Related PTSD[d]	125.77	100.65
SD	21.36	10.76
Suicide attempt	34.7%	5.2%
Violence[e]	10.28	9.75
SD	6.66	4.50
Brief MAST[f]	9.68	4.62
SD	9.59	7.91
DIS–drug abuse[g]	0.51	0.27
SD	0.92	0.57

Note. NVVRS = National Vietnam Veterans Readjustment Study; SD = standard deviation; MAST = Michigan Alcoholism Screening Test; DIS = Diagnostic Interview Schedule.
[a]Data for NVVRS based on reanalysis of data reported in Kulka et al. 1990a.
[b]Revised Combat Scale (Laufer et al. 1981).
[c]Keane et al. 1989a.
[d]Keane et al. 1988.
[e]Violent behavior measure from the NVVRS (Kulka et al. 1990b).
[f]Pokorny et al. 1972.
[g]Robins et al. 1981.

year after entry into the PTSD Clinical Teams Program ($N = 476$). Measurements were gathered through a series of structured interviews conducted at the time of entry to the program and at 4, 8, and 12 months thereafter.

Any attempt to track adjustment longitudinally is subject to the problem of missing data at one or more of the time points. Fortunately, a new approach to this problem, *random regression modeling*, has been developed by statistical researchers for use with incomplete longitudinal data (Gibbons et al. 1993). The random regression approach uses available data to make the best estimate of the missing data for each subject by imputing values and performing the desired analyses. We have used Program 5V of the BMDP statistical package (Schluchter 1988) for the analyses reported on in this chapter.

Indices of Adjustment

Because war-related PTSD is a persistent and disabling disorder for many veterans in this sample, outcomes were measured in multiple functional domains in addition to PTSD symptomatology. These domains included mental and physical symptoms; interpersonal relations and violent behavior; social contact; employment and income; VA compensation status; and involvement with the criminal justice system. The methods and measures of assessment for these domains are as follows.

PTSD, psychological symptoms, and medical problems.   PTSD symptoms were assessed by the Mississippi Scale for Combat-Related PTSD (Keane et al. 1988), and guilt reactions to war-zone experiences were assessed by the Guilt Inventory (Laufer and Frey-Wouters 1988). General psychological distress was assessed by the General Severity Index of the Brief Symptom Inventory (Derogatis and Melisaratos 1983) and the Psychiatric Symptoms Index from the Addiction Severity Index (ASI; McLellan et al. 1985). Suicide attempts were assessed as a dichotomous variable during the 30 days before both baseline and follow-up. The ASI Alcohol and Drug Indices were used to measure the severity of substance abuse problems. Medical difficulties were assessed with the ASI Medical Condition Index.

Interpersonal relations and violence. Interpersonal relations were assessed by use of the ASI Family Index, and violence, by a seven-item scale derived from the NVVRS reflecting a veteran's recent violent behavior (α = .80) (Kulka et al. 1990a).

Social contact and involvement, and employment and income. Social contact and involvement were assessed by use of the Social Participation Index of Katz and Lyerly (1963) and by a count of the number of different people to whom the veteran felt emotionally close. Employment was assessed by the number of days that the veteran worked during the preceding month.

VA compensation status. VA compensation was measured by an index specially constructed to encompass the full range of compensation levels. Veterans without service connection (i.e., compensation) received a value of 0; those who were service connected at less than 10% received a value of 1; those who were service connected at 10% or more but less than 50% received a value of 2; those who were service connected at 50% or more but less than 100% received a value of 3; and those who were service connected at 100% received a value of 4.

Criminal justice involvement. Current difficulties with the criminal justice system were assessed with the ASI Legal Difficulties Index.

Plan of Data Analysis

In studying the care of severely ill patients, it is as important to know when change occurs, and in what sequence, as it is to know the net magnitude of change. Preliminary analyses on partial data from this study suggested that there are two phases of change during the first year of PCT treatment: a movement phase (the first 4 months), in which significant changes occur, and a stabilization phase (months 4–12), during which gains are maintained but not extended (Fontana et al. 1993). Because of these preliminary indications of differential amounts of change during different phases of treatment, we took care to examine change during these two time frames.

Data analysis was conducted first by performance of two series of one-way random regression analyses. One series evaluated the significance of changes from the beginning of treatment to 4 months (the movement phase), and the other evaluated changes over the remainder of the year, across the three remaining time points (4, 8, and 12 months following intake). The statistical significance of change during each period was evaluated by use of Wald's chi-square.

In the second phase, these analyses were repeated as interactional random regression analyses in which six baseline characteristics and six treatment characteristics were dichotomized and examined as factors that might significantly affect the veterans' response to treatment. In clinical terms, these analyses determine whether the course of treatment differs for veterans who differ on certain key characteristics—for example, whether veterans with substance abuse problems in addition to PTSD, or veterans who are seeking compensation, show more or less change in their symptoms and social adjustment than other veterans). In statistical terms, these analyses examine the interaction of background and treatment characteristics with time course for each outcome measure. A significant interaction means that either the degree of change or the direction of the change is significantly different for veterans who differ on the characteristic in question.

Pretreatment Background Characteristics

The six background characteristics selected for examination were

1. Vietnam War service (88% of the sample) versus service in other eras
2. The possibility of secondary financial gain (i.e., veterans seeking to obtain [76.4%] vs. retain [13.7%] compensation vs. those who were not [9.9%])

3. Clinical prognosis (veterans with complicating clinical factors [94.8%] vs. others [5.2%])
4. Exposure to childhood physical or sexual abuse (15.4%)
5. Comorbid substance abuse (26%)
6. Availability of social support (divided at the median on a social support scale [$\alpha = .79$])

Participation in Treatment

Special attention was also paid to examination of the relationship between outcome and various aspects of PCT treatment. Data for these treatment measures were primarily derived from the Clinical Process Form (CPF), a structured clinical summary completed by PCT clinicians 2, 4, 8, and 12 months after each veteran entered treatment. Data on satisfaction were derived from patient interviews. Six treatment characteristics were hypothesized to be associated with greater improvement:

1. Regularity of attendance in therapy (58.5% of the sample)
2. Length of time in therapy (4 months or less [40%] vs. more than 4 months [60%])
3. Number of therapy sessions attended during the year (split at the median, 14 sessions)
4. Degree of direct attention to war traumas in therapy ("some or a lot" [53%] vs. "little or none" [47%] by clinician's rating)
5. Termination of therapy because goals had ostensibly been achieved, as judged by clinician (5.1%)
6. Satisfaction with current PTSD treatment (highly satisfied [50.1%] vs. satisfied [39.8%] vs. dissatisfied [10.2%])

Course of Treatment and Predictive Variables

Changes Over Time for All PTSD Clinical Teams Program Veterans Considered Together

Changes in adjustment, as assessed by changes in symptoms and social functioning, for the movement and stabilization phases are presented in Table 19–4. All but one instance of sig-nificant change occurred during the first 4 months, and that significant change occurred in half (7 of 14) of the clinical do-mains assessed. Significant, but small, decreases in PTSD symp-toms, and somewhat larger decreases in substance abuse, legal difficulties, and the propensity to violence, are evident. An in-crease was noted in the number of days worked for pay. These changes all indicate significant improvement in adjustment in a group of veterans who had been suffering from PTSD for an average of 21 years. There was also a significant increase in re-ceipt of VA compensation.

The one significant change observed during the remainder of the year was a decrease in the number of days worked, back toward the baseline level. Thus, although no significant contin-ued improvement occurred, little regression was noted either. With the exception of employment, veterans maintained the gains that they had achieved earlier. In general, then, these re-sults confirm the characterization of the two follow-up periods as movement and stabilization phases, respectively.

Variables Moderating Change

The interactions between change and the six background and six treatment characteristics described earlier in this section were screened for the number of significant tests that could have occurred by chance. Because there were 15 adjustment ar-eas, each of which was examined for two phases, there were a total of 30 tests for each stratification characteristic. To rule out significant tests that were likely to have occurred by chance, we insisted that at least three tests reach significance at $P < .05$ for any one characteristic before we considered the tests to in-dicate a nonchance relationship between that characteristic and the course of adjustment over time.

The vast majority of factors showed no relationship to mea-sures of clinical change beyond those due to chance. The three characteristics that did meet the standard of three significant tests were 1) current substance abuse, 2) regularity of atten-

Table 19–4. Means and random regression analyses for changes in symptoms and social functioning over time in the clinical sample seen by Department of Veterans Affairs PTSD clinical teams

Adjustment index measure	Movement phase			Stabilization phase			
	Baseline	4 months	χ^2	4 months	8 months	12 months	χ^2
Mississippi Scale for Combat-Related PTSD[a]	122.67	121.24	5.11[*]	121.46	120.81	121.30	NS
Guilt Inventory[b]	2.66	2.67	NS	2.65	2.66	2.69	NS
Brief Symptom Inventory[c]	2.08	2.09	NS	2.09	2.11	2.13	NS
Suicide attempt	0.03	0.04	NS	0.04	0.06	0.04	NS
Addiction Severity Index[d]							
Psychiatric Symptoms Index	0.54	0.52	NS	0.51	0.51	0.51	NS
Alcohol Index	0.11	0.08	17.56[**]	0.07	0.07	0.07	NS
Drug Index	0.03	0.02	11.37[**]	0.02	0.01	0.02	NS
Medical Condition Index	0.49	0.49	NS	0.48	0.49	0.46	NS
Family Index	0.25	0.24	NS	0.24	0.21	0.22	NS
Legal Difficulties Index	0.09	0.06	5.46[*]	0.06	0.06	0.06	NS

Violence[e]	9.38	6.38	132.75**	6.29	6.24	6.11	NS
Days worked	6.33	7.55	10.17**	7.63	7.21	6.74	6.99*
Number of people close to	10.93	10.60	NS	10.72	10.67	11.03	NS
Social participation[f]	11.31	11.17	NS	11.12	11.39	11.20	NS
Service connection[g]	1.21	1.29	19.65**	1.31	1.31	1.34	NS

Note. The means for each time point are displayed, as are the chi-square (χ^2) values for those changes that were significant at the .05 level or .001 level. The means for the "4 months" time point differ slightly between the movement and stabilization phases because the difference in inclusion of other time points contributed slight variations to the imputation of missing values. NS = not significant.

*P < .05; **P < .001.

[a]Keane et al. 1988.
[b]Laufer and Frey-Wouters 1988.
[c]Derogatis and Melisaratos 1983.
[d]McLellan et al. 1985.
[e]Violent behavior measure from the NVVRS (Kulka et al. 1990b).
[f]Katz and Lyerly 1963.
[g]Compensation.

dance in therapy, and 3) duration of participation in treatment. To minimize the chance that differences found for the stratification of these characteristics were artifacts of differences in the initial level of psychopathology or social maladjustment, we repeated the analyses for these three characteristics, covarying the influence of prognostic status, and initial scores on the Mississippi Scale for Combat-Related PTSD, the Brief Symptom Inventory, and the ASI Alcohol and Drug Indices. Inclusion of these covariates, however, did not change the results of any of the analyses. Patterns of change stratified by these three characteristics, when the covariates mentioned above were controlled, are presented below.

Current substance abuse.   Substance-abusing veterans improved more than non–substance-abusing veterans in terms of their alcohol and drug abuse during the movement phase and continued to improve more in terms of their drug abuse during the stabilization phase (Table 19–5). However, much of this difference between the two groups is a function of the fact that nonabusing veterans started at a "floor" level and had very little room to improve further.

In other areas of adjustment, the frequency of suicide attempts decreased among substance-abusing veterans to a level approximately the same as that among non–substance-abusing veterans during the stabilization phase. Also, substance-abusing veterans increased, overall, their frequency of participation in activities with others between 4 and 12 months, whereas the nonabusing veterans did not. In addition, from 4 to 12 months, substance-abusing veterans experienced a worsening in their PTSD symptoms, whereas nonabusing veterans did not. Guilt, general psychiatric distress, and legal problems distinctly increased in substance-abusing veterans between 4 and 8 months but declined again by 12 months. Although these findings might suggest that as veterans with active substance abuse problems reduce their use of alcohol or drugs they experience transient increases in PTSD and related symptomatology, empirical analysis did not support this interpretation since there was no signifi-

Table 19–5. Means and random regression analyses for significant changes in symptoms and social functioning over time in the clinical sample seen by Department of Veterans Affairs PTSD clinical teams by level of current substance abuse

Adjustment index measure	Substance abuse	Movement phase			Stabilization phase			
		Baseline	4 months	χ^2	4 months	8 months	12 months	χ^2
Mississippi Scale for Combat-Related PTSD[a]	Yes	125.59	123.02	NS	123.82	126.92	125.24	11.74**
	No	121.67	120.46		120.56	118.93	120.16	
Guilt Inventory[b]	Yes	2.85	2.78	NS	2.76	2.87	2.78	6.65*
	No	2.59	2.62		2.62	2.60	2.65	
Brief Symptom Inventory[c]	Yes	2.20	2.14	NS	2.17	2.31	2.21	8.56*
	No	2.04	2.07		2.07	2.05	2.11	
Suicide attempt	Yes	0.04	0.09	NS	0.09	0.10	0.03	6.97*
	No	0.03	0.03		0.03	0.05	0.04	
Addiction Severity Index[d]								
Alcohol Index	Yes	0.30	0.13	90.18**	0.12	0.15	0.15	7.13*
	No	0.05	0.06		0.06	0.05	0.04	
Drug Index	Yes	0.10	0.05	23.74**	0.05	0.03	0.03	9.17**
	No	0.01	0.01		0.01	0.01	0.01	

(continued)

Table 19–5. Means and random regression analyses for significant changes in symptoms and social functioning over time in the clinical sample seen by Department of Veterans Affairs PTSD clinical teams by level of current substance abuse (continued)

| Adjustment index measure | Substance abuse | Movement phase | | | Stabilization phase | | | |
		Baseline	4 months	χ^2	4 months	8 months	12 months	χ^2
Legal Difficulties Index	Yes	0.12	0.09	NS	0.08	0.13	0.10	6.57[*]
	No	0.07	0.05		0.05	0.04	0.04	
Social participation	Yes	11.04	11.23	NS	11.14	10.70	11.84	9.06[**]
	No	11.39	11.23		11.22	11.64	11.04	

Note.   *$P < .05$; **$P < .001$.
[a]Keane et al. 1988.
[b]Laufer and Frey-Wouters 1988.
[c]Derogatis and Melisaratos 1983.
[d]McLellan et al. 1985.

cant correlation between reduced substance abuse and increased PTSD symptoms. These temporary changes may have been related to the constructive reduction in the use of chemicals to numb awareness, and a concomitant increase in self-awareness and subjective distress.

Regularity of attendance at therapy.　Veterans who attended therapy regularly and those who did not both showed a reduction in violent behavior and an increase in the number of days worked in the movement phase (Table 19–6). Those who attended regularly, however, improved somewhat less than those who did not attend regularly. In the stabilization phase, however, veterans who did not attend therapy regularly showed a decline in the number of days worked, and by 12 months they worked no more days than veterans who attended therapy regularly.

Veterans who attended regularly showed a greater increase in the number of people they felt close to during the movement phase, whereas those who did not attend therapy regularly showed a decrease in the number of people they felt close to. At the end of the stabilization phase (1 year), however, the groups were comparable in this area as well.

Although regularity of attendance shows a statistically significant relationship with improvement in some areas, these findings vary from one measure to another, and their magnitudes are neither sustained nor impressive from a clinical perspective.

Duration of participation in treatment.　Veterans who stayed in treatment more than 4 months showed a decline in their family adjustment problems during the movement phase, whereas veterans who left treatment by 4 months showed an increase in family adjustment problems (Table 19–7). In the stabilization phase, however, veterans who stayed in treatment showed no further reduction in family stress, whereas those who had left treatment showed substantial improvement in family adjustment. In the realm of legal difficulties, veterans who left treatment by 4 months recorded significant improvement during the

Table 19–6. Means and random regression analyses for significant changes in symptoms and social functioning over time in the clinical sample seen by Department of Veterans Affairs PTSD clinical teams by regularity of attendance in therapy

Adjustment index measure	Regular attendance	Movement phase			Stabilization phase			
		Baseline	4 months	χ^2	4 months	8 months	12 months	χ^2
Violence[a]	Yes	8.49	5.96	4.62*	6.00	5.85	5.62	NS
	No	10.69	7.01		6.78	7.02	7.00	
Days worked	Yes	6.58	7.04	6.11*	6.97	7.30	6.50	8.45*
	No	5.89	8.30		8.55	6.95	6.77	
Number of people close to	Yes	10.55	10.97	8.23**	11.02	10.85	11.00	NS
	No	11.50	10.11		10.40	10.36	11.17	

Note.   *$P < .05$; **$P < .01$.
[a]Violent behavior measure from the NVVRS (Kulka et al. 1990b).

movement phase, whereas veterans who stayed in treatment manifested no change. Neither group had additional changes in clinical problems during the stabilization phase. These patterns suggest that veterans with legal difficulties may have come to a PCT for help in resolving these difficulties and then left treatment shortly after the resolution of these problems.

Patterns of change in employment in the two groups are quite different. Veterans who left treatment by 4 months increased their days worked substantially during the movement phase, whereas those who stayed in treatment made no change. This increase in the number of days worked observed among those who had left treatment tended to erode in the stabilization phase, although the number of days worked remained higher at the end of the year than at the beginning. Those who stayed in treatment continued to make no change in their employment during the stabilization phase. It is possible that being in treatment is negatively associated with employment, because work schedules conflict with attendance at therapy sessions. It is also possible that having an orientation of solving one's problems oneself contributes to both working more and leaving treatment.

Discussion and Conclusions

In this chapter we have examined the course of clinical change in a subgroup of veterans who suffer from severe PTSD as well as many other adjustment problems, and who have suffered from these problems for more than 20 years in the majority of cases. The analyses of clinical change revealed modest, but statistically significant, improvements during the first 4 months following program entry in 6 of 14 clinical domains: PTSD symptoms, alcohol abuse, drug abuse, legal problems, violent behavior, and employment. We have called this period the movement phase because of the diversity and significance of the changes observed. In contrast, the next 8 months were marked by a maintenance of gains, although there was some

Table 19–7. Means and random regression analyses for significant changes in symptoms and social functioning over time in the clinical sample seen by Department of Veterans Affairs PTSD clinical teams by length of treatment

Adjustment index measure	Length of treatment	Movement phase			Stabilization phase			
		Baseline	4 months	χ^2	4 months	8 months	12 months	χ^2
ASI–Family Index	Up to 4 mo	0.24	0.28	5.18*	0.27	0.21	0.18	9.83*
	>4 mo	0.26	0.22		0.22	0.22	0.24	
ASI–Legal Difficulties Index	Up to 4 mo	0.12	0.07	3.82*	0.06	0.09	0.07	NS
	>4 mo	0.06	0.06		0.06	0.05	0.05	
Days worked	Up to 4 mo	5.79	9.19	15.59**	9.32	7.60	7.11	8.21*
	>4 mo	6.67	6.87		6.84	6.94	6.43	

Note.   ASI = Addiction Severity Index (McLellan et al. 1985).
*P < .05; ***P < .001.

decline in employment effort back to baseline levels. We have, accordingly, termed this period the stabilization phase.

On the one hand, these results are impressive in that a group of veterans who had been seriously troubled for many years showed a significant improvement in response to treatment. On the other hand, the results are somewhat disappointing in that the magnitude of improvement was modest and did not extend to all of the domains examined. We believe these modest gains reflect more on the severity and chronicity of the problems faced by these veterans than on the quality of the treatment they received. As noted above, four of the six teams were led by nationally recognized experts in the treatment of PTSD, and the majority of clinicians on these teams had considerable experience in treating veterans with PTSD.

Interaction analyses undertaken to identify specific patient and treatment factors moderating improvement revealed few differences among veteran subgroups. Contrary to expectations, no relationship was identified between clinical change and 1) Vietnam War service, 2) the possibility for secondary gain from VA compensation payments, 3) good clinical prognosis, 4) history of child abuse, 5) current social support, 6) the number of therapy sessions attended, 7) attention to war trauma in treatment, 8) attainment of treatment goals according to the primary clinician's judgment, or 9) veteran's satisfaction with services. Veterans who had recently been abusing substances did show a somewhat different pattern of change from that found in non–substance-abusing veterans, including greater improvement in substance abuse problems and suicidality, but also some exacerbation of PTSD symptoms. Veterans who attended therapy regularly and who participated for more than 4 months also showed some significant differences in pattern of improvement, but these differences were generally small in magnitude and tended to dissipate by the end of the year.

It may be objected that the methodology used was insensitive to more impressive changes that may actually have taken place. Pre-post measures on instruments that are psychometrically sound are often quantitatively modest and may reflect only small increments of improvement when compared with patient or therapist global impressions of improvement. A recent demonstration of this phenomenon appeared in an important series of articles on the KOACH program, a treatment developed for Israeli soldiers of the Lebanon War (Shalev et al. 1992; Z. Solomon et al. 1992a, 1992b). In that program, reports indicate that treated soldiers were actually somewhat more symptomatic on psychometric measures after treatment, even though the soldiers themselves and their clinicians globally judged that they were feeling better and had improved. We believe that there is an important place for different types of outcome measures. Pre-post psychometric measures, however, are the most rigorous indices of change, as well as the most conservative.

The finding that treatment parameters (e.g., intensity and/or duration of treatment) were not associated with greater degrees of improvement might be taken as suggesting limited specific impact of treatment on clinical status. That improvement was observed through the first 4 months but not thereafter also suggests an attenuating impact of treatment. We believe that these data illustrate, above all else, the tenacity and severity of PTSD that has lasted for an average of 20 years. We also believe these findings have important implications for treatment.

First, these data confirm the existence of a group of veterans with severe and persistent PTSD who need treatment that is responsive to their unique clinical circumstances. It is often assumed that because PTSD is the result of a traumatic experience, it should be resolved or be resolvable by another intense, healing experience and that acceptance of the fact that symptoms may never dissipate amounts to defeatism. It must be remembered, however, that in the NVVRS, 98.9% of veterans diagnosed with current PTSD also met the criteria for another lifetime psychiatric disorder (Kulka et al. 1990, p. VI-19-1); a recent genetic study suggested that as much as one-third of the variance in PTSD symptomatology among Vietnam War veterans may be genetically determined (True et al. 1993). The data presented here and elsewhere (Friedman and Rosenheck, in press) suggest that for some PTSD patients, clinical expectations should be lowered and that a long-term supportive approach should be adopted, according to the principles outlined earlier in this chapter (see Table 19–2).

Second, because most improvement occurs early in treatment, it is possible that the intensity of treatment can or should be reduced after the first 4 months of involvement. This is, in fact, what happened in the PCT sample presented here. Using data from the subgroup with four completed interviews ($n = 331$), we found that these individuals had 13.4 PCT sessions in the first 4 months, 11.5 in the second 4 months, and 9.5 in the third 4 months. When total outpatient services were examined (PCT plus other psychiatric services), we again found a decline in use, from 26.3 to 21.9 to 18.5 sessions. These veterans thus continue to use services but at a reduced level, perhaps in response to their clinical improvement and/or their greater degree of clinical stability. Although it is possible that the reduction in intensity could be even greater, it is important to remember that vulnerable patients need to have support readily available to deal with the myriad crises that seem to erupt in their lives. We believe continuity and consistency of care are of paramount importance with these patients but that the exact intensity of treatment must be a matter of clinical judgment and negotiation with the client.

Third, and finally, it is time to turn our attention to considering the applicability of rehabilitative programs, such as those developed for the chronically mentally ill or for patients with severe substance abuse, to these veterans (Anthony et al. 1989; Leda et al. 1993; Liberman 1988; Stein and Test 1980). Social skills training, intensive case management, and vocational rehabilitation approaches developed for the treatment of schizophrenic or homeless mentally ill patients may be of value for veterans with chronic PTSD. This is not to deny that these veterans have PTSD or to minimize the impact on them of traumatic war experiences. It is, however, to recognize that after 20 years, a new set of treatment approaches may be of particular value to them.

As with many other efforts to treat people with severe and

persistent illnesses, we appear to be faced, once again, with the question, "Is the glass half empty or half full?" The best answer to this question is, of course, that from either perspective, there is not as much water in the glass as we would have liked. In this chapter, we have shown that there exists a population of veterans who do not recover from war-zone trauma and who need sustained assistance. We do not have and cannot realistically expect to have clinical tools powerful enough to fully or even largely relieve these veterans of their sufferings. But we have also shown that multimodal treatment delivered by committed specialists is associated with clinical improvement. Effecting such improvement is surely no small accomplishment, but it is also an accomplishment that suggests that there may be alternative avenues in the treatment of these veterans that have yet to be explored. Alertness to chronic, long-term PTSD in veterans of the Persian Gulf War in particular and of future wars in general should be increased.

References

Anthony WJ, Cohen M, Farkas A: Psychiatric Rehabilitation. Boston, MA, Psychiatric Rehabilitation Press, 1989

Archibald HC, Tuddenham RD: Persistent stress reaction after combat: a 20-year follow-up. Arch Gen Psychiatry 12:475–481, 1965

Boudewyns PA, Hyer LH: Physiological response to combat memories and preliminary treatment outcome in Vietnam veteran PTSD patients treated with direct exposure therapy. Behavior Therapy 21:63–87, 1990

Boudewyns PA, Hyer LH, Woods M, et al: PTSD among Vietnam veterans: an early look at treatment outcome using direct therapeutic exposure. Journal of Traumatic Stress 3:359–368, 1990

Cooper NA, Clum GA: Imaginal flooding as a supplemental treatment for PTSD in combat veterans: a controlled study. Behavior Therapy 20:381–391, 1989

Derogatis LR, Melisaratos N: The Brief Symptom Inventory: an introductory report. Psychol Med 13:595–605, 1983

Fontana A, Rosenheck RA: Traumatic war stressors and psychiatric symptoms among World War II, Vietnam theater, and Korean veterans, in Fontana A, Rosenheck RA, Spencer H: The Long Journey Home III: The Third Progress Report on the Department of Veterans Affairs PTSD Programs. West Haven, CT, Northeast Program Evaluation Center, Evaluation Division of the National Center for PTSD, Department of Veterans Affairs Medical Center, 1993, Appendix H

Fontana A, Rosenheck R, Spencer H: The Long Journey Home III: The Third Progress Report on the Department of Veterans Affairs PTSD Programs. West Haven, CT, Northeast Program Evaluation Center, Evaluation Division of the National Center for PTSD, Department of Veterans Affairs Medical Center, 1993

Friedman MJ, Rosenheck RA: PTSD as a persistent mental illness, in The Seriously and Persistently Mentally Ill: The State-of-the-Art Treatment Handbook. Edited by Soreff S. Seattle, WA, Hogrefe & Huber (in press)

Gibbons RD, Elkin I, Waternaux C, et al: Some conceptual and statistical issues in analysis of longitudinal psychiatric data. Arch Gen Psychiatry 50:739–750, 1993

Katz MM, Lyerly SB: Methods for measuring adjustment and social behavior in the community, I: rationale, description, discriminative validity and scale development. Psychol Rep 13:505–535, 1963

Keane TM, Caddell JM, Taylor KL: The Mississippi Scale for Combat-Related PTSD: studies in reliability and validity. J Consult Clin Psychol 56:85–90, 1988

Keane TM, Fairbank JA, Caddell JM, et al: A clinical evaluation of a scale to measure combat exposure. J Consult Clin Psychol 55:53–55, 1989a

Keane TM, Fairbank JA, Caddell JM, et al: Implosive (flooding) therapy reduces symptoms of PTSD in Vietnam combat veterans. Behavior Therapy 20:245–260, 1989b

Kulka RA, Schlenger WE, Fairbank JA, et al: The National Vietnam Veterans Readjustment Study: Tables of Findings and Technical Appendices. New York, Brunner/Mazel, 1990a

Kulka RA, Schlenger WE, Fairbank JA, et al: Trauma and the Vietnam War Generation: Report of Findings from the National Vietnam Veterans Readjustment Study. New York, Brunner/Mazel, 1990b

Laufer RS, Frey-Wouters E: War trauma and the role of guilt in post-war adaptation. Paper presented at the meetings of the Society for Traumatic Stress Studies, Dallas, TX, October 1988

Laufer RS, Yager T, Frey-Wouters E, et al: Legacies of Vietnam, Vol III: Post-War Trauma: Social and Psychological Problems of Vietnam Veterans and Their Peers. Washington, DC, U.S. Government Printing Office, 1981

Leda CL, Rosenheck RA, Medak S: First Progress Report on the Department of Veterans Affairs Veterans Industries/Therapeutic Residences Program. West Haven, CT, Northeast Program Evaluation Center, 1993

Liberman RP (ed): Psychiatric Rehabilitation of Chronic Mental Patients. Washington, DC, American Psychiatric Press, 1988

McLellan AT, Luborsky L, Cacciola J, et al: New data from the Addiction Severity Index: reliability and validity in three centers. J Nerv Ment Dis 173:412–423, 1985

Peniston EG: EMG bio-feedback assisted desensitization treatment for Vietnam combat veterans post-traumatic stress disorder. Clinical Biofeedback and Health 9:35–41, 1986

Perconte S: Stability of positive treatment outcome and symptom relapse in post-traumatic stress disorder. Journal of Traumatic Stress 2:127–136, 1989

Pittman RK, Altman B, Geenwald E, et al: Psychiatric complications during flooding therapy for posttraumatic stress disorder. J Clin Psychiatry 52:17–20, 1991

Pokorny A, Miller B, Kaplan H: The Brief MAST: a shortened version of the Michigan Alcoholism Screening Test. Am J Psychiatry 129:342–345, 1972

Robins LN, Helzer JE, Croughan J, et al: National Institute of Mental Health Diagnostic Interview Schedule: its history, characteristics, and validity. Arch Gen Psychiatry 38:381–389, 1981

Rosenheck RA, Fontana A: Long-term sequelae of combat in World War II, Korea and Vietnam: a comparative study, Individual and Community Responses to Trauma and Disaster: The Structure of Human Chaos. Edited by Ursano RJ, McCaughey BG, Fullerton CS. Cambridge, UK, Cambridge University Press, 1994, pp 330–359

Rosenheck RA, Massari LA: Wartime military service and utilization of VA health care services. Mil Med 158:223–228, 1993

Schluchter MD: 5V: unbalanced repeated measures models with structured covariance matrices, in BMDP Statistical Software Manual, Vol 2. Edited by Dixon WJ. Berkeley, University of California Press, 1988, pp 1081–1114

Scurfield R, Kenderdine S, Pollard R: Inpatient treatment for war-related post-traumatic stress disorder: initial findings on a longer-term outcome study. Journal of Traumatic Stress 3:185–202, 1990

Shalev A, Spiro SE, Solomon Z, et al: Positive clinical impressions, I: therapists' evaluations. Journal of Traumatic Stress 5:207–216, 1992

Silver S: Post-traumatic stress and the death imprint: the search for a new mythos, in Post-Traumatic Stress Disorder and the War Veteran Patient. Edited by Kelley WE. New York, Brunner/Mazel, 1985, pp 43–53

Solomon SD, Gerrity ET, Muff AM: Efficacy of treatments for posttraumatic stress disorder: an empirical review. JAMA 268:633–638, 1992

Solomon Z, Shalev A, Spiro SE, et al: Negative psychometric outcomes; self-report measures and a follow-up telephone survey. Journal of Traumatic Stress 5:225–246, 1992a

Solomon Z, Spiro SE, Shalev A, et al: Positive clinical impressions, II: participants' evaluations. Journal of Traumatic Stress 5:217–224, 1992b

Stein LI, Test MA: Alternative to mental hospital treatment, I: conceptual model, treatment program, and clinical evaluation. Arch Gen Psychiatry 37:392–397, 1980

Sutker PB, Thomason BT, Allain AN: Adjective self-descriptions of World War II and Korean prisoners of war and combat veterans. Journal of Psychopathology and Behavioral Assessment 11:185–192, 1989

True WR, Rice J, Eisen SA, et al: A twin study of genetic and environmental contributions to liability for posttraumatic stress symptoms. Arch Gen Psychiatry 50:257–264, 1993

Part V
Conclusion

20

The Effects of War on Soldiers and Families, Communities and Nations: Summary

Robert J. Ursano, M.D.
Ann E. Norwood, M.D.

In recent years the psychiatric and psychological literature on the effects of war has focused on posttraumatic stress disorder (PTSD), emphasizing the powerful effects of trauma on individuals. War is always a major life event that can reorganize a person's life, leading to the establishment of new goals and direction. For some individuals, however, war results in the development of painful symptoms that can impair the ability to work and to love.

The Persian Gulf War has reminded the world, the United States in particular, of the extent to which war involves not only those who are fighting but also the communities from which they come, their families, and an entire nation's commitment, resources, hopes, and fears. The Gulf War highlighted the technological advances in the ability to prepare for war, to wage war, and to transmit information about war. Never before had war been brought instantaneously into the homes of so many families so far away from the front. CNN brought the war to life in real time. The trauma of war does not begin when the bullets fly; it begins with the separations from home and the loss of family and community resources. In this war, it became clear that children can lose mothers as well as fathers, and communities can lose doctors and salesmen, all before any weapons have been fired.

The anticipation of war is an often overlooked stressor (Table 20–1). The mobilization of reserve forces in the U.S. was part of this anticipation and emphasized to the nation that this was a national war, not one limited to a small group of active-duty soldiers who are often thought of both as a part of and as apart from the rest of the nation.

The authors in this volume have focused on describing the war from this broad perspective, addressing the stressors associated with the war, the individuals and groups affected, and the long-term effects. Other volumes have described combat psychiatry, but the psychiatric problems of war are not limited to the combat theater or even to the combatants. The stress and trauma of war begin before the conflict and extend beyond the soldiers to families, communities, and the entire nation. In addition, the care and treatment of those who suffer psychiatric disorders continue well beyond the combat theater. How to provide the best psychiatric care in a world of rapid evacuation, of potential chemical casualties, and of families learning of family members' injury or death through the media before commanders are able to notify them is of great importance.

Table 20–1.   Stressors of anticipating war

Unexpected separation
Family disruption
Rapid deployment
Loss of parent
Loss of civic leaders and community members
Heavy logistical requirements
Rapid training
Exposure to new environments and environmental conditions
 (e.g., desert, heat)
Unknown future
Boredom/waiting

Stressors of War

The multiple stressors of the combat environment in the Persian Gulf War included the threat of chemical and biological warfare (CBW). The effectiveness of CBW is based on its capacity to induce terror. The recognition and management of the effects of such terror, as well as training in the management of the biological consequences of CBW, are a necessary component of psychiatric care in the combat theater. The protective clothing and protective shelters add both a sense of safety and an additional burden to those fighting. Chemical and biological agents cannot be seen and often are not detected until their deadly effects have begun to take hold. This inability to see the threat is an important aspect of the stress of the CBW experience that affects leaders and troops as well as civilians and influences their decision making and actions. Social support from family and friends may be of particular importance to maintaining manageable levels of anxiety. Active training (i.e., actual training exercises with the protective equipment) and active management of fatigue appear to be important elements in decreasing psychiatric distress and increasing the experience of safety in a CBW environment. CBW is a powerful threat that challenges community leaders as well as combat leaders to use their management skills to decrease the terror of individuals, groups, and communities.

Missile attacks bring their own experience of terror. In Israel, the fear of chemical weapons in SCUD missile attacks led to a large number of people incorrectly assuming that they had been exposed to CBW and flooding the emergency rooms. Over time, this response decreased. However, initially, a response such as this can easily overwhelm all treatment resources. The ability to provide advance warning of potential bombardments, which enabled Israeli citizens to take cover in sealed rooms and put on protective devices, was a very important intervention for managing the terror of the attacks. As in most studies of trauma, the resiliency of communities stands out over time. However, the management of the initial impact and the recovery process are important for all communities threatened by CBW.

The specific psychiatric effects of war trauma have been studied for many years. In the Civil War, perhaps the bloodiest war ever fought by the U.S., psychiatric casualties were described as "nostalgia." In World War I, the terms "shell shock" and "war neurosis" were used. It is now recognized that PTSD, depression, and substance abuse are well-documented effects of war.

Because the Gulf War was brief, there were not the feared number of combat stress disorder casualties. Had the war been more prolonged, and had CBW been used, the outcome might have been very different. Since World War II, it has been well documented that the number of psychiatric casualties is directly related to the intensity of combat. Thus, perhaps the most important psychiatric intervention in any war is that the war be made brief.

Shortly after their return from the Gulf War, a substantial number of veterans were reporting psychiatric symptoms, although the number who had symptoms that, over time, actually met the diagnostic criteria for PTSD appeared to be approximately 9%. More detailed knowledge of the effects of the Persian Gulf War awaits further study. Individuals exposed to death and the dead after Operation Desert Storm are at high risk. They have been shown to have elevated levels of intrusion and avoidance that have persisted, in those who could be followed, for more than 1 year. Past literature indicates that those who were wounded are also at increased risk.

Children are a special group who are vulnerable to multiple stresses of war, including being left by their parents as well as experiencing the direct effects of combat. Few data are available on the effects of Operations Desert Shield and Desert Storm on either children left behind by military parents or, more directly, the children of Kuwait, Iraq, and Israel who suffered the more direct effects of threat to life. Because the deployment was relatively short, one would expect the consequences on children left behind by military parents to be relatively mild. As in most studies, the effects of traumas and disasters on children depend greatly on the responses of the parent. Programs that provide support to families and to parents can be expected to have positive effects on the children. In addition, the return to normalcy following war, frequently built on the reestablishment of a school schedule, brings back an experience of safety that is accompanied by knowledge of what to expect rather than fear of the unexpected. Communities need outreach programs and contingency plans to provide this support and aid for children in times when war is possible.

No generation has escaped the experience of war: preparing for battle, leaving loved ones, conflict, and returning home. The return home is a major psychosocial event that actually begins before the return in the fantasies of the homecoming stirred in the returning soldiers, sailors, airmen, and marines (Table 20–2). These fantasies are built from communications with home, the experience of the separation, and the hopes and fears of the future. In addition, the returning soldier often expects some type of material reward, whether it is veterans' benefits, a medal, or community recognition. These expectations can have a critical impact upon how the veteran experiences the return home.

In addition, the receiving family and community, both of which have had to adjust to the separation, must now adjust to the return. The longer the war, and the longer the deployment, the greater the readjustment required both for the family and for the community. Those fathers who had become both father and mother during Operation Desert Storm, when their wives deployed to the Persian Gulf, had to relinquish not only the bur-

Table 20–2.   Structure of the recovery environment

Deployed servicemembers' fantasies of return home
Readjustment of roles: family, community, and society
Organization of the meaning of return
Deployed servicemember's fears of changes in the family
Family's fears of changes in the deployed servicemember

dens but the joys of this newly found role. Those mothers who had become both father and mother during their husbands' war deployment faced similar adjustment.

The reality of homecoming can be jarring or can facilitate the recovery process. Society—the family, the community, and the nation—plays a very important role in constructing the meaning of the return. Both formal and informal organizations help the reintegration of the veteran into society. The veteran and the spouse/family have similar fantasies, wishes, and fears of the reunion. Both wonder whether the father, mother, or spouse has been changed by war.

Preparation for War

Preparation for the Persian Gulf War involved a substantial portion of the U.S. population. Roughly one-third of the U.S. population has had an affiliation with the military at some time. The active-duty military, retired military, and their families include nearly 10 million members. The mobilization of reservists reached far into the communities of the nation. This was the first mobilization of the reserve and National Guard forces since World War II. More than 227,000 reservists and guard members were called up, and approximately half of these were deployed to the Persian Gulf or overseas. Families filled with hunger for information became "addicted" to the news.

The uniformed personnel of the 1990s are an all-volunteer force. The average military member is better educated and much more likely to be married and have children than his or her counterpart of the 1960s and 1970s. In the Vietnam War, 16% of those in-country were married with children; in the Gulf War, almost 60% were married with children. Women also now constitute approximately 10% of Americans serving in uniform. Therefore, the military spouse is also different from in previous eras: the spouse may be male or female. The military wife is now more likely to be working outside the home and to be less active in traditional volunteer activities.

Despite these structural changes, the stress of war remains a powerful event affecting the entire family. Families of active-duty reserve and National Guard members experienced the mobilization and fears of Operation Desert Storm. Nearly 23,000 single-parent military families were confronted with the deployment. Although it is not known how many of these parents had custody of their children, it is estimated that nearly 32,000 children were affected by the deployment of the single parent. Congressional hearings on this issue during the war emphasized that this will be an important issue for future wars. Operationally effective and actual, rather than "It'll never happen," family deployment plans are now critical. The separation of single parents from their children raised important issues for the entire society to confront. In times of war, the needs of children and the needs of the nation may be in conflict.

Information about the war was brought into homes instantaneously by television, providing the opportunity both for reassurance and for increased fear and distress. Self-help groups were an important source of support for military spouses who lived in communities with a substantial number of deployed military servicemembers. Family support programs for active-duty members were a consistent source of information and group support; however, reserve units and National Guard units were less likely to have such a centrally organized resource.

In Europe also, outreach programs for families of active-duty members who were deployed to the Persian Gulf were developed. There was substantial concern about mass casualties in a single unit and about how a small American community in Germany might respond to such news, which could reach them via CNN long before their community support units could individually talk to them and offer comfort and support. Families always want to decrease uncertainty with information. However, this information, such as the time of the unit's departure or, after deployment, its location, cannot always be provided.

Sensitive attention to the families' needs is part of the task of assuring the military member that his or her family is being cared for. Most often, the care of the family members left behind falls to the spouse of a military group's leader. Such a spouse may or may not be trained or particularly skilled in the needs of these tasks. Further attention to these individuals who are asked to carry the burden of providing support to the families of military members is needed in planning the support network for families in times of future war.

A high number of casualties were expected in the war, including casualties from CBW. Both the Department of Defense and the Department of Veterans Affairs (VA) developed contingency plans for the management of substantial numbers of psychiatric and wounded casualties. For the VA, this plan included the identification of key issues, the development of training plans, and rethinking the provision of psychiatric care to acutely rather than chronically war-traumatized veterans. These concerns formed a core backdrop to the development of VA educational plans. Reorienting to acute care is a critical element in the treatment of combat casualties, since one hopes to maximize their return to work and family even if they return to the U.S. in a patient role. The principles of military psychiatry, which include maximizing the individual's independence and autonomy and decreasing identification with the patient role, are important ingredients in the ongoing treatment of war casualties outside the battle theater.

Of course, for the soldiers themselves, there were extensive deployment stressors. Initially, soldiers were most concerned about the uncertainty of the duration of their deployment. In November and December 1990, this uncertainty was somewhat relieved by the announcement that the deployment would be "for the duration." Although this was not good news, it did relieve the additional burden of uncertainty, which enhanced the soldiers' perception that combat was the event that would mark the end point of their deployment and their imminent return home.

In most units, morale improved significantly between September and December of 1990. By December, camps were more structured and many of the basic needs of life were present. Typically, morale was rated as being just as high as it had been at their home stations. Morale during Operations Desert Shield/ Storm, as in all wars, was critically influenced by mail, showers, tents, rest areas, hot food, cold drinks, free time, and entertainment. Telephones were a mixed blessing. They provided contact with home, which could relieve distress and worry, but offered the opportunity to learn of critical events that increased the burden of the soldier who was deployed away from home where he or she could not affect what was occurring stateside. Soldiers viewed attention to their morale as a clear symbol of the caring and respect of their leaders. There were very few incidents of the usual measures of poor morale (i.e., disciplinary actions, sick call, accidents, intragroup conflicts). By December, most problems were family related. Rumors of a "Dear John letter" would echo through a unit. Cohesion was more variable in support units than in combat units. Reserve units were very much aware of the 180-day limit on their deployment. The anticipated stress of combat is a significant component of the psychological dimensions of war.

Treatment, Recovery, and Reintegration

Returning servicemembers from the Persian Gulf War faced a nation supportive of their actions and pleased to have them return. Rapid return home facilitates the return to family and community but also adds to the stress of reintegration as one moves from being in the desert one day to being at home at the dinner table in, for example, the Midwest the next day. For some servicemembers, the stress of the war persisted. Casualty assistance officers are an often-forgotten group who must manage the stresses of notifying loved ones of the death of their son/husband/father or daughter/wife/mother. Such tasks are emotionally draining. In the Army this is usually done by noncommissioned officers. The strong emotions of the grief-stricken family, the stress of obtaining timely and accurate information to convey to the family, and the experience of identifying with the lost victim increased the stress of this work. The intense media exposure added to the level of distress. Working with families over an extended period appeared to heighten the identification of the casualty assistance officer with the family and their grief process. The availability of more senior individuals and debriefings can lighten the burden of the casualty assistance officer and strengthen his or her ability to maintain a supportive, informative relationship with the family.

The problem of listening to the distress of others is also a prominent part of the experience of mental health workers who must aid the returning Gulf War soldiers. The ability to maintain one's empathic stance in the face of the realities of war is critical to the clinician's ability to hear the trauma of the war environment, the terror of battle injury, the fear of loss of one's identity, the inevitable anger, and the worries of returning home. The therapist's ability to be alert to his or her own conflicts, wishes, and fears is critical to maintaining a listening stance. Only through the clinician's awareness of his or her own sources of vulnerability can the therapist's empathy be maintained, whether that be in psychotherapy or in consultation with soldiers and family members.

The development of an effective consultation-liaison service for returning battle-injured servicemembers is a major challenge. Early identification, normalization of fears, anxieties, and anger, and provision of opportunities for debriefing are critical components to instituting a consultation-liaison outreach within a general medical hospital for patients returned from the battlefield. This area, although not widely written about, is central to tertiary care in modern warfare, where the patient may be rapidly evacuated far from the battlefront and may be surrounded by individuals with little knowledge of the battlefield itself or of the patient's unit or family.

The stressors reported by veterans surveyed at Ft. Devens, Massachusetts (see Chapter 18), confirmed that only a small percentage of deployed military members had experienced traditional heavy combat exposure stressors. However, many reported domestic stressors. Interestingly, the recall of combat stressors increased over time in the follow-up of the Ft. Devens group. The meaning of this increased level of recall and reporting warrants further study. The contributions of intervening stressors, of social context, and of reporting need to be examined. For prisoners of war, low rates of psychopathology similar to those seen in other deployed military groups were found following the Persian Gulf War. The brief time of captivity and the limited period of war helped maintain the prisoners' optimism of probable return home.

For those soldiers who returned to the U.S. with psychiatric illness, psychiatric treatment was begun in the medical centers. Little literature is available that describes the care and treatment of returned psychiatric casualties still in the acute phase of their illness. In the modern war theater, with rapid air evacuation to the States, care for this population will be of increasing importance. Maintaining basic principles of military psychiatric care to include normalization of experiences, expectation of recovery, and decrease in identification with patienthood is a central component of psychiatric care delivered away from as well as in the combat theater. The management of an inpatient milieu for combat psychiatric disorders requires particular attention to transference and countertransference issues.

The long-term effect of the Persian Gulf War on veterans is not yet known. However, studies of the long-term care of Vietnam War veterans provide important areas to be considered and lessons to be heeded. Although the level of psychiatric impairment from Operation Desert Storm at present appears to be low, certainly some individuals will be left with chronic residual effects and will require care for extended periods. Care in the first months of return may be most important to recovery and rehabilitation. Specific social skills training and vocational rehabilitation for veterans with chronic PTSD are indicated.

Directions

War in the modern world affects soldiers and family, communities and nations. It is an all-involving national event. The stress of war begins with its anticipation and includes the problems of rapid transportation, separation from loved ones, adaptation in extreme environments, and exposure to threats of life, new and frightening weapons, and death and the dead. The boredom of waiting and even the reunion home entail additional stressors that must be managed by soldiers and their nation. Because of rapid transportation and air evacuation, medical facilities outside the combat theater now must be prepared to provide acute psychiatric care for war casualties. The effects of rapid communication and deployment on families, nations, and individuals require ever-present attention to the evolving nature of the stressors of war. The literature on war and other human-made disasters can enhance our understanding of the traumatic effects of the chaos of human-made disasters on individuals and groups.

Understanding the demands of war requires broad conceptualization of the biological, psychological, and sociocultural events involved in moving from anticipation of war to reintegration home. The treatment of psychiatric casualties, consultation to communities exposed to the stresses of deployment and return, provision of outreach programs for war-injured veterans, and support to military families are all part of the modern requirements of psychiatric care in times of war.

Index

*Page numbers printed in **boldface** type refer to tables or figures.*